S0-EJQ-601

BIOLOGICAL RESPONSE MODIFIERS IN HUMAN ONCOLOGY AND IMMUNOLOGY

ADVANCES IN EXPERIMENTAL MEDICINE AND BIOLOGY

Recent Volumes in this Series

Volume 159
OXYGEN TRANSPORT TO TISSUE–IV
Edited by Haim I. Bicher and Duane F. Bruley

Volume 160
PORPHYRIN PHOTOSENSITIZATION
Edited by David Kessel and Thomas J. Dougherty

Volume 161
MYOCARDIAL INJURY
Edited by John J. Spitzer

Volume 162
HOST DEFENSES TO INTRACELLULAR PATHOGENS
Edited by Toby K. Eisenstein, Paul Actor, and Herman Friedman

Volume 163
FOLYL AND ANTIFOLYL POLYGLUTAMATES
Edited by I. David Goldman, Joseph R. Bertino, and Bruce A. Chabner

Volume 164
ADVANCES IN COAGULATION, PLATELET FUNCTION, FIBRINOLYSIS, AND VASCULAR DISEASES
Edited by Antonio Strano

Volume 165
PURINE METABOLISM IN MAN–IV
Edited by Chris H. M. M. de Bruyn, H. Anne Simmonds, and Mathias Müller

Volume 166
BIOLOGICAL RESPONSE MODIFIERS IN HUMAN ONCOLOGY AND IMMUNOLOGY
Edited by Thomas Klein, Steven Specter, Herman Friedman, and Andor Szentivanyi

BIOLOGICAL RESPONSE MODIFIERS IN HUMAN ONCOLOGY AND IMMUNOLOGY

Edited by

Thomas Klein
Steven Specter
Herman Friedman
and
Andor Szentivanyi

University of South Florida
Tampa, Florida

PLENUM PRESS • NEW YORK AND LONDON

Library of Congress Cataloging in Publication Data

International Symposium on Biological Response Modifiers in Human Oncology and Immunology (1982: Tampa, Fla.)
Biological response modifiers in human oncology and immunology.

(Advances in experimental medicine and biology; v. 166)
"Proceedings of an International Symposium on Biological Response Modifiers in Human Oncology and Immunology, held July 12-14, 1982, in Tampa, Florida."
Bibliography: p.
Includes index.
1. Cancer—Immunological aspects—Congresses. 2. Immunotherapy—Congresses. 3. Immune response—Regulation—Congresses. I. Klein, Thomas W. II. Title. III. Series.
RC268.3.I48 1982 616.99′4079 83-13410
ISBN 0-306-41391-4

Proceedings of an International Symposium on Biological Response Modifiers in Human Oncology and Immunology, held July 12-14, 1982, in Tampa, Florida

A Division of Plenum Publishing Corporation
233 Spring Street, New York, N.Y. 10013

Printed in the United States of America

ACKNOWLEDGEMENTS

The editors wish to extend appreciation to the members of the satellite symposium scientific organizing committee. Co-chairmen of the committee were: B. Serrou, Montpellier, France; C. Rosenfeld, Villejuif, France; H. Friedman, Tampa, USA. Committee members were: L. Chedid, Paris, France; J. Hadden, Tampa, USA; E. Hersh, Houston, USA; S. Kotani, Osaka, Japan; R. Oldham, Frederick, USA; A. Szentivanyi, Tampa, USA; Y. Yamamura, Osaka, Japan. Through the efforts of this committee, quality investigators were attracted to the meeting resulting in a successful and scientifically stimulating three-day conference.

The symposium was supported in part by corporate sponsors. We gratefully acknowledge the generous financial contributions from the following companies: Hoffman-LaRoche, Inc., Research Division, Nutley, NJ: Department of the Army, Medical Research and Development Command, Fort Detrick, MD; Merck Sharp & Dohme, Research Laboratories, Rahway, NJ; Pfizer, Central Research, Groton, CT; Wyeth Laboratories, Clinical Research & Development, Philadelphia, PA; The Upjohn Company, Cancer Research, Kalamazoo, MI; Smith Kline & French Laboratories, Research and Development, Philadelphia, PA; Newport Pharmaceuticals International, Inc., Newport Beach, CA; A. H. Robins, Richmond, VA; Alpha Biochemical Company, Washington, D. C.

Our thanks go also to the faculty of the Department of Medical Microbiology and Immunology, University of South Florida, and especially Dr. Steven Specter who contributed much to the management and efficient operation of the conference. Finally we express appreciation to Mrs. Lucy Penn for the typing and preparation of the manuscripts prior to publication.

PREFACE

The topic of biological response modifiers has attracted the attention of many biomedical investigators, including immunologists, oncologists, pharmacologists, microbiologists, and biochemists, as well as clinical practitioners of medicine. This has occurred mainly because of the realization that the complex system of cellular and humoral interactions culminating in a productive immune response is under exquisite regulatory control for normal immune responses and that loss of control may markedly influence the capability of a host to respond in a productive manner to the numerous immunologic "insults" encountered in the environment. Furthermore, biological response modification is considered by many to be a natural offshoot of the relatively new application of "immunotherapy" to cancer.

It is widely recognized that "immunotherapy" was practiced at the end of the last century and the beginning of this century when it was recognized that microbial infections were caused by distinct species of bacteria and that passive administration of serum containing antibody to these microbes or their products could, in many cases, favorably influence the outcome of an infectious process. Furthermore, in the area of infectious disease it became quite apparent that "vaccines" prepared from killed microorganisms, or products thereof, could render an individual specifically resistant to that microorganism and, in many cases, increase in a nonspecific manner resistance to other organisms. This became quite evident with the advent of the use of attenuated mycobacteria for vaccination against tuberculosis. The use of the attenuated bovine strain of Bacille Calmette-Guerin (BCG) ushered in an era of potential vaccination not only against a specific microbe but the induction of "nonspecific" immunity to other organisms. Nevertheless, it is quite evident that this idea of immunotherapy or immunomodulation in terms of infectious diseases was not pursued with much vigor because of the discovery of antibiotics. Thus, specific drugs were found to be not only effective in killing or inhibiting the growth of bacteria in vitro, but also in vivo. The "rediscovery" that BCG might be of some value in patients with certain malignancies, especially those of the lymphoid system, ushered in a new era of possible treatment of malignant disease by nonspecific immunotherapy.

There has been much criticism concerning immunotherapeutic approaches in cancer. There are both proponents and detractors for the idea that malignancies may be controlled by immunologic methods better than by more conventional methods such as surgery, radiation, and chemotherapy. There are also proponents of the idea that immunotherapy should be used as an adjunct treatment for cancer. Regardless of the view of investigators in this field, it is apparent that there are many approaches now being taken attempting to specifically and nonspecifically stimulate the immune response of patients with tumors with a wide variety of immunomodulating agents. Furthermore, it is quite evident that in many other disease states, including those induced by infectious agents, genetic disorders, etc., there may be marked diminution of immune competence either at the level of individual immunological pathways or at the level of immune cells. Similarly, there are many pathologic situations in which enhanced immune responses, or inappropriate responses, contribute to the disease state. Thus, there has been much interest in developing immunomodulating agents and biological response modifiers, not only for cancer but for other aspects of immunology.

Among those individuals concerned with immunomodulating agents are the immunopharmacologists who constitute a new group of investigators attempting to bridge the area between the two parental disciplines of immunology and pharmacology. In July 1982 the Second International Congress on Immunopharmacology was held in Washington, D. C. The organizers of the Congress proposed a specific satellite symposium be held in Tampa, FL, immediately following the Congress. The topic of the symposium was Biological Response Modifiers in Human Oncology and Immunology. This volume is based on the proceedings of that satellite symposium which brought together over 120 investigators from numerous countries to discuss in detail pros and cons of biological response modification in cancer and in the general field of human immunology. The volume consists of manuscripts derived from both symposium talks and contributed research papers involving both clinical and basic studies utilizing animal models.

The first chapter represents the keynote address presented by Dr. Y. Yamamura, President of Osaka University. Dr. Yamamura summarizes various forms of cancer immunotherapy, including studies employing microbial adjuvants, synthetic adjuvants, monoclonal antibodies, and cytokines. The introduction is followed by a major section of the volume dealing with biological response modifiers derived from leukocytes. This section begins with a consideration of the interferons. A great deal of new information is available concerning these substances and this is reviewed by Drs. Stewart and Stebbing. The next group of chapters deals with monoclonal antibodies, substances of great importance which were not even considered possible less than a decade ago. The utilization of monoclonal antibodies in cancer therapy is reviewed by Dr. Oldham and others. Thymosin and thymic extracts, which have been studied for nearly two decades as possible immunomodulating agents, are reviewed in a number of papers concerning cancer immunology. Dr. Talal's chapter on interleukin completes this section of the volume and discusses these interesting intermediary soluble molecules which have been described and examined in recent years as important mediators of a wide variety of immune responses, especially those considered to be mediated by T cells and macrophages.

The third section of the volume deals with biological response modifiers derived from microorganisms. A variety of microbial products and their potential usefulness is described. Dr. Kotani reviews in detail muramyl dipeptides and synthetic analogs which, in the last half dozen years or so, have been shown to have marked immunomodulatory effects. Subsequent chapters in this section deal with the influence of various other microbial products on tumor progression and immune status in a variety of clinical and animal studies.

Synthetic biological response modifiers are discussed in the fourth section of the volume. Included in this section are sulfur-containing compounds such as Imuthiol and other chemically defined drugs such as Isoprinosine and NPT 15392. A vast amount of information is reported concerning the effect of these substances on human and animal tumors as well as the effects on immune function. The subsequent section of the volume describes the acquired immunodeficiency syndrome (AIDS) including descriptions of the disease, the immune abnormalities involved and the potential for treatment with biological response modifiers. The volume is then completed with summaries of workshops on animal models for studying biological response modifiers and clinical models.

It appears likely that the broad range of topics discussed in this volume will focus attention on the extremely rapid evolution of the subject of biological response modifiers in human immunology. It appears somewhat unique that the bioscientists from many disciplines, including biochemistry, pharmacology, immunology, microbiology, etc., have focused their interest and attention on the exciting possibility of restoring immunoresponsiveness and/or reversing immunodeficiency in patients with diseases as diverse as cancer, autoimmunity and infections. It is hoped that publication of this series of papers will stimulate additional investigative work in the area of disease process alteration by biological response modifiers.

Thomas Klein
Steven Specter
Andor Szentivanyi
Herman Friedman

CONTENTS

IMMUNOSTIMULATION IN CANCER PATIENTS

Yuichi Yamamura[1] and Ichiro Azuma[2]

Osaka University, Yamada-oka, Suita, Osaka 565, Japan;[1]
Section of Chemistry, Institute of Immunological Science
Hokkaido University, Kita-ku, Sapporo 060, Japan[2]

INTRODUCTION

The studies on the cancer immunology and its application to the cancer immunotherapy in humans are attractive subjects for the immunologists and oncologists. However, in order to discuss the immunostimulation and its application to cancer patients, the following should be considered.

(1) Does the immunity against tumor cells really exist? Is it possible to detect the tumor-specific or tumor-associated antigen which is clearly different from normal cells?

(2) Is the immune response in cancer patients able to be cytotoxic to cancer cells? Does it show the suppressive effect on tumor growth and regress tumors?

(3) If it is possible, what kinds of effector cells should be stimulated.

(4) What is the most effective modality for the stimulation of effector cells?

Immune cells such as killer T lymphocytes, macrophages, and natural killer cells are known to be cytotoxic for tumor cells. Other T cell populations which augment or suppress killer T cells are also reported to associate with tumor immunology. In the case of cancer immunotherapy, it is very important to potentiate the amplifier T cells and eliminate the suppressor T cells. It may be very difficult to say how many cells and what kinds of immune competent cells are required for the development of the maximum cytotoxicity to tumor cells to induce the regression of tumors. It is highly dependent on the antigenic characteristics or number of cancer cells. The discrepancies obtained in *in vitro* experiments and in cancer patients has made it difficult to find out the effective treatment with immunological modalities.

In this keynote address, we would like to summarize the results on cancer immunotherapy which were obtained based on recent progress in basic immunology.

OVERVIEW ON CANCER IMMUNOTHERAPY WITH IMMUNOPOTENTIATOR

Under the term "cancer immunotherapy," many kinds of immunopotentiators are now being used in the treatment of various kinds of human cancers, however, there is no clear evidence that these immunopotentiators develop antitumor activity via immune response against cancer cells, and few clinical trials were confirmed to be effective statistically under the well-controlled randomized design.

Table 1 summarizes the various trials for cancer immunotherapy. Active cancer immunotherapy involves the induction of specific tumor immunity by immunization with tumor cells, modified tumor cells or their components. Adoptive cancer immunotherapy includes cancer treatment prevention of cancer by the stimulation of antitumor activity of cancer patients using passive transfer of antibodies to cancer cells, immune competent cells cytotoxic for tumor cells or cytokines such as lymphokines, lymphotoxins, interleukins and interferons. Nonspecific immunotherapy which stimulates the immune status of cancer patients using immunoadjuvants is the most popular modality for the treatment of cancer patients.

STIMULATION OF ANTITUMOR IMMUNITY WITH IMMUNOADJUVANTS

Initially, immunotherapy using immunoadjuvants such as living BCG, *Corynebacterium parvum*, and methanol-extracted residue of tubercle bacilli (MER) were widely employed for the treatment of human leukemia and malignant melanoma. More recently various kinds of living or killed bacterial cells, their fractions, polysaccharides prepared from various kinds of mushrooms, low molecular weight chemicals such as bestatin, levamisole, vitamin A derivatives, have been used in experimental tumor systems and clinical trials. However, some of these adjuvants were not evaluated as real immunopotentiators, and clinical effectiveness was not proved by well-controlled randomized trials. The Second International Conference on "Present Status in Human Cancer Immunotherapy" which was held in April, 1980 at the National Cancer Institute (United

Table 1. Cancer Immunotherapy

Active immunotherapy

(1) Tumor cells
(2) Modified tumor cells
(3) Tumor antigens
(4) Tumor vaccine + immunoadjuvants

Adoptive immunotherapy

(1) Antibody (monoclonal)
(2) Lymphocytes
(*In vitro* cultured with TCGF)
(3) T cell factors
(4) Transfer factors and immune RNA

Nonspecific immunotherapy

(1) Microbial preparations
(2) Polysaccharides
(3) Synthetic compounds
(4) Thymic factors
(5) Fat-soluble vitamins

States) played a very important role for the evaluation of cancer immunotherapeutics in human cancer treatment (32).

Previously we reported the adjuvant activity of BCG cell wall skeletons (BCG-CWS) especially the augmentation of cytotoxic killer T cells and macrophages and the prolongation of survival of tumor-bearing animals in experimental models and cancer patients (2, 35). We have also shown that the cell-wall skeleton of *Nocardia rubra* has a similar chemical structure to BCG-CWS and more potent adjuvant activity, but less toxicity than BCG-CWS (1, 25, 38). Sato and his coworkers at Chiba University have examined the efficacy of N-CWS on gastric cancer in a well-designed randomized trial (31). The patients in the control group received surgical operation and chemotherapy with mitomycin. Immunotherapy group patients were treated by intradermal injection of N-CWS in addition to surgical removal and chemotherapy. A total 118 patients in control group and 137 patients in N-CWS treated group were registered, and the survival periods of both groups were examined statistically. The analysis of background factors indicated that no significant difference existed between control and N-CWS treated groups in terms of sex, age, histological types, and macroscopic and pathological findings at the surgical operation. The prolongation of survival periods of all patients was not observed, however, the survival periods of patients with noncurative resected cases and with pathological stage IV showed statistically significant prolongation ($p < 0.01$) (Fig. 1). It is too early to obtain conclusions on the efficacy of N-CWS in patients with clinical stage I and curative resected cases, because most of these patients are still surviving.

Previously, McKneally's group (19) has reported that intrapleural injection of living BCG was effective for the prolongation of survival period of stage I lung cancer patients after surgical resection. However, cooperative clinical trial groups chaired by Mountain and Gail reported that surgical adjuvant therapy with intrapleural injection of living BCG in the non small cell lung cancer patients with stage I was not effective statistically for the prolongation of survival period (24).

We have applied N-CWS for the immunotherapy of lung cancer. We compared by randomized trial the survival period of lung cancer patients of the control group which received conventional therapies such as surgical resection, radiotherapy and chemotherapy, with that of the immunotherapy group which received N-CWS in addition to the conventional therapy. Statistically significant prolongation of survival period was not observed in all cases at different stages, however, the survival period of small cell carcinoma patients, especially in clinical stage III and IV, was prolonged significantly ($p < 0.05$) (Fig. 2) (36). The efficacy of N-CWS on patients with malignant pleurisy was also significant ($p < 0.05$) in the prolongation of survival period and disappearance of pleural effusion (37). These results suggest that the well-designed randomized trial is essential for the evaluation of immunopotentiators, and also indicate that these immunopotentiators cannot be expected to be effective on all cases of different kinds of cancers, cell types, and clinical stages.

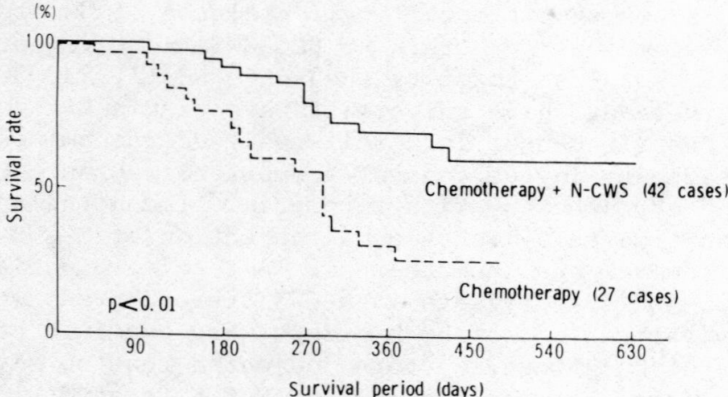

Fig. 1. Effect of N-CWS on gastric cancer patients. (Noncurative resection cases).

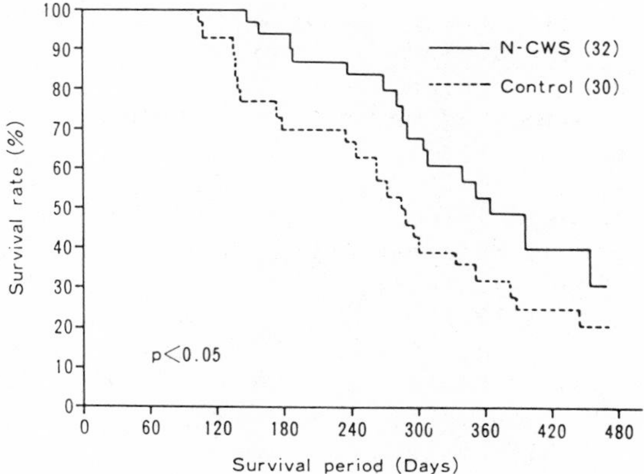

Fig. 2. Effect of N-CWS on small cell carcinoma stage III and IV of lung cancer patients.

Although immunoadjuvants are very effective in experimental cancer systems, their clinical effectiveness is often lacking. The nonspecific immunotherapy with immunoadjuvants may be useful as adjuvant therapy in combination with other modalities for the cancer treatment.

IMMUNOMANIPULATION WITH SYNTHETIC COMPOUNDS

As described above, bacterial whole cells have been used as immunoadjuvants. However, the methods for standardization and quality control of these agents is difficult and chemical purification of immunoadjuvants is being pursued. Umezawa and his group (33) are now trying to evaluate the clinical effectiveness of bestatin which is the inhibitor of leucinaminopeptidase and aminopeptidase B. Bestatin is now applied for the immunotherapy of cancer such as malignant melanoma, bladder cancer and squamous cell carcinoma. Randomized trials on melanoma are showing promising results.

Previously, Ellouz et al. (5), Lederer et al. (14) and Kotani et al. (13) have clearly shown that the minimum structural requirement for the adjuvant activity of mycobacteria cell wall is N-acetylmuramyl-L-alanyl-D-isoglutamine, so-called MDP (muramyldipeptide). MDP was shown to have potent adjuvant activity for the development of delayed-type hypersensitivity and humoral antibody production _in vivo_ when it was given as water-in-oil emulsion together with antigen. However, MDP could not stimulate tumorcidal cytotoxic effector cells _in vivo_, and showed no antitumor activity in any experimental tumor system _in vivo_. We have chemically synthesized various kinds of MDP derivatives and their antitumor activity was examined in syngeneic transplantable tumor systems (30, 34). We have already shown that the cell-wall skeleton of Mycobacteria, Nocardia and Corynebacteria contained so-called mycolic acids which are α-branched-β-hydroxy long chain fatty acid and mycolic acid may play some important role in the physicochemical characteristic (lipophylicity) of cell-wall skeletons. We synthesized 6-O-mycoloyl-MDP (Fig. 3a) by the introduction of mycolic acid into 6-OH position of muramic acid residue of MDP, and these synthetic 6-O-mycoloyl-MDP derivatives were shown to have potent adjuvant activity for the induction of delayed-type hypersensitivity and killer T cells to tumor cells, but were less active for the enhancement of humoral antibody formation *in vitro*. 6-O-mycoloyl-MDP showed tumor suppression and regression activity in mice and guinea pig tumor systems, however, it was less active than BCG-CWS or N-CWS. By further investigations on the chemical synthesis of MDP derivatives, we found that 6-O-quinonyl-MDP derivative (Fig. 3b) had similar antitumor activity as BCG-CWS in experimental tumor system (30). 6-O-quinonyl-MDP is now being examined for efficacy in clinical applications in human cancer. Recently, Fidler's group (7, 8) has reported that MDP encapsulated into liposome has potent adjuvant activity on macrophage activation and also on the inhibition of cancer metastasis in experimental models. This new approach reported by Fidler may prove to be of importance in the development of newer cancer immunopotentiators.

CANCER IMMUNOTHERAPY WITH MONOCLONAL ANTIBODY

Cancer immunotherapy with specific monoclonal antibody against tumor cells is one of the most fascinating approaches in the field of cancer therapy. The most dramatic clinical effects was obtained with patients of recurrent B cell lymphoma by Levy's group. Malignant B cell lymphoma is the cell clone carrying unique immunoglobulin on the cell surface. This unique immunoglobulin variable region, so-called idiotype, will be useful as the tumor-specific cell-surface marker of malignant B lymphoma cell. Hatzubai et al. (9) and Miller and Levy (22) induced immunoglobulin production in B lymphoma cells by hybridization with murine myeloma cells and obtained monoclonal immunoglobulins. They immunized mice with these immunoglobulins and prepared anti-idiotype antibody against the immunoglobulin derived from the B cell lymphoma cells. The monoclonal antibody thus obtained was shown to react specifically to human malignant B lymphoma which was used for immunization, and remarkable tumor regression was observed in the patient by the intravenous injection of the monoclonal anti-idiotype antibody. Levy's group (20, 21) also has treated adult T cell leukemia patients by using mouse monoclonal antibody which react with human T cell surface marker Leu-1 antigen. By the administration of mouse monoclonal antibody, dramatic disappearance of circulating leukemia cells was observed, however, they returned to pretreatment level over the ensuing 24 hrs. Schlossman's

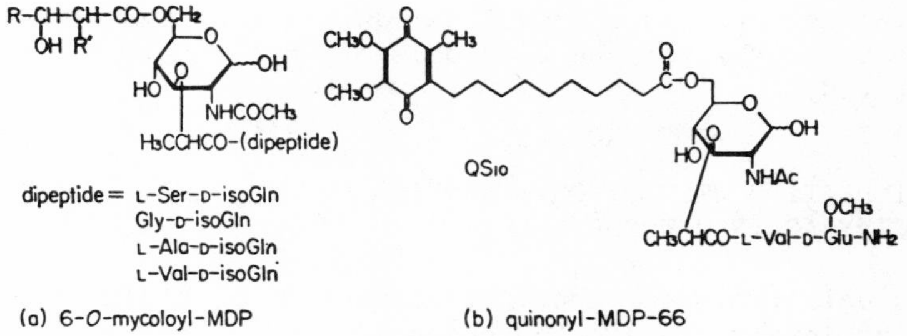
R-CH-CH-CO-OCH2
OH R'
O
OH
HO
NHCOCH3
H3CCHCO-(dipeptide)
dipeptide = L-Ser-D-isoGln
Gly-D-isoGln
L-Ala-D-isoGln
L-Val-D-isoGln
(a) 6-O-mycoloyl-MDP
CH3O
CH3
CH3O
QS10
OH
HO
NHAc
OCH3
CH3CHCO-L-Val-D-Glu-NH2
(b) quinonyl-MDP-66

Fig. 3. Chemical structures of acyl-MDP derivatives.

group (28, 29) has also treated patients with mouse monoclonal antibody against common acute lymphoblastic leukemia antigen (CALLA) and malignant lymphoma and observed clinical improvement in patients. Magnani et al. (17) have applied monoclonal antibody against solid gastrointerstinal cancer. It is interesting that the antigen which reacts with specific monoclonal antibody against human colon carcinoma is monoasialoganglioside.

Previously, Old's group reported that a preparation of mouse monoclonal antibody R24 against human melanoma cells reacted with human melanomas and astrocytomas, but not other tumor cells and normal cells. However, recent results reported by Old's group indicate that the antigenic character recognized by melanoma specific monoclonal antibody R24 and GD3 ganglioside, and this glycolipid was detected in normal cells, but a large amount of GD3 was present on malignant melanoma cell surface (27). Another approach for the treatment of cancer with monoclonal antibody is the conjugation of chemotherapeutic agents, ricin or diphtheria toxin to monoclonal antibody (23). These immunotoxins are expected to kill specifically the tumor cells. Although these approaches offer promise for the cancer therapy, the following problems have yet to be solved. (1) the circulating tumor antigen may combine with monoclonal antibody and inhibit or modulate their activity. (2) At the present time, mouse monoclonal antibody are used for treatment. The repeated intravenous injections of these foreign proteins may induce allergic reaction in patients, and the induction of antibody against monoclonal antibody may block its antitumor activity.

Another approach was made by Irie's group (10, 11). They have reported that the antibody against malignant melanoma associated antigen, so-called "oncofetal antigen," was detected in the sera of the patients with malignant melanoma, and that the antibody titer in patients sera correlated with the prognosis of the patients. Recently, Irie et al. have established a cell line from patients peripheral lymphocytes by E. B. virus transformation which secretes monospecific antibody against oncofetal antigen. This group is now planning to apply serotherapy to malignant melanoma patients by using monospecific anti-oncofetal antibody.

It is suggested that monoclonal antibody against tumor cells will also be useful for the diagnosis of cancer as well as cancer treatment (18).

IMMUNOSTIMULATION WITH CYTOKINES WHICH DEVELOP CELL-MEDIATED CYTOTOXICITY AGAINST TUMOR CELLS

Clinical trials for cancer treatment with partially purified or recombinant interferon are now being widely carried out. Although the antitumor activity of the antiviral agent, interferon, is not yet confirmed in experimental tumor systems and clinical trials, clinical applications of interferon, are being done with much expectation, sometimes extravagant expectation. As reported by Gutterman and his cooperative group (6) recombinant or partially purified human interferon showed partial tumor regression in approximately half of advanced cancer patients, however, side effects such as fever, chills, myalgia, headache, fatigue, reversible leukopenia and granulocytopenia were observed.

The recent development of techniques for expansion of human lymphoid cells *in vitro* to large numbers using T cell growth factor (TCGF, Interleukin 2) has provided new possibilities for identifying, isolating and expanding of autologous human lymphoid cells cytotoxic for tumors. For this purpose, Rosenberg's group (15, 16) has established the method of production and partial purification of TCGF of mouse and human. Cytotoxic T cell lines and clones have been developed with specific cytotoxic reactivity to selected mouse tumors such as murine lymphoma, FBL-3, and appropriately sensitized lymphocytes which are subsequently expanded in TCGF are capable of curing mice with disseminated lymphoma. Lymphoid cells sensitized to tumor antigens are derived by *in vivo* immunization followed by *in vitro* boosting. Following growth in TCGF, these cells are capable of curing mice with disseminated tumors. Similar experimental results were obtained by Cheever's group (3, 4). On the basis of these results, preliminary experiments exploring the *in vivo* injection of cells expanded in TCGF or TCGF alone into humans have been performed by Rosenberg and his group.

Very recently, Kishimoto and his group (12, 26) at Osaka University, succeeded in the establishment and characterization of a human T hybrid cell secreting human TCGF. Cell fusion was made between an azaguanine-resistant T-cell line selected from a human T-leukemia cell line (CCRF-CEM) with T lymphocytes from normal human peripheral blood stimulated with concanavalin A. One of the established hybrid clones, 24A, possessing characteristics of T cells secreted human TCGF. The culture supernatants induced the proliferation of concanavalin A stimulated murine T cells and supported the proliferation of TCGF-dependent human cytotoxic T cells. Experimental antitumor activities by adoptive transfer of TCGF treated lymphoid cells and clinical application of this human TCGF, obtained by hybridoma is now being attempted. The culture supernatant from the other hybrid clone, 55-A, showed helper activity in the induction of cytotoxic T cells but did not show any TCGF activity. The result proved the presence of the killer helper factor other than TCGF. Many hybrid clones have been established in these experiments and several other lymphokines involved in the proliferation or differentiation of T or B lymphocytes or in the activation of macrophages have been identified. Isolation and characterization of homogeneous lymphokines obtained from hybrid clones will provide powerful tools for the potentiation of immune responses against cancer.

SUMMARY

It is interesting to treat cancer patients by the potentiation of their depressed immune status. There are many immunopotentiators which showed potent antitumor activity in experimental tumor systems *in vivo* and *in vitro*, however, which were not always effective in well-designed controlled clinical trials. At the present time, we should say that cancer immunotherapy is not the first modality for cancer treatment and we should be careful not to miss more effective modalities for the treatment of cancer patients by the overestimation of cancer immunotherapy. Further extensive studies will be required to establish new modalities such as the development of more effective immunostimulation which is cytotoxic to tumor cells and the exploration of combined immunostimulation by using more than two immunotherapies, or immunotherapy combined with other cancer therapeutic modalities.

REFERENCES

1. Azuma, I., T. Taniyama, F. Hirao and Y. Yamamura. 1974. Antitumor activity of cell wall skeletons and peptidoglycolipids of mycobacteria and related microorganisms in mice and rabbits. Gann 65: 493.

2. Azuma, I., and Y. Yamamura. 1979. Immunotherapy of cancer with BCG cell-wall skeleton and related materials. Gann Monogr. Cancer Res. 24: 121.

3. Cheever, M. A., P. D. Greenberg and A. Fefer. 1981. Specific adoptive therapy of established leukemia with syngeneic lymphocytes sequentially immunized *in vivo* and *in vitro* and nonspecifically expanded by culture with interleukin 2. J. Immunol. 126: 1318.

4. Cheever, M. A., P. D. Greenberg, A. Fefer and S. Gillis. 1982. Augmentation of the anti-tumor therapeutic efficacy of long-term cultured T lymphocytes by in vivo administration of purified interleukin. J. Exp. Med. 155: 968.

5. Ellouz, F., A. Adam, R. Ciorbaru and E. Lederer. 1974. Minimal structure requirements for adjuvant activity of bacterial peptidoglycan derivatives. Biochem. Biophys. Res. Commun. 59: 1317.

6. Gutterman, J. U., S. Fein, J. Quesada, S. J. Horning, J. L. Levine, R. Alexanian, L. Bernhardt, M. Kramer, H. Speigel, W. Colburn, P. Trown, T. Merigan and Z. Dziewanowska. 1982. Recombinant leukocyte A interferon: Pharmacokinetics, single dose tolerance and biologic effects in cancer patients. Annals of Int. Med. (in press).

7. Fidler, I. J., S. Sone, W. E. Fogler and J. L. Barnes. 1981. Eradication of spontaneous metastases and activation of alveolar macrophages by intravenous injection of liposomes containing muramyl dipeptide. Proc. Natl. Acad. Sci. USA 78:1680.

8. Fidler, I. J., S. Sone, W. E. Fogler, D, Smith, D. G. Braun, L. Tarcsay, R. J. Gisler and A. J. Schroit. 1982. Efficacy of liposomes containing a lipophilic muramyl dipeptide derivative for activating the tumoricidal properties of alveolar macrophages *in vivo*. J. Biol. Response Modifiers (in press).

9. Hatzubai, A., D. G. Malone, R. Levy. 1981. The use of a monoclonal anti-idiotype antibody to study the biology of a human B cell lymphoma. J. Immunol. 126:2397.

10. Irie, R. F., P. C. Jones, D. L. Morton and N. Sidell. 1981. *In vitro* production of human antibody to a tumour-associated foetal antigen. Br. J. Cancer 44: 262.

11. Jones, P. C., L. L. Sze, P. Y. Liu, D. L. Morton and R. F. Irie. 1981. Prolonged survival for melanoma patients with elevated IgM antibody to oncofetal antigen. J. Natl. Cancer Inst. 66: 249.

12. Kaieda, T., M. Okada, N. Yoshimura, S. Kishimoto, Y. Yamamura and I. Azuma. 1982. A human helper T cell clone secreting both killer helper factor(s) and T cell-replacing factor(s). J. Immunol. 129: 46.

13. Kotani, S., Y. Watanabe, F. Kinoshita, T. Shimono, I. Morisaki, T. Shiba, S. Kusumoto, Y. Tarumi and K. Ikenaka. 1975. Immunoadjuvant activities of synthetic N-acetylmuramylpeptides or amino acids. Biken J. 18: 105.

14. Lederer, E. 1982. Immunomodulation by muramyl peptides: Recent developments. Clin. Immunol. Newsletter 3: 83.

15. Lotze, M.T., E. A. Grimm, A. Mazumder, J. L. Strausser and S. A. Rosenberg. 1981. Lysis of fresh and cultured autologous tumor by human lymphocytes cultured in T-cell growth factor. Cancer Res. 41: 4420.

16. Lotze, M. T., B. R. Line, D. J. Mathisen and S. A. Rosenberg. 1980. The in vivo distribution of autologous human and murine lymphoid cells grown in T cell growth factor (TCGFP: Implications for the adoptive immunotherapy of tumors. J. Immunol. 125: 1487.

17. Magnani, J. L., M. Brockhaus, D. F. Smith, V. Ginsburg, M. Blaszcayk, K. F. Mitchell, Z. Steplewski and H. Koprowski. 1981. A monosialoganglioside is a monoclonal antibody-defined antigen of colon carcinoma. Science 212: 55.

18. Marx, J. L. 1982. Monoclonal antibodies in cancer. Science 216: 283.

19. McKneally, M. F., C. Maver, L. Lininger, H. W. Kausel, J. B. McIlduff, T. M. Older, E. D. Foster and R. D. Alley. 1981. Four-year follow-up on the Albany experience with intrapleural BCG in lung cancer. J. Thorac. Cardiovas. Surg. 81: 485.

20. Miller, R. A. and R. Levy. 1981. Response of cutaneous T cell lymphoma to therapy with hybridoma monoclonal antibody. Lancet 2: 226.

21. Miller, R. A., D. G. Maloney, J. McKillop, and R. Levy. 1981. In vivo effects of murine hybridoma monoclonal antibody in a patient with T-cell leukemia. Blood 58: 78.

22. Miller, R. A., D. G. Maloney, R. Warnke, and R. Levy. 1982. Treatment of B-cell lymphoma with monoclonal anti-idiotype antibody. New Eng. J. Med. 306: 517.

23. Moller, G. (ed.). 1982. Antibody Carriers of Drugs and Toxins in Tumor Therapy. Immunol. Rev., Vol. 62.

24. Mountain, C. F. and M. H. Gail. 1981. Surgical adjuvant intrapleural BCG treatment for Stage I non-small cell lung cancer. J. Thorac. Cardiovasc. Surg. 82: 649.

25. Ogura, T., M. Namba, Y. Yamamura and I. Azuma. 1979. Immunotherapeutic effect of BCG and Nocardia rubra cell-wall skeletons on syngeneic tumors in rats. In W. D. Terry and Y. Yamamura (eds.) Immunobiology and Immunotherapy of Cancer. Elsevier North/Holland Publishers, New York.

26. Okada, M., N. Yashimura, T. Kaieda, Y. Yamamura and T. Kishimoto. 1981. Establishment and characterization of human T hybrid cells secreting immunoregulatory molecules. Proc. Natl. Acad. Sci. USA 78: 7717.

27. Pukel, C. S., K. O. Lloyd, L. R. Travasos, W. G. Dippold, H. F. Oettgen and L. J. Old. 1982. G_{D3} a prominent ganglioside of human melanoma. J. Exp. Med. 155: 1133.

28. Ritz, J., J. M. Pesando, J. Notis-McConarty, H. Lazarus and S. Schlossman. 1980. A monoclonal antibody to human acute lymphoblastic leukaemia antigen. Nature 283: 583.

29. Ritz, J., J. M. Pesando, S. E. Sallan, L. A. Clavell, J. Notis-McConarty, P. Rosenthal and S. F. Schlossman. 1981. Serotherapy of acute lymphoblastic leukemia with monoclonal antibody. Blood 58: 141.

30. Saiki, I., Y. Tanio, M. Yamawaki, M. Uemiya, S. Kobayashi, T. Fukuda, H. Yukimasa, Y. Yamamura and I. Azuma. 1981. Adjuvant activity of quinonyl-N-acetylmuramyldipeptides in mice and guinea pigs. Infect. Immun. 31: 114.

31. Sato, H., T. Ochiai, H. Sato, R. Hayashi, K. Watanabe, T. Asano, K. Isono and T. Tanaka. 1982. Result of randomized clinical trial of immunotherapy with Nocardia rubra-CWS. J. Jap. Surg. Soc. (in Japanese) (in press).

32. Terry, W. D. and S. T. Rosenberg (ed). 1982. Immunotherapy of Human Cancer. Excepta Medica, Amsterdam.

33. Umezawa, H., T. Aoyagi, H. Suda, M. Hamada and T. Takeuchi. 1976. Bestatin, an inhibitor of aminopeptidase B, produced by actinomycetes. J. Antibiot. 29: 97.

34. Yamamura, Y., I. Azuma, K. Sugimura, M. Yamawaki, M. Uemiya, S. Kusumoto, S. Okada and T. Shiba. 1976. Adjuvant activity of 6-O-mycoloyl-N-acetylmuramyl-L-alanyl-D-isoglutamine. Gann 67: 867.

35. Yamamura, Y., M. Sakatani, T. Ogura and I. Azuma. 1979. Adjuvant immunotherapy of lung cancer with BCG cell wall skeleton (BCG-CWS). Cancer 43: 1314.

36. Yamamura, Y., T. Ogura, M. Sakatani, F. Hirao, S. Kishimoto, K. Furuse, M. Kawahara, M. Fukuoka, M. Takada, O. Kuwahara and N. Ogawa. 1982a. Randomized controlled study on adjuvant immunotherapy for unresectable lung cancer with Nocardia rubra cell wall skeleton. Gan to Kagakuryoho (in Japanese) (in press).

37. Yamamura, Y., T. Ogura, M. Sakitani, F. Hirao, S. Kishimoto, K. Furuse, M. Kawahara, M. Fukuoka, M. Takada, O. Kuwahara, H. Ikegami, S. Nakamura and N. Ogawa. 1982b. Clinical effect of Nocardia rubra cell wall skeleton (N-CWS) on lung cancer with malignant pleural effusion. Gan to Kagakuryoho (in Japanese) (in press).

38. Yamamura, Y., K. Yasumoto, T. Ogura and I. Azuma. 1981. *Nocardia rubra* cell wall skeleton in the therapy of animal and human cancer. In E. M. Hersh (ed.), Augmenting Agents in Cancer Immunology. Raven Press, New York.

INTERFERONS: SEVERAL QUESTIONS AND FEW ANSWERS

William E. Stewart II

Department of Medical Microbiology and Immunology
University of South Florida College of Medicine
Tampa, Florida (USA)

INTRODUCTION

A number of clinical trials are presently ongoing to test the utility of interferons (IFNs) as antiviral and antitumor agents; several tabulations of these have appeared and, in sum, these show that more trials are warranted (Reviewed in Ref. 1). Rather than reiterate these spotty pilot studies, I should like to consider the few key questions which should focus on the status of IFN trials.

Questions

1. How effective is IFN in cancer?
2. What are "maximum tolerated doses" for IFNs?
3. How can IFNs be evaluated in combination therapy with other cytotoxic agents?
4. The last question is of particular concern to me personally. IFNs have been studied now for 25 years and I personally have been studying them for 20 years, yet for the last several years now I keep asking myself, "How did a nice antiviral substance like IFN get mixed up with a bunch of immunologists and oncologists"?

To start by answering the last question first, it is appropriate to point out that the original rationale for using IFN in cancer patients was based on extrapolation from the scientific data. In the late 60's and early 70's, several workers had demonstrated that several virally-induced tumors of mice could be inhibited by the, supposedly, antiviral activity of IFN (Reviewed in Ref. 1 and 2).

Therefore, in the early 70's Hans Strander, Karolinska Hospital, on the assumption that osteogenic sarcoma was likely to be a virally-induced tumor of man, started injecting human leukocyte-derived α IFN preparations into post-operated osteogenic sarcoma patients (3). Although his rationale - that continued virus activity might be involved in metastasis and, therefore, IFN should prevent this as a prophylactic anti-viral agent - in this case seems doubtful, his data in these cancer patients started to look promising by 1975 (4). As a consequence, IFNs began to be tested in limited numbers of patients with other cancers, even though there was no reason to suspect viral involvement in most of these (5-8).

Fortunately, continued basic lab work was hurrying along in parallel with these clinical trials, not so much to find reasons for planning trials of this antiviral substance in cancer patients, but rather to find new rationalizations why IFN might be giving the even moderately positive results being seen in some of the patients.

First, by the late 70's, we were able to show, *beyond a doubt*, that IFN *per se* would inhibit growth of transformed cells (9) (and did so presumably better than it inhibited normal cells). Thus, we had a more palatable reason for using IFN in cancer patients than if it were solely an antiviral agent. With this activity of IFN as a supposed prognosticator of IFN's antitumor effect, many simplifiers were rushing to look for an *in vitro* correlate of IFN utility in cancer patients. It was suddenly proposed that cancer patients being considered for IFN therapy be screened to see if their tumor cells responded to IFN's cell growth inhibitory effect *in vitro*; if not, no need to waste IFN on them.

However, Ion Gresser and his colleagues muddied this picture by showing that IFN could exert an antitumor effect in mice injected with tumor cells that were *completely resistant* to IFN *in vitro* (10) (either to its antiviral or cell-growth-inhibitory activity) because these cells lacked IFN receptors (11). This meant, of course, that IFN was acting not as either a direct antiviral substance or as a direct anticellular substance, but was acting indirectly on the tumor cells, that is: as a Biological Response Modifier (BRM).

Indeed, it was subsequently found, with much rejoicing, that IFNs could augment NK cell activity (12) and, once again, the "true" antitumor mechanism of IFNs appeared to have been discovered. It now appears that IFNs can activate macrophages and can do nearly anything that can be measured biologically (Reviewed in Ref. 1). To date, no single consistent correlate has been identified to account for IFN as an antitumor agent.

IFN IN COMBINATION THERAPY

To answer the question about using IFN in combination therapy with other cytotoxic agents, several complexities must be considered. First, can the direct actions of IFNs be exerted in the system if the cytotoxic agent has affected the target cells? We know from *in vitro* studies that cells treated with cytotoxic substances fail to respond fully to IFN's antiviral action (13). On the other hand, *in vitro* studies suggest that the cytostatic activity of IFN might be enhanced in conjunction with other cytotoxic substances (14). It is, therefore, difficult to predict what to expect with combined therapy in terms of the direct actions of IFNs. In regard to the *indirect* effects of IFNs, as with all the other BRMs, cytotoxic removal or reduction of effector cell populations would likely diminish the merits of the therapy.

Of course, to accurately assess IFN in combination therapy would require that we use it at the *optimal* dose. To date no one knows what is the optimal dose for any IFN in any disease. So far, it has been given on the following dose rationales:

1) amounts available
2) precedence
3) "maximum tolerated doses".

Each of these three "reasons" for dosage determination deserves lengthy comment, but I shall spare you my soap-box routine. Briefly, however, initially Strander gave 3-million units 3 times a week because that was the maximum amount of IFN he could get for his trials (3). Subsequently, several workers used that dosing because there was a precedent for it (6-8), but it soon became evident that 10-million or 30-million daily might be better, *if* it were available in such quantities (7).

MAXIMUM TOLERATED DOSES OF IFN

The *maximum tolerated dose* concept has come into concern. With the availability of very highly purified natural IFNs and recombinant-derived IFNs, it has been substantiated that IFN induces several so-called "side" effects, notably fever, fatigue and blood element alterations (15). The so-called MAXIMUM TOLERATED DOSE of IFN has been quoted by some workers to be about 30-100 million units (16). This, of course, requires a definition of "tolerated", which must be balanced against the severity of the disease involved, as well as such considerations as how compromised the patient might already be due to other cytotoxic drugs, etc.

I submit that no patient injected with IFN to date has yet received an amount of IFN anywhere nearly approaching the amounts of IFN that is routinely produced by our own bodies during any number of systemic acute viral infections. For example, patients injected with 30-million units of α IFN achieve a fairly even distribution of the IFN through the bloodstream with peak blood levels being only a few hundred units/ml and these IFN levels last only a few hours and then disappear (Reviewed in Ref. 1). However, children with measles, mumps, etc., have IFN blood levels in the 1,000's of units/ml and such levels last and are TOLERATED for days (17). Incidentally, the "side-effects" of IFN injections resemble the prodromal symptoms of most of these systemic viral infections.

Another point to consider in terms of IFN dose determinations is the marked heterogeneities of IFNs. The variety of α IFN forms that occur naturally (18) and the enormous numbers that can be generated as fused protein hybrids (19), each have importantly distinct biological properties. Thus, one form of α IFN (perhaps to be produced as a patented product by Company A) might have significantly different properties from another α IFN (the product of Company B). They might have identical levels of activities in vitro antiviral assays, yet one might be much more potent than the other in terms of cell-growth-inhibition (or NK cell enhancement or inhibition), thereby giving completely different effects and/or "side" effects at otherwise seemingly similar dose levels. Therefore, rather than determining the optimal dose of IFNs as a BRM group, it will likely be necessary to determine such dose for each individual IFN.

EFFECTIVENESS OF IFN IN CANCER

The clinical data with IFN to date are still preliminary. Negative results don't mean anything; positive results mean they can be improved once we know more about optimal doses, routes, etc. There have been several anecdotal trials giving complete responses (See Ref. 1). There have been some controlled trials that have also shown encouraging responses (21). The osteosarcoma trial data are holding up more than 5 years now (22). Laryngeal papillomas invariably give complete responses to α IFNs (but not to β IFN) (23). Jordan Gutterman's breast cancer results have been substantiated by the American Cancer Society collaborative trials (25). Alpha IFNs have given complete responses in several Kaposi's sarcoma patients (25). Beta IFN has given complete responses in some patients with nasopharyngeal carcinomas (26). Also, the uncontrolled studies showing cures of various warts (as reported by the Yugoslavs nearly a decade ago) (27) have now been confirmed in controlled trials (21,25). It seems likely that IFNs will be of some use in the control of cancers, but years of work remain to determine the required base-level information for its rational use.

SUMMARY

Interferons, which have been studied for many years as antiviral agents, are now receiving considerable attention as antitumor and immunomodulatory agents. The data to date are sufficiently interesting to warrant further studies on several fronts. Clearly, the results that have been obtained so far tend to pose more questions than they answer.

REFERENCES

1. Stewart II, W. E. 1981. The Interferon System, 2nd Edition, Springer-Verlag, Vienna-New York.

2. Gresser, I. 1972. Antitumor effect of interferon. Adv. Cancer Res. 16: 97-140.

3. Strander, H., K. Cantell, P. A. Jakobsson, U. Nilsonne, G. Soderberg. 1974. Exogenous interferon therapy of osteogenic sarcoma. Acta Orthop. Scand. 45: 958-967.

4. Strander, H., K. Cantell, S. Ingimarsson, P. A. Jakobsson, U. Nilsonne, G. Soderberg. 1977. Interferon treatment of osteogenic sarcoma: a clinical trial. Fogarty Intern. Center Proc. 28: 377-380.

5. Strander, H. 1977. Interferons: anti-neoplastic drugs? Blut 35: 277-288.

6. Merigan, T. C., K. Skoro, J. H. Breeden, R. Levy, S. A. Rossenberg. 1978. Preliminary observations on the effect of human leukocyte interferon in non-Hodgkins lymphoma. N. Engl. J. Med. 299: 1444-1453.

7. Hill, N. O., L. Loeb, A. Pardue. 1978. Leukocyte interferon production and its effectiveness in acute lymphatic leukemia. J. Clin. Hematol. Oncol. 8: 66-70.

8. Ikic, D., Z. Markic, V. Orelic, B. Rode, P. Nola, K. Smudj, M. Knezevic and D. Jusic. 1981. Application of human leukocyte interferon in patients with urinary bladder papillomatosis, breast cancer and melanoma. Lancet I: 1022-1024.

9. Stewart II, W. E., I. Gresser, M. G. Tovey, M. T. Bandu and S. LeGoff. 1976. Identification of the cell-multiplication-inhibitory factors in interferon preparations as interferons. Nature 262: 300-303.

10. Gresser, I., C. Maury and D. Brouty-Boye. 1972. On the mechanism of the antitumor effect of interferon in mice. Nature 239: 167-168.

11. Gresser, I., M. T. Bandu and D. Brouty-Boye. 1974. Interferon and cell division. IX. Interferon-resistant L1210 cells: characteristics and origin. J. Natl. Cancer Inst. 52: 553-559.

12. Trinchieri, G., D. Santoli and H. Koprowski. 1978. Spontaneous cell-mediated cytotoxicity in humans: role of interferon and immunoglobulins. J. Immunol. 120: 1849-1860.

13. Lockart, R. Z. 1964. The necessity for cellular RNA and protein synthesis for viral inhibition from interferon. Biochem. Biophys. Res. Commun. 15: 513-518.

14. Chany, C., F. Fournier and S. Rousset. 1971. Potentiation of the antiviral activity of interferon by actinomycin D. Nature New Biology 230: 113-114.

15. Scott, G. M., J. Wallace, D. A. J. Tyrreu, K. Cantell, D. S. Sechar and W. E. Stewart II. 1982. An interim report on studies on the toxic effects of human leukocyte-derived interferon-alpha. J. Interferon Res. 2: 127-130.

16. Merigan, T. C. 1981. Personal communication.

17. Petralli, J. K., T. C. Merigan and J. R. Wilbur. 1965. Circulating interferon after measles vaccination. New Engl. J. Med. 273: 198-201.

18. Stewart II, W. E. and J. Desmyter. 1975. Molecular heterogeneity of human leukocyte interferon. Virology 67: 68-78.

19. Streuli, M., A. Hau, W. Bou, W. E. Stewart II., S. Nagata and C. Weissmann. 1981. Target cell specificity of two species of human interferon produced in *E. coli* and hybrid molecules derived from them. Proc. Nat. Acad. Sci. USA. 78: 2848-2852.

20. Stewart II, W. E., P. DeSomer, V. G. Edy, K. Paucker, K. Berg and C. A. Ogburn. 1975. Distinct molecular species of human interferons: leukocyte and fibroblast. J. Gen. Virol. 26: 327-333.

21. Pazin. G. J., M. Ho, H. Hoverkos, J. A. Armstrong, M. Breinig, H. Wechsler, A. Arvin, T. Merigan and K. Panteu. 1982. Effects of interferon-alpha on human warts. J. Interferon Res. 2: 235-244.

22. Strander, H. 1982. 3rd Annual International Congress for Interferon Research, Miami, Florida, November 1982.

23. Strander, H. 1977. Administration of exogenous interferon into patients with neoplastic diseases. Fifth Aharon Katzir-Katchalsky Conference. Rehovot, Israel.

24. Borden, E. and collaborators. 1981. Second Annual International Congress for Interferon Research, San Francisco, California, October 1981.

25. Krown, S. 1982. 3rd Annual International Congress for Interferon Research. Miami, Florida, November 1982.

26. Nietheimmer, D. 1981. Personal communication.

27. Ikic, D., S. Smerdel, E. Soos and D. Jusic. 1975. Preliminary study of the use of interferon on condylomata acuminata in women, pp. 223-225. Proc. Symp. Clin. Use of Interferons. Yugoslav. Acad. Sci.

INTERFERON HYBRIDS: PROSPECTS FOR THERAPY

Nowell Stebbing

AMGen, Inc., 1900 Oak Terrace Lane, Thousand Oaks
CA (USA)

INTRODUCTION

Recombinant DNA techniques have led to determination of the structure of human interferons and production of individual molecular species of interferon free from other species and other proteins simultaneously induced in human cell cultures. Comparison of the properties of different molecular species of interferon and molecular hybrids between the various species has indicated the extent to which the various biological properties of interferons may be separated. This information provides a basis for considering the design of particular molecular constructions of interferons with particular desired properties. The production of hybrid interferons from different genes with common restriction enzyme sites provides a method for producing desirable analogs. The current data are here reviewed with respect to potential clinical utility of such materials.

STRUCTURE OF HUMAN INTERFERONS

The structure of eleven human leukocyte interferons (IFN-αs) has been determined by molecular cloning and these consist of 165 or 166 amino acid residues (1-3). Hybridization of DNA probes to the human genome indicates the existence of up to 16 distinct genetic loci for leukocyte interferons (2). Each IFN-α subtype differs from other subtypes in about 20 amino acid residues and the overall homology between all the known IFN-α sequences is 52%. A consensus sequence for these IFN-αs is shown in Figure 1. All but one of the IFN-αs contain 4 cysteine residues (IFN-αD contains 5) and the two disulphide bridges shown in Figure 1 are known to exist in IFN-αA, whose structure has been most extensively studied (4, 5). IFN-αA

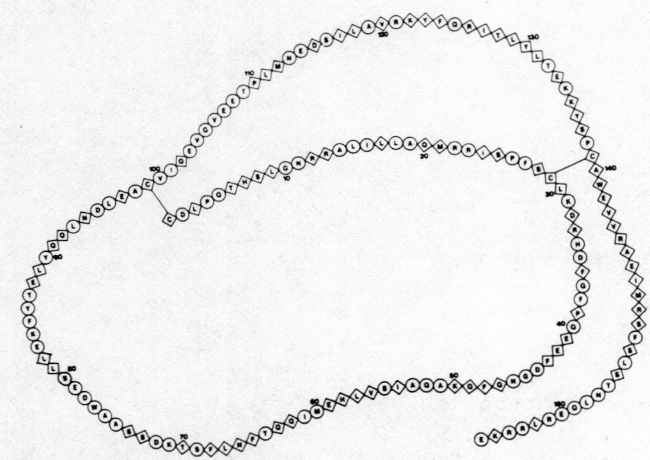

Fig. 1. Consensus sequence of human leukocyte interferons. Residues in squares are common to all known IFN-α subtypes. The standard single letter code is used for designating amino acids. The disulphide bridges are for IFN-αA. (4).

contains 165 residues (residue 44 is taken as a gap in the comparative data summarized in Figure 1). So far, only one IFN-β_1 (IFN-β_1) has been detected by recombinant DNA methods and only one gene has been identified by hybridization to the human genome (2).

The cloned fibroblast interferon contains 166 amino acid residues and shows some homology with the IFN-αs: 38/166 amino acid positions are common between IFN-β_1 and all the known IFN-αs. Evidence for additional IFN-β_1 genes comes from production in mouse/human hybrid cells of oocyte translatable mRNA which does not hybridize with an IFN-β_1 probe and synthetizes interferon neutralized only by antibody to human IFN-β_1(6). Human immune interferon (IFN-γ) consists of 146 amino acid residues with no apparent homology to IFN-αs or IFN-β_1 and there also appears to be only one gene for IFN-γ (7).

The human IFN-αs do not seem to be glycosylated in their natural form (8) and no glycosylation sites occur in the known human IFN-α species. IFN-β_1 contains one known glycosylation site and naturally appears to contain approximately 18 percent carbohydrate (9). In its natural form IFN-γ appears to be glycosylated and there are two known glycosylation sites (7) IFN-β_1 contains only three cysteines: there is no cysteine near the N-terminus, as occurs for all the IFN-αs. However, it is likely that IFN-β_1 contains a disulphide bridge which is essential for antiviral activity (10). Whether other biological properties of IFN-β_1 are thus lost is unknown. IFN-γ contains two cysteines, at positions one and three and these do not seem to be involved in any intramolecular structure.

Despite absence of glycosylation when expressed in bacteria, cloned human IFN-β_1 and IFN-γ have biological properties comparable to those of the natural interferon preparations.

The homology between IFN-αs at the nucleotide level is even greater than at the amino acid level and common restriction enzyme sites occur in the genes for the various IFN-α subtypes. A common BglII site occurs in the genes for IFN-αA and -αD at a position corresponding to amino acid residue 61 and a PvuII site occurs in the genes for several IFN-α subtypes at a position corresponding to amino acid residue 91. These common restriction enzyme sites have allowed construction of hybrids such as IFN-αAD(Bgl) : the first subtype indicated alphabetically is the source of the N-terminal fragment and the second, the source of the C-terminal fragment and the site of recombination is designated by the abbreviation for the restriction site involved (Figure 2). In addition to the IFN-αA and -αD hybrids, indicated in Figure 2, a series of hybrids, involving the common PvuII site, have been formed with IFN-αA, -αD and other IFN-α subtypes (IFN-αB, -αF, -αG) (11). A BglII or Sau3A restriction site at a position corresponding to residue 150 in IFN-αA, -αD and -αI has allowed construction of other hybrids, also indicated graphically in Figure 2. These hybrids contain 165 or 166 amino acid residues, depending on whether or not they contain the N-terminal portion of IFN-αA and these materials allow examination of the effect of varying the C-terminal 15 amino acid residues.

BIOLOGICAL PROPERTIES OF HUMAN INTERFERONS

Individual leukocyte interferon subtypes show distinct antiviral effects against different viruses in various mammalian cell cultures (13-15). The hybrid interferons also have distinct antiviral activity (12; see also Figure 2) and in the case of IFN-αA and -αD, mixtures have additive effects, whereas the -αAD hybrids have greater activity than the parental subtypes and the -αDA hybrids have much lower activity. These observations have been confirmed using highly purified materials and a notable feature of IFN-αAD(Bgl) is its high activity in mouse cells (14) and against infections of mice (16). IFN-αAD(Bgl) also shows activity against the L1210 leukemia in BDF$_1$ mice (17) and these properties have allowed investigation of antiviral and antitumor effects in rodents.

In addition to their antiviral and antitumor effects, interferons have also been found to modulate a number of cellular and humoral immune responses and, at the biochemical level, several effects leading to inhibition of protein synthesis have been observed. Some of the known effects of interferons are listed in Table 1. Causal relations between the various effects of interferons remain unclear and the relation of in vitro and cell culture effects to antiviral and antitumor effects in vivo is also not established.

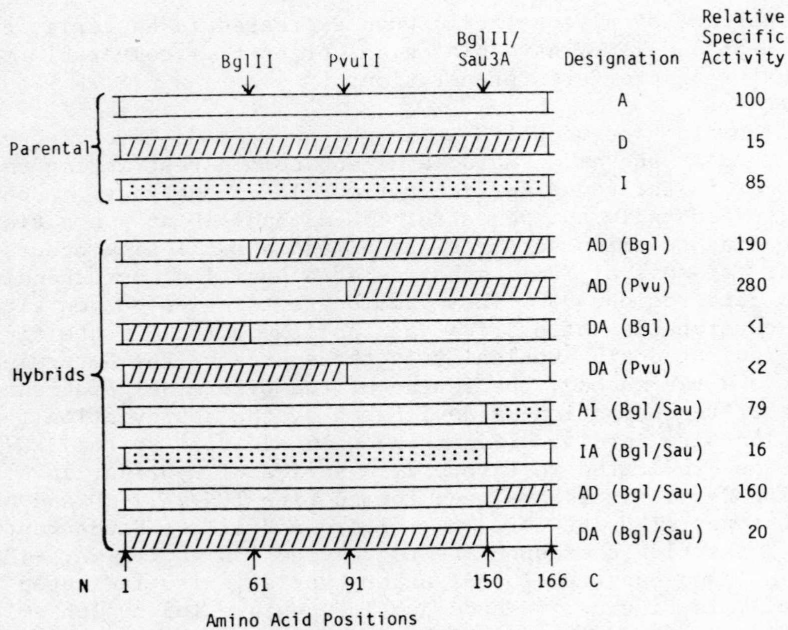

Fig. 2. Schematic representation and designation of hybrid IFN-αs. IFN-αA and hybrids incorporating the N-terminus of IFN-αA contain 165 residues. The relative specific activities relative to IFN-αA are from in vitro coupled transcription/translation of the genes (see 12). The absolute specific activity of IFN-αA is 10^8 U/mg protein. BglII, PVuII, and BglII/Sau3A refer to restriction enzyme sites.

Without doubt some of the biological properties of interferons are, in part at least, independent while others are secondary to primary effects, perhaps on protein synthesis or cell membranes. Although the independent effects of interferons may not be due entirely to distinct molecular domains it should be possible to construct derivative proteins which retain some of the biological properties and lack others. Successful screening of derivative interferons for desired properties will be facilitated by understanding which properties may be inherently linked and those that may be independent. Studies with recombinant DNA derived materials have indicated effects which are independent and some which may be dependent.

Antiviral effects observed in fibroblast cultures appear to be unreleated to antiviral effects in vivo, that is, viruses resistant to interferon in cell cultures may still be affected in vivo (18). Also, efficacy against a virus responsive in cell cultures may be destroyed by suppression of macrophages in vivo (19). Moreover, the cloned human interferon subtype, IFN-αA, is as effective against HSV-1 infection of the rabbit eye as highly potent buffy coat

Table 1. Properties of interferons associated with antiviral and antitumor activities

---

Biochemical/Intracellular Effects

Synthesis of 2'5'-oligo A and activation of RNase F
Stimulation of protein kinase activity
Cytoskeleton effects
Suppression of the P-450 mono-oxygenase system

Immunological Effects

Stimulation of NK cell activity and maturation of precursors
Leukopenia
Suppression of antibody synthesis
Stimulation of Fc receptor sites
Stimulation of antibody dependent cellular cytotoxicity

interferon preparations (20) although IFN-αA has a poor activity in rabbit cell cultures (14).

In the case of HSV-1 infections indirect mechanisms appear to be important for in vivo efficacy (20). However, in monkeys and mice there is a correlation between cell culture and in vivo efficacy of various interferons (12, 16, 21). Nevertheless, it should be noted that in monkeys dose-response studies indicate that IFN-αD is more effective against EMC virus infections than IFN-αA although IFN-αA has a considerably higher specific activity against this virus in cell cultures (12). Antitumor effects occur against tumor cell lines selected for resistance to antiproliferative effects of interferons (22). The nature of the indirect effects mediating antiviral and antitumor effects is uncertain, but the hybrid, IFN-αAD(Bgl), does not stimulate mouse NK cells against L1210 as target cells (15). Efficacy post tumor inoculation indicates an antibody dependent mechanism and antibody dependent cell mediated cytotoxicity may be important for antitumor effects.

IFN-αA causes leukopenia in rhesus monkeys but not squirrel monkeys (23). However, antiviral effects have been demonstrated with this interferon in both species (18, 21) indicating that leukopenia is not intrinsically linked with antiviral effects. Suppression of P-450 metabolism in the mouse occurs only with interferons which show antiviral activity, against EMC virus at least (24). Suppression of P-450 may arise simply because of inhibition of protein synthesis which will readily affect a major, rapidly turning over set of proteins such as those of the P-450 system in hepatocytes. In mice and hamsters, IFN-αA has no antitumor effects but the efficacy of cyclophosphamide is abrogated by simultaneous treatments (17). Clearly IFN-αA is exerting some biological effect in this situation but suppression of P-450 does not seem to be involved (17). It is possible that IFN-αA suppresses an immune response essential for the antitumor activity of cyclophosphamide and a suppressor cell activity seems most probable (25).

STURCTURE/ACTIVITY RELATIONS

Although the studies just reviewed indicate interferon functions which may be separable there is as yet no definitive data relating particular activities with structural domains. Binding of interferons to cellular receptors is likely to be a critical factor determining all subsequent biological effects. Receptor binding studies indicate that the leukocyte and fibroblast interferons bind to the same cellular receptors (26). However, events leading to antiviral activity cannot simply be sequalae to receptor binding because different IFN-α subtypes have different activities against the same viral infection of the same cell types (12, 14). Presumably other molecular domains result in specific effects leading to the different properties of the different interferons and receptor binding must be distinct from activation of mechanisms leading to biological effects (27).

Studies with hybrid leukocyte interferons indicate that both the N- and C-terminal portions of the leukocyte interferons are involved in receptor binding (12, 28). These studies involved the IFN-αAD(Bgl) and -αDA(Bgl) hybrids, shown in Figure 2. The IFN-αAD(Bgl/Sau) hybrid includes only the 15 C-terminal residues of IFN-αD and shows antiviral activity comparable to that of IFN-αAD(Bgl). The IFN-αIA and IFN-αDA hybrids have low activity (Figure 2). Thus the C-terminal 15 amino acids clearly have dramatic effects on activity of these interferons. However, limited proteolytic cleavage of IFN-αA, resulting in loss of the C-terminal 13 residues results in a material retaining nearly all antiviral, cell binding and antibody binding activity (5). Moreover, active interferons lacking the 10 C-terminal amino acids have also been isolated from induced human cell cultures (29). The BglII/Sau3A site at residue 150 of IFN-αA has been used to construct a gene which codes for a derivative (IFN-αA-11) lacking the last 11 amino acid residues. Curiously, this interferon has greatly reduced antiviral activity (3). Presumably folding of IFN-αA-11 during synthesis results in a structure distinct from that obtained by post translation cleavage of the C-terminus.

Although the C-terminal 13 residues of IFN-αA appear to be unnecessary for activity, at least when removed after synthesis, the majority of the rest of the molecule seems to be essential. Neither trypsin or cyanogen bromide fragments nor reconstituted mixtures of fragments have antiviral or cell binding activity (5). The _cys_ 29 to _cys_ 138 disulphide bond appears to be essential for activity

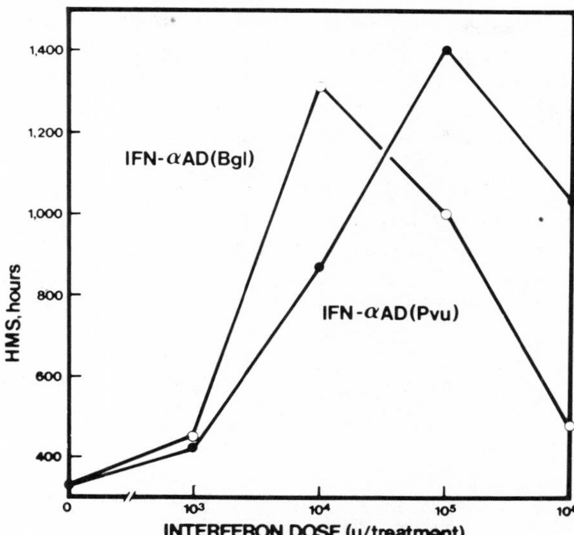

Fig. 3. Dose response of efficacy of IFN-αAD(Bgl) and IFN-αAD(Pvu) against the L1210 Leukemia in BDF_1 mice. All interferons given once daily on days 1 to 12 post tumor inoculation at the doses indicated and the harmonic mean survival (HMS) time determined after 60 days (30).

because limited oxidation products are only active if this bond is maintained (5). That the other disulphide, cys 1 to cys 98 is not essential was implied by the activity of fusion proteins lacking cys 1 (1).

At least one of the two tryptophans in IFN-αA appears to be important for activity, that is, chemical modification of the tryptophans greatly reduced antiviral, antigenic and cell receptor binding activity (5). The formation of hybrids with the same N- and C-termini but different internal sequences allows determination of the role of other residues. The three IFN-αAD hybrids, shown in Figure 2, illustrate this approach and in this case most extensive pharmacological data exist for IFN-αAD(Bgl) and IFN-αAD(Pvu). The only differences between these two materials are the differences between IFN-αA and -αD between residues 61 and 91 and these are at positions 68, 79 and 85 (30). These residues are thr, asp, cys in IFN- AD(Bgl) and ser, thr, tyr in IFN-αAD(Pvu). In mouse cells these two interferons show a difference in specific activity of about five fold. However, only IFN-αAD(Bgl) shows significant protection of EMC infected mice and this hybrid interferon appears to be much more potent than IFN-αAD(Pvu) against the L1210 leukemia in mice. However, in the tumor system the two hybrids show different dose response curves (see Figure 3). Above 10^4 U/treatment IFN-αAD(Bgl) shows decreasing efficacy whereas the efficacy of IFN-αAD(Pvu) only decreases at doses over 10^5 U/treatment (30). The interferon doses are units determined on MDBK cells for which the specific activities and hence the amounts of the materials are very similar (30). The differences between the two curves shown in Figure 3 would be even greater for interferon titers on human or mouse cells.

IFN-αAD(Bgl) causes suppression of mouse P-450 metabolism (24) with predictable effects on the activity of hexabarbital and acetaminophen, both of which are metabolized by P-450 (31). However, IFN-αAD(Pvu) does not affect metabolism of hexabarbital or acetaminophen (30). The pharmacokinetics in rats of these two hybrid interferons are different. Although nephrectomization decreases clearance of interferons from the plasma, this effect is much more prominent for IFN-αAD(Pvu) than IFN-αAD(Bgl). All these differences arise from the three amino acid residue differences between these very similar materials.

Because of the potential clinical importance of the negative interaction between cyclophosphamide and interferon, it seemed important to determine whether the effect occurs with natural interferons. In addition, because relatively high interferon doses were used, the effect of a lower interferon dose was investigated. The data, in Figure 4, show that in the mouse L1210 system interferon doses of 500 U/treatment cause enhanced rather than decreased antitumor effects with cyclophosphamide, regardless of whether natural mouse interferon or IFN-αAD(Bgl) was used.

FUTURE DEVELOPMENTS

The construction of hybrid interferons has provided an initial method for probing structure/activity relationships of interferons. Most current data relates to IFN-αs because they are a family of related genes with common restriction enzyme sites. Related genes have not yet been identified by recombinant DNA methods for IFN-β_1 and IFN-γ. However, with the data obtained for IFN-αs from molecular hybrids, it should be possible to predict desirable structures for particular purposes such as particular virus infections or tumors. These new analogs may be most conveniently produced by complete synthesis of genes rather than elaborate construction of hybrid genes. Complete gene synthesis may also be applicable to constructing analogs of IFN-β_1, and IFN-γ and the properties of such analogs may also be used to design particularly desirable materials.

The initial goal of structure/activity studies includes analysis of the extent to which known effects of interferons, such as those listed in Table 1, can be dissociated. The properties of clinical significance also need to be ascertained, in addition to factors which might augment efficacy. Pharmacokinetics and drug interactions are likely to be important. However, the construction of novel

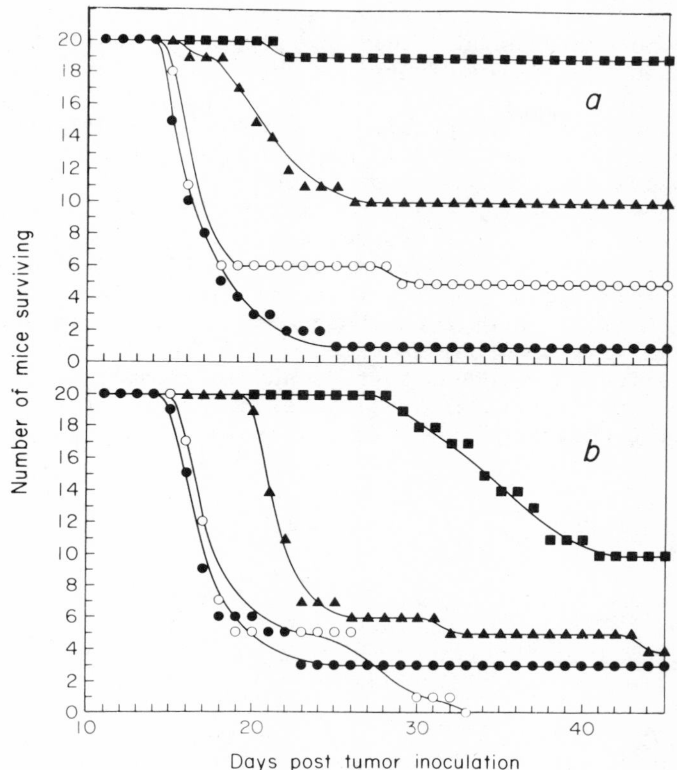

Fig. 4. Effects of (a) IFN-αAD(Bgl), (b) mouse interferon in combination with cyclophosphamide against the L1210 Leukemia in BFD_1 mice. Interferon (500 U/treatment) given once daily on days 1 to 12 post tumor inoculation alone (○), and in combination with cyclophosphamide (■). Cyclophosphamide, 0.5 mg/treatment given on days 1 to 3 post tumor inoculation. Cyclophosphamide alone (▲), and saline controls (●). All treatments i.p. (S. H. Lee, H. Chiu, and N. Stebbing, unpublished).

interferons presents the obvious danger that the new materials will show antigenicity. This problem has already arisen with natural preparations of IFN-α and $-\beta_1$ and individual IFN-α subtypes. The cause of this problem needs to be assessed before a solution for synthetic interferons can be determined. Despite the difficulties of devising and selecting novel hybrid interferons for clinical use, the potential advantages are very significant. The interferons are highly potent agents with numerous properties whose contribution to overall clinical effects will be difficult to determine. Natural materials, as with other therapeutic agents, are likely to be replaced by more specific agents designed for specific diseases and purposes.

Pharmacological assessment of existing members of gene families and hybrid molecules should indicate properties which may be removed without losing desired antiviral or antitumor effects, as discussed here. Understanding the relation of cell culture to in vivo effects of interferons remains a problem of considerable practical as well as theoretical interest. It is perhaps remarkable that the hybrid interferon IFN-αAD(Bgl), with pronounced activity in mouse cells, has also shown antiviral and antitumor activity in mice comparable to mouse interferon. Furthermore, effects on P-450 and in vivo drug interactions appear to be very similar for IFN-αAD(Bgl) and mouse interferon. It seems unlikely that this arises from coincidental construction of an interferon whose entire amino acid sequence is closely similar to a mouse interferon. Further studies with hybrid interferons in heterologous systems should greatly extend our understanding of the structure/activity relations of interferons and assist in the design of novel materials for particular clinical indications.

REFERENCES

1. Nagata, S., H. Tiara, A. Hall, L. Johnsrud, M. Streuli, J. Escodi, W. Boll, K. Cantell, and C. Weissmann. 1980. Synthesis in *E. coli* of a polypeptide with human leukocyte interferon activity. Nature 284: 316-320.

2. Goeddel, D. V., D. W. Leung, T. J. Dull, M. Gross, R. M. Lawn, R. McCandliss, P. H. Seeburg, A. Ullrich, E. Yelverton, and P. W. Gray. 1981. The structure of eight distinct cloned human leukocyte interferon cDNAs. Nature 390: 20-26.

3. Franke, A. E., H. M. Shepard, C. M. Houck, P. W. Leung, D. V. Goeddel, and R. M. Lawn. 1982. Carboxy terminal region of hybrid leukocyte interferons affects antiviral specificity. DNA (in press).

4. Wetzel, R., L. J. Perry, D. A. Estell, N. Lin, H. L. Levine, B. Slinker, F. Fields, M. J. Ross, and J. Shively. 1981. Properties of a human alpha interferon purified from *E. coli* extracts. J. Interferon Res. 1: 381-390.

5. Wetzel, R., H. L. Levine, D. A. Estell, S. Shive, J. Finer-Moore, R. M. Stroud, and T. A. Bewley. 1982. Structure-function studies on human alpha interferon. *In* T. Merigan and R. Friedman (eds.), Chemistry and biology of interferons: Relationship to therapeutics. UCLA Symp. Mol. Cell. Biol. 25, Academic Press, New York (in press).

6. Pitha, P. M., D. L. Slate, N. B. K. Raj, and R. H. Ruddle. 1982. Human β_1 interferon gene localization and expression in somatic cell hybrids. Mol. Cell. Biol. 2: 564-570.

7. Gray, P. W., D. W. Leung, D. Pennica, E. Yelverton, E. Najarian, C. C. Simonsen, R. Derynck, P. J. Sherwood, D. M. Wallace, S. L. Berger, A. D. Levinson, and D. V. Goeddel. 1982. Expression of human immune interferon cDNA in E. coli and monkey cells. Nature 295: 503-508.

8. Allen, G., and K. H. Fantes. 1980. A family of structural genes for human lymphoblastoid (leukocyte-type) interferon. Nature 287: 408-411.

9. Harkins, R. N., P. E. Hass, W. H. Kohr, B. B. Aggarwal, P. K. Weck, and S. Apperson. 1982. Structural and biological properties of purified bacteria derived human fibroblast interferon. Proc. Natl. Acad. Sci. (in press).

10. Shepard, H. M., D. Leung, N. Stebbing, and D. V. Goeddel. 1981. A single amino acid change in human fibroblast interferon (IFN-β_1) abolishes antiviral activity. Nature 294: 563-565.

11. Weck, P. K., S. Apperson, E. Hamilton, and N. Stebbing. 1982. Biological properties of genetic hybrids of bacteria-derived human leukocyte interferons. J. Cell. Biochem. Suppl. 6: 104.

12. Weck, P. K., S. Apperson, N. Stebbing, P. W. Gray, D. Leung, H. M. Shepard, and D. V. Goeddel. 1981. Antiviral activities of hybrids of two major human leukocyte interferons. Nucleic Acids Res. 9: 6153-6166.

13. Masucci, M. G., R. Szigeti, E. Klein, G. Klein, J. Gruest, L. Montagnier, H. Taira, A. Hall, S. Nagata, and C. Weissmann. 1980. Effect of interferon-α_1 from E. coli on some cell functions. Science 209: 1431-1435.

14. Weck, P. K., S. Apperson, L. May, and N. Stebbing. 1981. Comparison of the antiviral activity of various cloned human interferon-α subtypes in mammalian cell cultures. J. Gen Virol. 57: 233-237.

15. Lee, S. H., S. Kelley, H. Chiu, and N. Stebbing. 1982. Stimulation of natural killer cell activity and inhibition of proliferation of various leukemic cells by purified human leukocyte interferon subtypes. Cancer Res. 42: 1312-1316.

16. Weck, P. K., E. Rinderknecht, D. A. Estell, and N. Stebbing. 1982. Antiviral activity of bacteria derived human leukocyte interferons against encephalomyocarditis virus infection of mice. Infect. Immun. 35: 660-665.

17. Stebbing, N., P. K. Weck, J. T. Fenno, S. Apperson, and S. H. Lee. 1981. Comparison of the biological properties of natural and recombinant DNA derived human interferons, p. 25-33. In E. DeMaeyer, G. Galasso and H. Schellekens (eds.), The biology of the interferon system. Elsevier/North Holland.

18. Schellekens, H., W. Weimar, K. Cantell, and L. Stitz. 1979. Antiviral effect of interferon in vivo may be mediated by the host. Nature 278: 742.

19. Stebbing, N., K. M. Dawson, and I. J. D. Lindley. 1978. Requirement for macrophages for interferon to be effective against encephalomyocarditis virus infection in mice. Infect. Immun. 19: 5-11.

20. Smolin, G., N. Stebbing, M. Friedlender, R. Friedlender, and M. Okumoto. 1982. Natural and cloned human leukocyte interferon in herpes virus infections of rabbit eyes. Arch. Ophthamol. 100: 481-483.

21. Stebbing, N., P. K. Weck, J. T. Fenno, D. A. Estell, and E. Rinderknecht. 1982. Antiviral effects of bacteria derived human leukocyte interferons against encephalomyocarditis virus infection of squirrel monkeys. Arch. Virol. (in press).

22. Gresser, I., C. Maury, and D. Brouty-Boye. 1972. Mechanisms of the antitumor effect of interferon in mice. Nature 239: 167-168.

23. Stebbing, N., S. H. Lee, B. J. Marafino, P. K. Weck, and K. W. Renton. 1982. Activity of cloned gene products in animal systems. In F. Ahmad, J. Schultz and E. E. Smith (eds.), From gene to protein: Translation into biotechnology. Academic Press, New York (in press).

24. Singh, G., K. W. Renton, and N. Stebbing. 1982. Homogeneous interferon from E. coli depresses hepatic cytochrome P-450 and drug biotransformation. Biochem. Biophys. Res. Commun. 106: 1256-1261.

25. Hengst, J. C. D., M. B. Mokyr, and S. Dray. 1981. Cooperation between cyclophosphamide tumoricidal activity and host antitumor immunity in the cure of mice bearing large MOPC-315 tumors. Cancer Res. 41: 2163-2167.

26. Branca, A. A., and C. Baglioni. 1981. Evidence that types I and II interferons have different receptors. Nature 294: 768-770.

27. Chany, C. 1976. Membrane-bound interferon specific cell receptor system: role in the establishment and amplification of the antiviral state. Biomedicine 24: 148-157.

28. Streuli, M., A. Hall, W. Boll, W. E. Stewart, S. Nagata, and C. Weissmann. 1981. Target cell specificity of two species of human interferon-α produced in *Escherichia coli* and of hybrid molecules derived from them. Proc. Nat. Acad. Sci. 78: 2848-2852.

29. Levy, W. P., M. Rubinstein, J. Shively, V. D. Valle, C. Y. Lai, J. Moschera, L. Brink, L. Gerber, S. Stein, and S. Pestka. 1981. Amino acid sequence of a human leukocyte interferon. Proc. Nat. Acad. Sci. 78: 6186-6190.

30. Lee, S. H., P. K. Weck, J. Moore, S. Chen, and N. Stebbing. 1982. Pharmacological comparison of two hybrid recombinant DNA derived human leukocyte interferons. *In* T. Merigan and R. Friedman (eds.), Chemistry and biology of interferons: Relationship to therapeutics. UCLA Symp. Mol. Cell. Biol. 25, Academic Press, New York (in press).

31. Moore, J. A., B. J. Marafino, and N. Stebbing. 1982. Influence of various purified interferons on pharmacological effects of drugs in mice. J. Path. (in press).

IMMUNOREGULATION BY LYMPHOKINES: IMMUNE INTERFERON AND LYMPHOTOXIN INDUCTION OF LYMPHOKINE ACTIVITY IN HUMAN PERIPHERAL BLOOD LEUKOCYTE CULTURES

C. H. Robbins

Genentech, Inc., 460 Point San Bruno Boulevard, South San Francisco, California, (USA)

INTRODUCTION

Immune responses to tumors are highly complex, with the final outcome dependent upon the interaction of several effector mechanisms within the immune system. Treatment of tumors, as well as other forms forms of immunological disease, has been based on use of nonphysiological agents that nonspecifically alter immunocompetent cell function. The ability of natural products of the immune system to affect immune function has been documented in many studies, in vivo and in vitro (1,2,3). Lymphokines, a group of regulatory substances produced by activated lymphocytes, have potential for development into powerful immunomodulatory tools. Research into mechanisms of lymphokine action has been hampered by lack of sufficient quantities of high purity. The number and properties of chemically distinct lymphokines is unknown. The various induction schemes used to produce lymphokines for study rarely yield a single bioactivity, and there is a strong probability that the interaction of several lymphokines is necessary to successfully modulate an immune function. Supernatants of mitogen-induced human peripheral blood lymphocyte (PBL) cultures contain several lymphokine activities. Analysis of kinetic studies has suggested a correlation in the appearance in culture supernatants of lymphotoxin activity (LT) and immune interferon (Im-IF). The interaction between LT and Im-IF was investigated in a serum-free human PBL culture system.

METHODS

Lymphotoxin used in these experiments was derived from

RPMI-1788, a human B cell line, provided by Dr. B. Aggarwal (Genentech). The cultures were grown in serum-free medium which was collected after 48 hr incubation. The preparations used in this study were purified at least one hundred fold, and had a titer of 4000 units/ml.

The immune interferon provided by Dr. E. Rinderknecht (Genentech) was produced by monkey COS-7 cells transfected with a plasmid containing the gene for human Im-IF. Serum-free culture supernatants were collected, and a partial purification procedure for Im-IF followed. The resulting preparation had a titer of 6000 units/ml, and no contaminating LT or macrophage migration inhibitory factor (MIF) activity. The IF activity was identified as Im-IF by antibody neutralization, pH 2 and SDS treatment (L. May, Genentech).

Antibody (Ab) to leukocyte IF was obtained from NAIAD, and antibody to fibroblast IF from Dr. Neidhammer. These were used at a 1:10 dilution. Antibody to murine Im-IF was the kind gift of Dr. H. M. Johnson (University of Texas Medical Branch, Galveston, TX), and antimurine L-cell IF Ab was provided by Dr. Meyers (NIH). The Ab to RPMI-1788 was prepared in rabbits, and each milliliter of antibody neutralized 84 units of LT. Anti-Im-IF Ab was provided by V. Anicetti (Genentech). This Ab was raised in rabbits from material purified from human PBL cultures, and neutralized 20 units Im-IF with a titer of 1:2000.

Cell Culture

Human peripheral blood leukocytes were obtained by leukophoresis. These cells were separated on ficoll-hypaque gradients and washed two times. The cells were cultured in 96-well microtiter plates (Costar) at a density of 5 x 10^6/ml, 200 μl/well. Culture medium was RPMI-1640, without serum and antibiotics. Cell viability was 97% or greater at start of culture. Cultures were set up with individual wells for each time point, so that culture volume and cell density were constant throughout incubation. Samples were harvested and spun in a microfuge, and the supernatants assayed for LT and IF activity.

Assays

LT activity was measured in an assay developed by Anna Hui, (Genentech). Briefly, mouse L929 fibroblast monolayers were grown in 96-well microtiter plates and exposed to mitomycin C. LT samples were added in serial dilutions across the plate, with an internal standard run on each plate. After a 48 hour incubation at 37°C, the monolayers were stained with crystal violet. The optical density in the center of each well was read by a Dynatek plate reader and an end-point determined as 50% cytopathic effect (CPE) compared with controls.

The antiviral activity of the samples was measured as cytopathic effects on HELA human fibroblast cell monolayers grown in 96-well microtiter plates. Serial dilutions of the samples were added to confluent monolayers of HELA cells and incubated for 18 hours. Vesicular stomatitis virus (VSV) was added, and 16 hours later the plates were stained with crystal violet. Values determined by this method are expressed as units relative to the NIH leukocyte IF standard G-023-901-527. Assays for murine IF activity involved murine H-2 cell line and EMC virus.

Interferon Characterization

In order to characterize interferon, samples were incubated for 1 hour at 4°C with 0.1% SDS, and then dialyzed overnight in PBS at 4°C. Alternatively, samples were brought to pH 2 with 1N HCl, held for 24 hours, at 4°C and then brought to pH 7.4 by 3N NaOH. Antibody neutralizations involved the mixing of 20 μl volumes of sample and antisera and incubation overnight at 4°C.

RESULTS AND DISCUSSION

Our studies of the mitogen stimulation of human PBL cultures have suggested a correlation between the production of LT and Im-IF. The data presented here show that these two lymphokines are related in their production. As shown in Table 1, PBL produced significant IF titers within 15 hours of commencing incubation with RPMI-1788-derived LT. The IF activity was still present in the culture

Table 1. Lymphotoxin (LT) Induction of IF Activity in Human PBL Cultures[1]

	IF (units/ml)			
	Hours of Incubation			
Treatment	15 hrs.	24 hrs.	48 hrs	72 hrs.
Control	9	9	7	7
512 units/ml LT	1083	1833	3667	8000
1024 units/ml LT	1750	3167	3667	3500

[1] Human PBL were cultured in the presence and absence of cell-line derived LT. Supernatants were harvested at indicated timepoints and assayed for IF activity. Both doses of LT resulted in significant increases in IF titer of the culture supernatants.

supernatants 72 hours after culture initiation. This induced IF activity showed significant antiviral titers in HELA, but not on MDBK cells (Table 2). Also, this activity was sensitive to heat, SDS and pH 2 treatment. Antibody to human Im-IF completely neutralized the induced IF activity, while Ab to human leukocyte and fibroblast IF had no effect on the antiviral activity. These results characterize the induced IF as Im-IF.

Cloned human Im-IF preparations were used to examine IF induction of LT activity. Human PBL incubated with 160 to 320 units/ml of Im-IF showed significant titers of LT in the culture supernatants by 15 hours of incubation (Table 3). Donor variation in the titers of LT produced was high. However, in all cases, LT titers in the Im-IF treated cultures exceeded control levels. This IF-induced LT activity was neutralized by Ab to 1788-derived LT (Table 4). This demonstrates that 1788-derived LT and Im-IF induced PBL-derived LT have common determinants relating to their in vitro cytotoxic activity.

Table 2. Characterization of the Interferon (IF) Activity Induced in PBL cultures by Lymphotoxin (LT)[1]

	Interferon Activity (units/ml)	
Treatment	LT-induced IF	Im-IF Control
Assay on HELA	687	250
Assay on MDBK	8	8
56°C, 1 hour	82	47
0.1% SDS, 1 hour	6	6
pH 2, 24 hours	6	6
% neutralization by:		
anti-LeIF	0%	-
anti-FIF	2%	-
anti-Im-IF	100%	92%

[1] Human PBL were cultured with 256 units/ml of LT. Supernatants were collected after 24 hours. These supernatants were treated as described below, then assayed to determine which class of IF was being induced. These results indicate that LT induces Im-IF activity in human PBL cultures. Three other trials gave similar results. Im-IF control was a partially purified sample of cloned Im-IF (Dr. E. Rinderknecht, Genentech).

Table 3. Im-IF Induction of LT Activity in PBL Cultures[1]

	LT (units/ml)		
	Hours of Incubation		
Treatment	15 hrs	24 hrs	48 hrs
Control	16	48	48
160 units/ml Im-IF	128 (.001)[2]	544 (.02)	1024 (.001)
320 units/ml Im-IF	96 (.05)	544 (.02)	1024 (.001)

[1] Human PBL were incubated plus or minus Im-IF. Supernatants were harvested and assayed for LT activity. Results are expressed as the mean of two experiments. All donor PBL showed levels of LT activity above control when treated with Im-IF. However, donor variation in response led to large standard deviations from the mean.

[2] Indicates P value derived from Student's t-test.

Table 4. LT Activity Induced by Im-IF is Neutralized by Antibody to Cell Line Derived LT[1]

	LT (units/ml)			
Treatment	-Ab	+Ab	% Neutra-lization	P
Control	16	16	-	-
160 μ/ml Im-IF	1024	75	93	.001
320 μ/ml Im-IF	1024	53	95	.001

[1] Human PBL's were cultured with Im-IF for 24-48 hours. The culture supernatants were assayed for LT in the presence and absence of antibody to LT. The antibody itself does not affect the LT assay system. Antibody sufficient to neutralize 2048 units LT/ml was added in each case.

As shown in Table 5, treating PBL cultures with two different doses of LT resulted in supernatant LT activity exceeding the LT titer added at initiation of culture. This excess LT activity (a 2-4.5 fold increase over treatment titer) appeared within the first 15 hours of culture. These results show that LT induces production of additional LT activity, as well as Im-IF (Table 1).

The converse experiment is shown in Table 6. Human PBL incubated with either 160 or 320 units/ml of cloned Im-IF produced IF exceeding the treatment titer by a factor of 2.3 - 26.6. These results indicate that Im-IF induces not only LT activity (Table 3) but also additional IF activity.

The observations reported here suggest a complex relationship between the two lymphokines, LT and Im-IF. These activities appear to be capable of autoinduction, as well as inducing each other. Once pure preparations of these lymphokines are available, it will be possible to further delineate the nature of this interaction and prove conclusively that the observed supernatant lymphokine activities were induced solely by the added LT or Im-IF.

Table 5. LT Induction of LT Activity in Human PBL Cultures[1]

	LT (units/ml)			
	Hours of Incubation			
Treatment	15 hrs	24 hrs	48 hrs	72 hrs
Control	32	32	64	64
512 units/ml LT	1088 (.05)[2]	1920 (.05)	1152 (.02)	2304 (.02)
1024 units/ml LT	2304 (.01)	1536 (.01)	2304 (.02)	2304 (.02)

1 Human PBL were incubated plus/minus LT. Supernatants were harvested at indicated times and assayed for LT activity. Results are expressed as the mean of four experiments. LT titers in excess of the LT added to the culture system were found in both dose treatments.

2 Indicates P value derived from Student's t-test.

Table 6. Im-IF Induction of IF Activity in Human PBL Cultures[1]

Treatment	IF (units/ml) Hours of Incubation 15 hrs	24 hrs	48 hrs	72 hrs
Control	8	8	8	8
160 units/ml Im-IF	1047	1667	4250	3667
320 units/ml Im-IF	833	1333	4125	2388

1 Human PBL were incubated plus or minus Im-IF. Supernatants were harvested at indicated times and assayed for IF activity. Results are expressed as the mean of four experiments. In all but 2 out of the 24 supernatants assayed, IF activity was in excess of that added at culture initiation.

SUMMARY

Supernatants of mitogen-induced human PBL cultures contain several lymphokine activities. Analysis of kinetic studies has suggested a correlation in the appearance in culture supernatants of lymphotoxin (LT) and immune interferon (Im-IF). We investigated this interaction between LT and Im-IF in the serum-free human PBL culture system. Partially purified LT was derived from a normal cell line, RPMI 1788. This LT, which had no contaminating IF activity, induced production of significant levels of IF activity as early as 15 hours after initiation of culture. This induced IF activity was identified as Im-IF by criteria of pH 2, SDS and heat sensitivity, as well as neutralization by AB to Im-IF. LT activity, in excess of the units added to the culture, was also measured in the LT-induced cultures.

In another group of experiments, partially purified human Im-IF, produced by expression of a cloned gene in monkey COS-7 cells, was added to human PBL cultures. This Im-IF, at concentrations of 160 and 320 units/ml, caused induction of LT activity. The induced LT activity was neutralized by AB raised to 1788-derived LT. Im-IF treated cultures also contained IF activity in excess of the titers added to the cultures. These results would suggest an interaction between LT and Im-IF at the level of production by lymphoid cells.

REFERENCES

1. Papermaster, B. W., C. D. Gilliland, J. E. McEntire, N. D. Rodes and P. A. Dunn. 1981. In vivo biological studies with lymphoblastoid lymphokines, p. 289-299. In A. L. Goldstein and M. A. Chirigos (eds.), Lumphokines and thymic hormones: Their potential utilization in cancer therapeutics. Raven Press, New York.

2. Geczy, C., A. G. Geczy and A. L. de Weck. 1976. Antibodies to guinea pig lymphokines. J. Immunol. 117: 66-72.

3. Khan, A., E. S. Martin, K. Webb, D. Weldon, N. O. Hill, J. Duvall and J. M. Hill. 1982. Regression of malignant melanoma in a dog by local injections of a partially purified preparation containing human α-lymphotoxin. Proc. Soc. Exp. Biol. Med. 169: 291-294.

MONOCLONAL ANTIBODIES AS ANTICANCER AGENTS

Robert K. Oldham

National Cancer Institute, Division of Cancer Treatment
Biological Response Modifiers Program, Frederick
Cancer Research Center, Frederick, MD (USA)

INTRODUCTION

A major problem with current modalities of cancer treatment has been the lack of specificity of the treatment for the cancer cell. It is well known that the therapeutic/toxic ratio is low for anticancer drugs and for radiation therapy. A major advance in the treatment of cancer could be heralded by the development of a class of agents that have a greater degree of specificity for the tumor cell. The technique of hybridization of an immortal myeloma cell line with an antibody-producing B cell as developed by Kohler and Milstein in the late 1970's provided a technique by which monoclonal antibodies could be produced in virtually unlimited quantities (1). Since the technique involved the selection of single cells and the clonal expansion of a single hybrid between the antibody-forming cell and the myeloma cell, this technique makes available, for the first time, monoclonal antibodies for use in cancer biology. Since most of the monoclonal antibodies developed against human tumor cells have been made in mice by immunizing the mouse with human tumor cells or extracts thereof, these monoclonals are mouse immunoglobulins and represent the way a mouse cell sees a human tumor cell. While there are many difficulties with respect to using mouse immunoglobulins as therapeutic reagents in man, this technique may provide one route around the problem of immunogenicity of tumors in man. It is possible that the mouse will recognize antigenic determinants on the human tumor cell <u>not recognized</u> by the patient's own immune system or not recognized well by that immune system. If this turns out to be the case, we will have a mechanism for developing specific monoclonal reagents defining antigenic specificities on the tumor cell which may be unique and cancer specific though nonimmunogenic in the primary host. Therefore, investigations into mouse monoclonal antibody may be important even given the future availability of human-derived monoclonal antibodies and even with the potential toxicities of mouse immunoglobulin reagents.

While the use of antibody alone is proceeding well in clinical trials throughout the United States, the use of animal tumor models will be very important in attempting to assess immunoconjugates and utilizing these conjugated reagents in cancer therapeutics. We have recently reviewed the animal tumor models that have been used for antibody studies (2, 3). There are clearly many models which may have great relevance to the design and development of improved immunoconjugated reagents for therapeutic use. Currently being tested are conjugates of monoclonal antibody to drugs, toxins, and radioisotopes. Each of these reagents carries its own therapeutic capabilities as well as its own intrinsic toxicities. However, each has the potential for enhanced therapeutic specificity given the conjugation to the antibody molecule and its inherent specificity for the antigenic site on the tumor cell. While many problems remain to be defined as to the class of immunoglobulin, the purification of antibody, the route and schedule of administration, the immune reactions to the mouse immunoglobulin, and as to the use of immunoconjugates, this field is the most fertile field for laboratory and clinical investigation of cancer-specific reagents. In this report, some of the ongoing clinical trials with monoclonal antibody will be reviewed in an attempt to discuss the possibilities and the problems with these trials. Some preliminary data on a particular guinea pig model for the development of immunoconjugates will also be presented.

MONOCLONAL ANTIBODY TRIALS IN MAN

The use of monoclonal antibodies in man has recently been reviewed (4, 5). While most of these trials involved individual patients or very small series of patients, early indications are that monoclonal antibody alone can have therapeutic effects in certain human malignancies. There have been preliminary results reporting the use of monoclonal antibody in a few solid tumors such as melanoma and gastrointestinal cancer (6), but the larger number of patients treated thus far have had leukemia or lymphoma (5, 7-12). Some of these early trials have been designed to approach preliminary questions that have been raised with respect to the feasibility of monoclonal antibody therapy and the rationale for the therapy and the rationale for the use of these reagents (Table 1).

Antibody trials in human T cell leukemia and lymphoma have been attempted using monoclonal antibodies with some T cell specificity. There are now a large number of antibodies that react

Table 1. Rationale for phase 1 monoclonal antibody (MoAb) serotherapy trials.

1. Determine toxicity of MoAb serotherapy in carefully monitored dose escalation trials.

2. Determine optimal dosage with reference to toxicity, and biological effects.

3. Determine clinical response to MoAb therapy.

4. Determine immune response to murine MoAb.

5. All of the above are essential preliminary data on MoAb prior to use of MoAb conjugated to drugs and toxins.

with most circulating T cells (examples would be T101 and anti-Leu-1 antibodies with the specificities shown in Table 2). Utilizing the anti-Leu-1 antibody, Miller and co-workers recently reported this antibody's ability to transiently drop the leukemic cell count in the peripheral blood of a patient with circulating malignant T cells (8). While the antibodies were effective in causing sharp drops in the white blood cell counts, the therapeutic effects were brief, lasting sometimes only hours before the leukemic cell count rose back to previous levels. However, another patient with cutaneous T cell lymphoma with skin plaques and enlarged lymph nodes was treated with anti-Leu-1 and partial responses in the skin lesions and lymph nodes were seen, accompanied by a sustained reduction in circulating malignant T cells (10). This was accomplished using repeated intermittent monoclonal antibody therapy. The mechanisms for the therapeutic effects in these patients are not clear. Possibilities include complement-mediated cytotoxicity, antibody dependent cell-mediated cytotoxicity, and direct antiproliferative effects. These investigators believe that the reticuloendothelial system is playing a major role and that some form of antibody coating of circulating cells is important in removing circulating blast cells. The precise mechanism for the therapeutic effects seen in the skin infiltrations is simply not clear at this point. Further studies are underway by these and other investigators with the use of anti-T cell reagents in both T cell leukemias and lymphomas and in T antigen bearing chronic lymphocytic leukemia (CLL). These trials should be of value in defining the role of anti-T cell monoclonal antibody alone in the treatment of these leukemias and lymphomas. It is already clear that there are certain problems implicit in the use of antibody alone in these therapeutic trials. As is shown in Table 3, many of these problems have possible solutions and in the context of these therapeutic trials these problems are being identified and the solutions being investigated.

Table 2. Specificities of T101 and anti-Leu-1 antibodies

Reactivity with normal and malignant cells	
T Lymphocytes	+
B Lymphocytes	-
Monocytes	-
Granulocytes	-
Non-B Non-T ALL	-
T-ALL	+
B-CLL	+
T-CLL	+
Sezary Cell Leukemia	+

Table 3. Problems with monoclonal antibody (MoAb) therapy

Problem	Possible Solutions
Antigenic modulation	Not all antibodies cause modulation; use 2 MoAb recognizing same antigen (different epitopes) or different antigens; choose different antigen
Release of free antigen	Plasmapheresis over immunoabsorbent column; schedule MoAb treatmemts 3 days apart
Antimouse antibodies	Human antibodies, low dose cyclophosphamide, plasmapheresis with immunospecific absorption
Non-sustained reduction of leukemic cells	Repeated intermittent MoAb infusions
Bone marrow neoplastic cells not affected	Conjugate MoAb to drugs or toxins

A more specific approach in the use of monoclonal antibody therapy has been described by Miller and co-workers (11). One of their patients with lymphoma became resistant to cytotoxic drugs and to interferon. In the laboratory, an anti-idiotype monoclonal antibody had been developed which was specific for the idiotype on the surface membrane of his lymphoma cells. Some of the characteristics of this individual patient trial are listed in Table 4. Circulating idiotype was detected prior to therapy but with continued monoclonal antibody therapy the idiotype was reduced and finally disappeared as circulating antibody appeared in the circulation. Subsequent to the appearance of circulating antibody, a clinical response occurred which progressed to a complete clinical response during the course of continued intermittent anti-idiotype monoclonal antibody therapy. Based on the most recent information available, this patient is still in complete remission in excess of one year after completing therapy. It has been pointed out that the histological type of lymphoma involved in this case was initially a favorable histology nodular lymphoma with a large number of T cells in the tumor bed. At the time of therapy the histology had changed to an unfavorable diffuse histology. Again, Miller and co-workers have postulated that the T cell might be involved along with antibody-coated tumor cells in the genesis of this clinical response. Monoclonal anti-idiotype antibodies are being prepared for further clinical trials to attempt to confirm this striking and intriguing observation.

Although large numbers of monoclonal antibody trials are being initiated, only a few trials have been underway for a sufficient period of time to have reported any results. Some of the trials

Table 4. Anti-idiotype MoAb serotherapy.

1. Non-secreting human lymphoma cells were fused with a murine HAT-sensitive myeloma line to produce a heterohybridoma.

2. This hybridoma secreted the monoclonal Ig found on the surface membrane of the human lymphoma cells.

3. 100 μg of this Ig injected intraperitoneally in CFA was used to immunize BALB/c mice followed by a second immunization on day 7 of 100 μg intravenously. Fusion was performed on day 10.

4. A murine hybridoma was selected that secreted an anti-idiotype MoAb (IgG_{2b}) recognizing the human lymphoma cells.

5. Complete tumor regression followed courses of serotherapy.

where results have been reported and some where patients are still accruing are listed in Table 5. Based on these preliminary trials using mouse-derived monoclonal antibodies, it is clear that these mouse immunoglobulin reagents can be given to man without severe acute toxicity. Clinical trials investigating different doses and schedules of administration are under way to determine the optimal way to give intravenous antibody alone in these phase I trials. Certain conclusions can be drawn based on these preliminary studies (Table 6). A major difficulty with antibody alone appears to be that of antigenic modulation, where apparent loss of the antigen involved in the reaction can occur within a few minutes to an hour or two after exposure to antibody. This modulation does appear to be temporary, with return of the antigen in many cases within 24 to 36 hours. While modulation may be a limiting problem for antibody alone, it may be a less limiting factor for immunoconjugates, where the initial conjugation and toxicity to the tumor cell may occur prior to or during modulation. In fact, it has been postulated that modulation may be a mechanism by which an immunoconjugated molecule could gain entrance into the cell. There are many approaches to enhance the efficacy of monoclonal antibody (Table 7), and many of these are being tried in animal tumor models and even in preliminary trials in man.

The Biological Response Modifiers Program has two monoclonal antibody trials in the early stages of development. The first trial

Table 5. Monoclonal antibody (MoAb) serotherapy trials.

Institution	Disease	MoAb	Reference
Sidney Farber	Lymphoma	Ab89	(12)
Sidney Farber	ALL	J-5	(7)
Stanford	T-CLL	LEU-1	(8)
Stanford	CTCL	LEU-1	(10)
Stanford	Lymphoma	Anti-idiotype	(11)
U. of Pennsylvania	GI	17-1A	(6)
U. California, San Diego	CLL	T101	(9)
National Cancer Institute-BRMP	CLL, CTCL	T101	-

Table 6. Conclusions from monoclonal antibody (MoAb) serotherapy trials.

1. Intravenous murine-derived MoAb can be given safely by prolonged infusion (>1 hr.) without immediate side effects.
2. Bronchospasm and hypotension have followed rapid infusion.
3. Dosages from 1 mg to 1500 mg can be given safely.
4. A sustained decline in leukemic cells requires multiple bi-weekly MoAb treatment over many weeks.
5. Skin lesions and lymph nodes can regress following MoAb treatment.
6. There has been no reduction in the bone marrow leukemia cells.
7. Antigenic modulation sometimes occurs following MoAb treatment.
8. Free antigen may be detected in the serum following MoAb treatment.
9. Antimouse antibodies may develop following MoAb therapy.

Table 7. Possible approaches to enhancing the efficacy of monoclonal antibody (MoAb) therapy.

1. Infuse more than one MoAb directed toward different epitopes on the same antigen.
2. Infuse more than one MoAb directed toward different antigens on the same cell.
3. Infuse more than one MoAb using different subclasses (IgG_1, IgG_2, IgM, etc.).
4. Develop polyclonal heteroantisera raised to MoAb purified antigens (different epitopes, different subclasses).
5. Immunoconjugate MoAb to drugs, toxins, and isotopes.

involves the use of T101 antibody in the treatment of patients with T antigen-bearing chronic lymphocytic leukemia and in patients with T cell leukemias and lymphomas. This trial is underway and results similar to those previously reported are being seen. A second trial using the 9.2.27 monoclonal antibody with a high degree of specificity for melanoma is about to be initiated. This trial involves the use of an IgG_{2a} monoclonal antibody recognizing the 250K antigen on the surface of melanoma cells (13). Both of these trials are phase I trials where escalating doses will be utilized to determine the biologic effects of these monoclonal reagents.

ANIMAL TUMOR MODELS

As is apparent from our recent review (2) of the animal tumor models that have been used in the evaluation of antibody therapy, there are many animal tumor models available for investigators interested in therapeutic trials of monoclonal antibody. Our interest has centered on the guinea pig model using the line 10 hepatoma in Sewell-Wright strain 2 guinea pigs (14-16). Previous studies using this syngeneic transplantable guinea pig model have shown that a majority of these animals can be cured of regional lymph node and micrometastatic disease with immunizations composed of BCG or its subcomponents admixed with irradiated tumor cells (14). While this active specific immunotherapy is effective at low tumor burdens and even has some efficacy at moderate tumor burdens, we felt that the addition of monoclonal antibody might prove efficacious in this model (15). Preliminary investigations were initiated to see what effect monoclonal antibody alone might have in this transplantable tumor model. A monoclonal antibody was raised against the line 10 tumor by immunizing BALB/c mice with viable line 10 cells and fusing the splenic lymphocytes to a P3X63-NS1-1 mouse myeloma line (16). The D3 clone of these fusions has produced a monoclonal antibody of the IgG1 class. This monoclonal antibody has specificity for line 10 cells and does not react significantly with normal cells or with a control tumor designated line 1 (Table 8). In vitro, using radioimmunoassay, immunofluorescence with flow cytometry, and immunoperoxidase staining, this antibody showed striking specificity for the line 10 tumor cells with little or no reactivity with any of the normal tissues tested (17). In vivo localization of the antibody was shown by external radioimaging and by immunohistologic techniques. Radioimaging demonstrated specific localization in the line 10 tumor (as opposed to normal tissues and the histologically similar but antigenically distinct line 1 tumor) by injecting ^{125}I-D3 antibody into tumor-bearing guinea pigs. Immunohistochemical studies revealed excellent localization to the tumor cells, and after 48 hours the only normal tissue where antibody could be demonstrated was the kidney. Even there, the specific localization was much higher for tumor than for the renal cells and no apparent kidney toxicity was seen in these animals. When monoclonal antibody alone was given to

Table 8. D3 monoclonal antibody specificity for cancer cells vs. normal guinea pig tissues

Antibody Dilution	Tissues (CPM ^{125}I-protein A Bound)*					
	Liver	Spleen	Kidney	Brain	L1	L10
1/5,000	735	3914	194	0	841	97,470
1/50,000	0	0	0	137	252	82,186

*P3 ascites background subtracted.

guinea pigs bearing the line 10 tumor, some diminution in tumor growth could be demonstrated but this was at best marginal. Because of the excellent localization and the lack of therapeutic effects with antibody alone, we began to investigate an immunoconjugate in this model. Animal tumor models are excellent vehicles for the testing of immunoconjugates as one can assess both the toxicity and the therapeutic efficacy in the model to better determine the type of immunoconjugate that might be most effectively applied in man. As is shown in Figure 1, excellent killing of a diphtheria toxin A chain conjugate to the D3 monoclonal antibody was seen at very low concentrations when the immunoconjugate was used to treat line 10 tumor cells in vitro. Subsequent to these studies, which also demonstrated that this effect was specific for the line 10 cell and

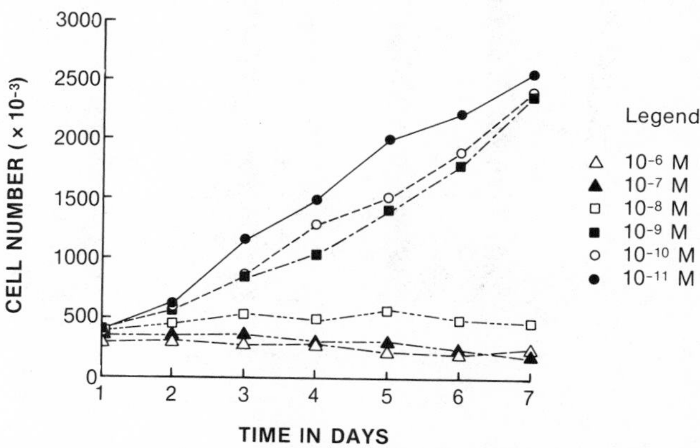

Fig. 1. Growth kinetics in vitro with D3 diphtheria toxin A chain. Visual assay of cell number after treatment with varying concentrations of immunoconjugate based on the molarity of the immunoconjugate.

was not seen with control normal cells nor with line 1 cells, the D3 diphtheria A chain conjugate was given intravenously in a preliminary study to guinea pigs bearing dermal line 10 tumors. As is illustrated in Figure 2, there was some initial reduction in tumor size of palpable tumors and a clear therapeutic effect of the conjugate by virtue of the demonstration of a slower outgrowth of the tumors in the treated animals compared to the controls. In these preliminary experiments only a single dose of conjugate was given, and after the initial therapeutic effect the treated animals did manifest tumor growth and subsequently died from progressive tumor growth. However, these early indications, along with the results reported by many others (2, 3), would indicate that immunoconjugates should be investigated as potential anticancer therapeutic agents.

CONCLUSIONS

The use of monoclonal antibody and its conjugates in the treatment of cancer is in a very early stage. While it is clear that much needs to be done to clarify many of the issues surrounding the use of antibody alone or conjugates of the antibody with other toxic substances, it has already been demonstrated in both animal

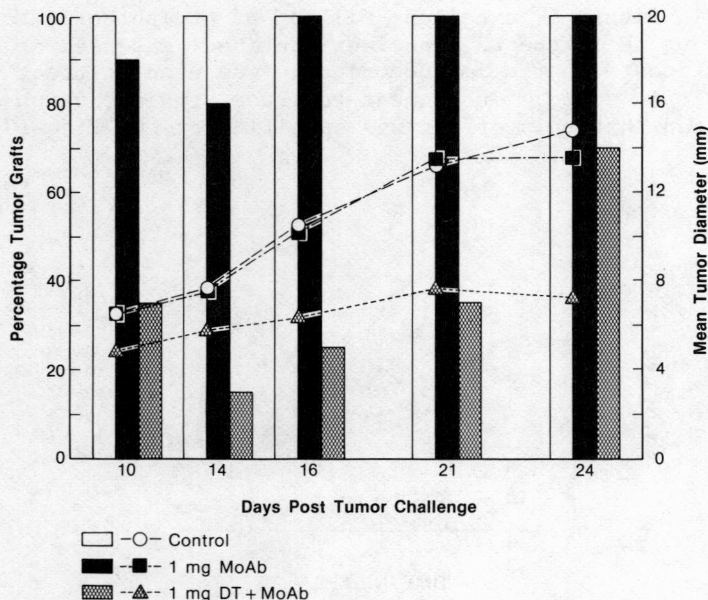

Fig. 2. In vivo study of D3 diphtheria toxin A chain conjugate in guinea pigs bearing dermal line 10 hepatocarcinoma. Bars represent the mean tumor diameter in millimeters.

tumor models and in man that antibody alone and antibody conjugated with drugs, toxins, and radioisotopes can have therapeutic effects. The potential for the use of monoclonal antibodies in cancer therapeutics seems enormous given the specificity that is inherent to the antibody-antigen reaction. There is the possibility of being able to better utilize the xenogeneic reagents developed in mice, rats, and sub-human primates for the treatment of cancer in man. These reagents may have the advantage of recognizing tumor cells which may be nonimmunogenic in man but which carry antigenic structures which are immunogenic in the xenogeneic species. An additional possibility is that even in man these tumors are immunogenic but the antibody response is quantitatively ineffective in controlling tumor growth and metastasis. If this can be demonstrated, then the antibody-forming cells can be isolated from the patient and human-human hybridomas developed producing homologous monoclonal antibody which may also be of therapeutic value.

Extensive phase I trials are needed to document the biologic effects and the toxic effects of antibody alone prior to proceeding to conjugate studies in man. These studies should investigate a wide dose range of antibody administered by different schedules utilizing reagents from different xenogeneic sources and of different antibody classes. These antibody-containing reagents should be prepared in a highly purified state, and trials using antibody fragments might also be initiated to improve our understanding of the role of antibody alone in man. Subsequent studies should utilize monoclonal antibody of human sources when this is available, and after appropriate animal model studies have been completed preliminary studies with immunoconjugates will be initiated. An interesting model in man for the <u>early</u> use of immunoconjugates might be in the bone marrow transplantation situation. Here one can treat the bone marrow for remaining tumor cells with an immunoconjugate and reinfuse the bone marrow after appropriate cleansing with very little risk of infusing significant quantities of the antibody conjugate in vivo. In this way, one may be able to assess, in a preliminary way, the value of immunoconjugates in man even before the therapeutic/toxic ratio of these reagents has been extensively investigated in phase I trials. While much work needs to be done to define the role of monoclonal antibody in the treatment of cancer, the future seems very bright, and this is the area of cancer biology that deserves the greatest emphasis for the development of new therapeutic reagents in the coming years.

REFERENCES

1. Kohler, G., and C. Milstein. 1975. Continuous cultures of fushed cells secreting antibody of predefined specificity. Nature (London) 256: 495.

2. Foon, K. A., M. I. Bernhard, and R. K. Oldham. 1982. Monoclonal antibody therapy: Assessment by animal tumor models. J. Biol. Resp. Modif. (in press).

3. Sherwin, S. A., K. A. Foon, and R. K. Oldham. 1983. Animal tumor models for biological response modifier therapy: An approach to the development of monoclonal antibody therapy in humans. In: S. Carter (ed.), Principles of cancer chemotherapy. McGraw Hill, New York (in press)

4. Rosenberg, S. A., and W. D. Terry. 1977. Passive immunotherapy of cancer in animals and man. Adv. Cancer Res. 25: 323.

5. Ritz, J., and S. F. Schlossman. 1982. Utilization of monoclonal antibodies in treatment of leukemia and lymphoma. Blood 59: 1.

6. Sears, H. F., B. Atkinson, J. Mattis, C. Ernest, D. Herlyn, Z. Steplewski, P. Häyry, and H. Koprowski. 1982. Phase-1 clincial trial of monoclonal antibody in treatment of gastrointestinal tumors. Lancet 1: 762.

7. Ritz, J., J. M. Pesando, S. E. Sallan, A. Clavell, J. Notis-McConarty,, P. Rosenthal, and S. F. Schlossman. 1981. Serotherapy of acute lymphoblastic leukemia with monoclonal antibody. Blood 58: 141.

8. Miller, R. A., D. G. Maloney, J. McKillop, and R. Levy. 1981. In vivo effects of murine hybridoma monoclonal antibody in a patient with T-cell leukemia. Blood 58: 78.

9. Dillman, R. O., D. L. Shawler, R. E. Sobol, H. A. Collins, J. C. Beauregard, S. B. Wornsley, and I. Royston. 1982. Murine monoclonal antibody therapy in two patients with chronic lymphocytic leukemia. Blood 59: 1036.

10. Miller, R. A., and R. Levy. 1981. Response of cutaneous T cell lymphoma to therapy with hybridoma monoclonal antibody. Lancet 2: 226.

11. Miller, R. A., D. G. Maloney, E. R. Warnicki, and R. Levy. 1982. Treatment of B cell lymphoma with monoclonal anti-idiotype antibody. N. Engl. J. Med. 306: 517.

12. Nadler, L. M., P. Stashenko, and R. Hardy. 1980. Serotherapy of a patient with a monoclonal antibody directed against a human lymphoma-associated antigen. Cancer Res. 40: 3147.

13. Morgan, A. C., Jr., D. R. Galloway, and R. A. Reisfeld. 1981. Production and characterization of monoclonal antibody to a melanoma specific glycoprotein. Hybridoma 1: 27.

14. Hanna, M. G., and L. C. Peters. 1978. Immunotherapy of established micrometastases with *Bacillus Calmette*-Guérin tumor cell vaccine. Cancer Res. 38: 204.

15. Hanna, M. G., and M. E. Key. 1982. Immunotherapy of metastases enhances subsequent chemotherapy. Science 217: 367.

16. Bernhard, M. I., K. A. Foon, G. C. Clarke, W. L. Christensen, L. Hoyer, M. G. Hanna, Jr., and R. K. Oldham. 1982. Guinea pig line 10 hepatocarcinoma model for monoclonal antibody serotherapy. I. Characterization of monoclonal antibody and description of antigen (submitted).

17. Key, M. E., M. I. Bernhard, K. A. Foon, R. K. Oldham, and M. G. Hanna. 1982. Guinea pig line 10 hepatocarcinoma model for monoclonal antibody serotherapy. II. *In vitro* localization of a monoclonal antibody in normal and malignant tissues (submitted).

TREATMENT OF A MURINE LEUKEMIA WITH CHLORAMBUCIL BOUND MONOCLONAL ANTIBODIES

Burton Feinerman[1], Ronald D. Paul[2], Gregg Feinerman

Papanicolaou Cancer Research Institute[1] and Department of Microbiology and Immunology, University of Miami School of Medicine[2], Miami Florida (USA)

INTRODUCTION

Metastasis is the major concern in the management of cancer (1). While standard chemotherapy has shown promise in the treatment of certain kinds of tumors, its utility has been limited due to toxicity to normal cells (2-3). Recent advances in experimental immunobiology, tumor immunology and cancer metastasis have increased our knowledge concerning the host's immune response to tumors and the regulation of tumor growth (4-5). These advances have also initiated new approaches in the diagnosis and treatment of cancer (6).

It is known that some tumors express antigens that distinguish them from normal cells (7-8). The knowledge of tumor specific transplantation antigens has led to the production of antibodies specific for various types of tumors and the attempt to use these antibodies for diagnosis and/or treatment. In general, success has been variable with the use of antisera, although some inhibition of tumor growth has been reported (9-10).

In this report, we present studies in which microgram quantities of monoclonal antibodies specific for a normal murine lymphocyte differentiation antigen (Thy 1), and bound with the cytotoxic alkylating agent chlorambucil, were used in the treatment of a murine lymphocytic leukemia. Therapeutic potential of this treatment was assessed early during the course of the disease by flow cytometric cell cycle analysis of tumor cells from experimental mice.

METHODS

Animals And Tumor

DBA/2 mice, 8-12 weeks old, were used throughout these studies. Mice were obtained from Simonson Laboratories and housed in our animal facilities for at least 1 week prior to use. The tumor used was a lymphocytic leukemia (P388), which was sustained in vivo by serial passage in DBA/2 mice. In all experiments mice were injected intraperitoneally (i.p.) with 1 x 10^5 P388 cells on day 0.

Binding Of Chlorambucil To Antibody

Monoclonal antimouse Thy 1, Lyt 1 and Lyt 2 were purchased from the Becton-Dickinson Monoclonal Antibody Center (Mountain View, CA). Rabbit antimouse immunoglobulin was generously provided by the Division of Biological Carcinogenesis Branch of the National Cancer Institute, from stocks supplied by the Frederick Cancer Center. Chlorambucil, p-(di-2-chloroethyl) aminophenylbutyric acid, was purchased from Burroughs Wellcome. Chlorambucil was bound to monoclonal antimouse Thy 1 by the method described by Israels and Linford (11). Briefly, antimouse Thy 1 and chlorambucil, were mixed at a concentration ratio of 10:1 and incubated overnight with gentle stirring at 4°C. Under these conditions, 90% of the available chlorambucil binds to immunoglobulins. The antibody-chlorambucil conjugates are then separated from free chlorambucil by exhaustive dialysis for 72 hours in phosphate buffered saline (pH 7.0) at 4°C.

DNA Staining And Analysis Of P388 Cells

Experimental mice were sacrificed by cervical dislocation. The ascitic fluid was collected from individual animals by three consecutive washes of the peritoneal cavity with 2 ml volumes of phosphate buffered saline. The collected P388 cells were washed three times with phosphate buffered saline and counted using a Coulter Cell Counter (Coulter Electronics, Hialeah, FL). One x 10^6 P388 cells from each experimental animal were then stained in a hypotonic propidium iodide/citrate solution according to the method described by Krishan (12). One to two x 10^3 stained P388 cells from each sample were analyzed in a Becton-Dickinson Fluorescence Activated Cell Sorter (FACS III). In this instrument, single cells in a fluid stream are excited by an argon ion laser beam (wavelength 488 nm). The emitted fluorescence is intercepted by a series of filters and photomultiplier tubes and converted to an electrical signal which is stored in a Nuclear Data multichannel pulse height analyzer as a DNA histogram. Quantitative cell cycle analyses of DNA histograms were performed by employing the technique of Barlogie (13).

RESULTS

The Effect of In Vivo Immunoglobulin Administration On The Growth of P388 Cells

Preliminary studies in this laboratory had demonstrated that approximately 70% of the ascitic cells from P388 tumor bearers stained positively with FITC conjugated monoclonal anti-Thy 1 antibody. Since this tumor appeared to be of the T cell lineage, a battery of antibodies specific for murine T cell differentiation antigens were administered to test their effect on tumor growth. The results of these studies are presented as the percent of P388 cells which are resting or in interphase (GoG1) and the percent of cells either actively synthesizing DNA or in mitosis (S + G2M). The data in Table 1 indicates that the percent of cells in GoG1 and S + G2M from animals treated with anti-Thy 1, Lyt 1 or Lyt 2 antibodies did not differ from that of mice injected with PBS or animals given antimouse Ig, the negative control group.

Table 1. The Effect of In Vivo Immunoglobulin Administration on the Cell Cycle of P388 Cells

		% of P388 cells in:[3]	
Group[1]	Treatment[2]	GoG1	S + G2M
1	PBS	62.2 ± 3.6	37.8 ± 3.6
2	Anti-Thy 1 (20 μg)	56.0 ± 5.5	44.0 ± 5.5
3	Anti-Lyt 1 (20 μg)	55.0 ± 2.8	45.0 ± 2.8
4	Anti-Lyt 2 (20 μg)	59.3 ± 2.5	40.7 ± 2.5
5	Antimouse Ig (100 μg)	57.5 ± 5.0	42.5 ± 5.0

[1] Mice were injected i.p. with 1 x 10^5 P388 cells on day 0.

[2] Mice were injected i.p. with 20 μg of either anti-Thy 1, Lyt 1 or Lyt 2 on days 0, 2, 4 and 6. Controls received either PBS or 100 μg of antimouse Ig.

[3] Mice were sacrificed on day 13. P388 cells were harvested and stained with propidium iodide. 1-2 x 10^3 cells from each sample were analyzed in the FACS III. Results are expressed as the mean percent of cells ± 1 S.D., in each phase of the cell cycle and are representative of 3-5 animals per experimental group.

The total number of tumor cells recovered from animals administered anti-T cell antibodies is shown in Table 2. The data indicate that total cell recovery in these experimental groups was not diminished in comparison to the total cell recovery from control mice (Groups 2, 3 and 4 compared to Groups 1 and 6).

The Effect of Chlorambucil Bound Anti-Thy 1 On The Growth of P388 Cells

Since the previous studies had shown no effect of anti-Thy 1, Lyt 1 or Lyt 2 administration on the growth of P388 cells, additional experiments were designed to test the effects of anti-Thy 1 antibodies bound with the cytotoxic agent chlorambucil, on the cell cycle of P388 cells. The results of these studies are presented in Table 3. It is evident from the data, that administration of chlorambucil bound anti-Thy 1 antibodies, had a mildly perturbing effect on the cell cycle of P388 cells. This is reflected in an increase in the percent of cells in GoG1 and a decrease in the percent of cells in S + G2M, when compared to mice injected with PBS. This change in the percent of cells in GoG1 and S + G2M was not seen in mice administered either anti-Thy 1 antibodies or chlorambucil alone.

Table 2. The Effect of In Vivo Immunoglobulin Administration on P388 Cell Recovery from Tumor Bearing Mice

Group[1]	Treatment[2]	Total number of cells recovered[3] x 10^6
1	PBS	371 ± 47
2	Anti-Thy 1 (20 μg)	421 ± 35
3	Anti-Lyt 1 (20 μg)	468 ± 44
4	Anti-Lyt 2 (20 μg)	402 ± 39
5	Anti-mouse Ig (100 μg)	345 ± 134

[1] As in Table 1.

[2] As in Table 1.

[3] Mice were sacrificed on day 13. P388 cells were recovered by repeated peritoneal washings and counted on a Coulter Cell Counter. Results are expressed as the mean number of cells recovered ± 1 S.D. of 3-5 animals per experimental group.

Table 3. The Effect of Chlorambucil Bound Anti-Thy 1 on the Cell Cycle of P388 Cells

Group[1]	Treatment[2]	% of P388 cells in:[3]	
		GoG1	S + G2M
1	PBS	67.2 ± 3.2	32.8 ± 3.2
2	Anti-Thy 1	70.0 ± 2.2	30.0 ± 2.2
3	Anti-Thy 1-chlorambucil	79.9 ± 4.4	20.1 ± 4.4
4	Chlorambucil	69.7 ± 4.7	30.3 ± 4.7

[1] Mice were injected i.p. with 1 x 10^5 P388 cells on day 0.

[2] Mice were injected i.p. with anti-Thy 1 (33.3 μg), anti-Thy 1 (33.3 μg) bound to chlorambucil (1.26 μg), or chlorambucil alone (1.26 μg) on days 0, 1, 2, 3, 4 and 5.

[3] Mice were sacrificed on day 6. P388 cells were harvested and stained with propidium iodide. 1-2 x 10^3 cells from each sample were analyzed in a FACS III. Results are expressed as the mean % of cells, ± 1 S.D., in each phase of the cell cycle and are representative of 3-5 animals per experimental group.

The total number of tumor cells recovered from mice treated with chlorambucil bound anti-Thy 1 antibodies were also lower than that recovered from mice injected with PBS (Table 4). This difference in cell recovery was not evident in mice treated with anti-Thy 1 antibodies or chlorambucil alone.

DISCUSSION

The objectives of the present study were to demonstrate the therapeutic potential of using monoclonal antibodies as vehicles for drug delivery. Initial experiments indicated that treatment with monoclonal anti-Thy 1, Lyt 1 or Lyt 2 had no effect on the P388 cell cycle or the number of leukemia cells recovered from experimental animals. This is in contrast to some reports stating significant improvement with monoclonal antibody therapy in the treatment of murine leukemias (9-10). However, there have been similar results by other investigators, pointing out the limited success of treatment with monoclonal antibody alone (14).

Table 4. The Effect of Chlorambucil Bound Anti-Thy 1 Antibody Administration on P388 Cell Recovery from Tumor Bearing Mice

Group[1]	Treatment[2]	Total number of cells recovered[3] x 10^6
1	PBS	29.3 ± 4.4
2	Anti-Thy 1	19.9 ± 5.5
3	Anti-Thy 1-chlorambucil	10.0 ± 2.8
4	Chlorambucil	26.0 ± 9.2

[1] As in Table 3.

[2] As in Table 3.

[3] Mice were sacrificed on day 6. P388 cells were recovered by repeated peritoneal washings and counted on a Coulter Cell Counter. Results are expressed as the mean number of cells recovered, ± 1 S.D., and are representative of 3-5 animals per experimental group.

When mice were treated with chlorambucil bound anti-Thy 1 monoclonal antibodies, the effect was strikingly different. Cell cycle analysis of leukemia cells harvested from these mice revealed that fewer cells were synthesizing DNA or actively dividing, and a greater number of cells were resting, as compared to cells taken from mice injected with anti-Thy 1 antibodies or chlorambucil alone. This alteration of the cell cycle correlated well with a decrease in tumor burden in anti-Thy 1-chlorambucil treated mice.

These studies point to the advantages that may result from targeting even small amounts of a cytotoxic agent with monoclonal antibodies. Obviously, more extensive, long range studies must be completed to fully realize the benefits of this type of treatment. However, it is likely that this technique may overcome some of the problems such as antigenic modulation and toxicity to normal cells, that are encountered by treatment with antibodies or chemotherapy alone. Further investigations in this field should be aided by the continued development of monoclonal antibodies to tumor specific or associated antigens.

SUMMARY

Mice bearing a murine T cell leukemia (P388) were treated with a battery of monoclonal antibodies specific for normal T cell differentiation antigens. Therapy was evaluated during the early course of disease by DNA cell cycle analysis and recovery of leukemia cells from tumor bearing mice. This form of therapy was shown to be ineffective. However, treatment with chlorambucil bound monoclonal antibodies was shown to be effective in reducing the number of leukemia cells undergoing DNA synthesis and mitosis, in addition to diminishing the tumor burden as compared to control mice. The potential benefits of this form of therapy are discussed.

REFERENCES

1. Zeidman, I. 1981. Metastasis, an overview, p. 1-28. In J. Marchalonis, M. Hanna and I. Fidler (eds.), Cancer Biology Vol. 2. Marcel Dekker, New York.

2. Clarysse, A. M., W. J. Cathey, G. E. Cartwright et al. 1969. Pulmonary disease complicating intermittent therapy with methotrexate. JAMA 209: 1861-1864.

3. Anderson, E. E., O. E. Cobb, J. F. Glenn. 1967. Cyclophosphamide hemorrhagic cystitis. J. Urol. 97: 857-858.

4. Poste, G. and I. J. Fidler. 1980. The pathogenesis of cancer metastasis. Nature 283: 139-146.

5. Hersh, E. M., J. U. Gutterman and G. M. Mavligit. 1975. Cancer and host defense mechanisms. In H. L. Ioachin (ed.), Pathobiology annual. Academic Press, New York.

6. Wright, P. W. and I. D. Bernstein. 1980. Serotherapy of malignant disease. Prog. Exp. Tumor Res. 25: 140.

7. Lausch, R. N. and F. Rapp. 1974. Tumor specific antigens and re-expression of fetal antigens in mammalian cells. Prog. Exp. Tumor Res. 19: 45.

8. Thomson, D. M. P. 1975. Soluble tumour-specific antigen and its relationship to tumour growth. Intl. J. Cancer 15: 1016.

9. Ritz, J., J. M. Pesando, J. Notis McConasty, L. A. Clavell, S. E. Sallan and S. F. Schlossman. 1981. Use of monoclonal antibodies as diagnostic and therapeutic reagents in acute lymphoblastic leukemia. Cancer Res. 41: 4771-4775.

10. Kirch, M. E. and U. Hammerling. 1981. Immunotherapy of murine leukemias by monoclonal antibody. I. Effect of passively administered antibody on growth of transplanted tumor cells. J. Immunol. 127: 805-810.

11. Israels, L. G. and J. H. Linford. 1963. Binding of chlorambucil to proteins, p. 399. In Proceedings of the fifth Canadian cancer research conference. Academic Press, New York.

12. Krishan, A. 1975. Rapid flow cytofluoreometric analysis of mammalian cell cycle by propidium iodide staining. J. Cell Biol. 66: 188-193.

13. Barlogie, B., B. Drewinko, D. A. Johnston et al. 1976. Pulse cytophotometric analysis of synchronized cells in vitro. Cancer Res. 36: 1176-1181.

14. Bernstein, I.D. et al. 1980. Monoclonal antibody therapy of mouse leukemia, p. 275-291. In R. H. Kennet, T. J. McKearn and K. B. Bechtol (eds.), Monoclonal antibodies. Hybridomas: a new dimension in biological analysis. Plenum Press, New York.

IMMUNE RESPONSE IN STRAIN 2 GUINEA PIGS TO THE SYNGENEIC L2C LEUKEMIA

Manuel J. Ricardo, Jr.[1] and Daniel T. Grimm[2]

Bowman Gray School of Medicine of Wake Forest University[1]
Department of Microbiology and Immunology, Winston-Salem, North Carolina, and The University of Tennessee[2]
Center for the Health Sciences, Department of Pediatrics
Memphis, Tennessee (USA)

INTRODUCTION

The L2C leukemia is a transplantable acute B lymphoblastic leukemia that arose spontaneously in a female strain 2 guinea pig (1). The presence of immunoglobulin (Ig) and complement receptors on the surface of L2C tumor cells has established the B lymphocyte lineage of this leukemia (2). Five closely related mutant sublines of the L2C leukemia have been described (3) and are presumed to be derived from the same stem cell on the basis of cytogeneic analyses (4). The sublines share a common IgM idiotypic (id) determinant(s) and can be classified into two major groups, those that have detectable immune-associated antigens (Ia) on their cell surface and those that lack detectable Ia antigens on the basis of serological analysis (3). The presence of Ia antigens is apparently important in eliciting immunity against the tumor because effective L2C tumor protection is induced in normal strain 2 guinea pigs when immunized with Ia^+ L2C tumor cells in adjuvant, but not generally with Ia^- L2C tumor cells (3). However, immunization with Ia^+ L2C cells protects the strain 2 guinea pigs against any of the 5 sublines. The latter finding supports the early observations made by Gross (5) that some strain 2 guinea pigs, when given a small dose of viable L2C tumor cells, developed resistance to a secondary challenge of L2C inoculum that produced fatal disease in syngeneic animals not previously given L2C tumor cells. Taken together, these results indicate that a tumor-associated transplantation antigen(s) (TATA) is present on L2C lymphoblasts. The IgM id determinants on the L2C cell surface have been implicated as a TATA for this tumor (6).

In this investigation, immunity against the L2C leukemia was evaluated simultaneously both at the humoral and cell-mediated level. Attention was focused in assessing the specificity of the L2C antibodies and L2C T effector cells in order to evaluate the antigens that could function as tumor-associated antigens (TAA). The results suggest that, with respect to humoral immunity, the IgM id determinant may function as a TAA, but that with regard to cell-mediated immunity the participation of the IgM id determinant was not apparent.

METHODS

Animals

Strain 2 and strain 13 guinea pigs were obtained from our own colony and were 6 months of age when used. Strain DHCBA guinea pigs were obtained from California Institute of Technology, Pasadena, CA. Rabbits were purchased through the Division of Animal Resources, Bowman Gray School of Medicine, Winston-Salem, NC.

Cells

The Ia^+ and Ia^- sublines of the L2C leukemia were maintained by subcutaneous (s.c.) serial passage of 10^7 viable tumor cells. Sixteen days after implant, the guinea pigs were exsanguinated by cardiac puncture and the leukemia cells were harvested from the blood by density centrifugation as described previously (7).

Guinea pig hepatocarcinoma cells were maintained in male strain 2 guinea pigs by intraperitoneal serial passage of 4×10^7 L1 cells or 10×10^7 L10 cells. The respective tumor cells were harvested from ascites fluid 14 days post implantation.

T lymphocytes were purified from guinea pig blood and lymphoid tissues as described previously (8). Enrichment of B lymphocytes was done by removing the adherent cells and T lymphocytes from lymph node and spleen cell suspensions. The adherent cells were removed by adherence to sterile plastic culture dishes and the T lymphocytes by E-rosetting followed by density centrifugation.

Tumor Protection

Normal strain 2 guinea pigs were immunized in the footpads with 10^7 Ia^+ leukemia cells emulsified in complete freund's adjuvant (CFA). Two weeks after primary immunization, the guinea pigs were challenged s.c. with 10^7 viable leukemia cells in medium 199 (GIBCO, Grand Island, NY). Guinea pigs that were protected against the leukemia were given four additional challenges of leukemia cells every two weeks. Sera were obtained from the protected guinea pigs and assayed for L2C antibody activity. The spleens from the protected guinea pigs also were harvested and assayed for cytotoxicity against the L2C tumor cells.

Iodination of Proteins

Staphylococcal protein A (Pharmacia Fine Chemicals, Inc., Piscataway, NJ) and guinea pig IgG1 were labeled with iodine-125 (100 mCi/ml, Amersham Radiochemical, Arlington Heights, IL) by the chloramine-T method as described previously (9).

Purification of Ig

Guinea pig IgG1 and IgG2 isotypes were fractionated by ion-exchange chromatography (8). The respective isotype fractions were adjusted to the original serum volume before they were used. Ig fractions from the other immune sera were purified on protein A-Sepharose columns as described previously (10). The respective $F(ab')_2$ fragments were obtained after digestion with pepsin (9).

Protein A Radiobinding Assay

Aliquots (50 μl) of the L2C immune sera (final dilution 1:8 in medium 199) were incubated with 10^5 viable L2C tumor cells for 45 min at 4^oC in medium 199 containing 20 mM sodium azide (50 μl). After the incubation period, the cells were washed 3 times with the same medium and 20,000 cpm of ^{125}I-protein A (sp. act. 85 μCi/μg) in 50 μl of medium 199 containing 10 mM sodium azide was added to the 50 μl of tumor cell suspensions. The incubation was done at 4^oC for 45 min. The unbound protein A was removed by washing the tumor cells 3 times with the same medium and the radioactivity in the cell pellet was determined.

Preparation of Antisera

The guinea pig strain combination 13 anti-2 was used to elicit the anti-Ia alloantiserum according to a previous procedure (10). The B.1 alloantiserum was elicited in DHCBA strain guinea pigs immunized with lymphoid cells from strain 13 guinea pigs as described previously (11). Strain 13 and strain 2 guinea pigs are histocompatible at the B locus.

Antibody to β_2 microglobulin (β_2m) was elicited in rabbits immunized in the footpads with 1 mg of purified guinea pig β_2m. Purification of β_2m from the urine of L2C-bearing guinea pigs was done on columns (2.4 x 100 cm) of Sephadex G-100 equilibrated with 0.01M Tris-HCl in 1.0 M NaCl, pH 8.0. Anti-λ id and anti-Fabμ id antisera were elicited in rabbits as described previously (12).

Inhibition of Antibody Binding

Binding inhibition experiments were performed by incubating 10^5 L2C tumor cells in 50 µl of medium 199 containing 20 mM sodium azide with 50 µl (diluted 1:5) of the appropriate $F(ab')_2$ reagent (see Table 2). Subsequently, the tumor cells were washed 3 times with the same medium, resuspended in 50 µl of medium and incubated with 50 µl of the various L2C immune sera (diluted 1:4) for 45 min at 4°C. Afterwards, the cells were handled as described in the protein A binding assay. Alternatively, the L2C cells were treated first with the $F(ab')_2$ reagents as described above and then with the ^{125}I-IgG1 (38,000 cpm, sp. act. 150 µCi/µg) immunoglobulin fractions that contained anti-L2C antibodies. After the incubation period (45 min at 4°C), the tumor cells were washed 3 times with medium 199 containing 10 mM sodium azide and the radioactivity in the cell pellet was determined.

Cytotoxicity Assay

Splenocytes were harvested from leukemia protected guinea pigs 2 weeks after the last in vivo challenge with L2C tumor cells. Single cell suspensions were prepared and aliquots of some of the cell suspensions (5 x 10^7 cells/ml) were treated with a 1:10 dilution of rabbit antiguinea pig T cell antiserum and guinea pig complement to remove the T cells before culture. Cytotoxic activity was elicited in vitro by incubating 10^7 splenocytes with 10^5 mitomycin C treated Ia^+ L2C cells. After the 5 day incubation period the splenocytes were washed and used in the chromium-51 release assay. Cytotoxic assays were carried out in microculture wells containing 10^4 chromium-51 labeled target cells and 10^6 effector splenocytes. The isotopic content of the culture supernatants was determined after the 16 h culture period at 37°C and 5% CO_2 atmosphere. The percentage of chromium release was determined according to the formula $\frac{I-N}{R-N}$ x 100, where I was the chromium released by immune spleens; N, the chromium released by nonimmune spleens; and R was the chromium released by freezing and thawing the labeled L2C target cells.

Inhibition of Cytotoxicity

The L2C target cells used in the inhibition experiments were treated with fresh glutaraldehyde (0.005%) for 5 minutes at 4°C either before or after the incubation with the respective $F(ab')_2$ reagents. This procedure prevented the surface antigens on L2C cells from capping and did not affect the lysis of the L2C target cells by immune splenocytes. In experiments where the L2C target cells were exposed to the $F(ab')_2$ reagents was done at 4°C for 45 minutes in the presence of 10 mM sodium azide. The cytotoxicity assay employing these target cells was performed as described earlier.

RESULTS

The syngeneic L2C immune sera known to contain detectable L2C antibodies were reacted with normal guinea pig lymphoid cells and malignant guinea pig cells in order to establish the cellular specificity of the L2C antibodies. The results given in Table 1 demonstrate that the L2C antibodies bind only to L2C tumor cells and not the L-1 and L-10 hepatocarcinoma tumor cells or normal B and T cells of guinea pig origin. The antibodies bound equally well to Ia^+ and Ia^- L2C leukemia cells. Furthermore, the L2C reactivity was not removed when immune serum was absorbed with normal guinea pig B cells and hepatocarcinoma cells.

Molecular Specificity of The Syngeneic L2C Antibodies

Binding competition experiments were performed using $F(ab')_2$ antibody fragments specific for known surface antigens on L2C tumor cells in order to establish the molecular specificity of the L2C antibodies. The data presented in Table 2 shows that

Table 1. Reactivity of L2C antibodies with normal and malignant guinea pig cells

Cell	Anti-L2C Serum	^{125}I-Protein A Bound (CPM)[a]
Normal B Cells	+[b]	862 ± 96
Normal T Cells	+	781 ± 79
Ia^+ L2C	+	5,779 ± 268
Ia^+ L2C	–	768 ± 53
Ia^- L2C	+	5,213 ± 32
Ia^- L2C	–	834 ± 78
L-1	+	919 ± 102
L-10	+	722 ± 53
Ia^+ L2C	+[c]	5,367 ± 276

[a] CPM is counts per minute and the values represent the mean radioactivity bound for three experiments, each done in triplicate. Standard error is given by ±.

[b] The (+) sign signifies that the cells were incubated with the antiserum. The (-) sign indicates that the cells were not exposed to the antiserum.

[c] Immune serum that was absorbed sequentially with L-1, L-10 and normal guinea pig B cells.

Table 2. Effect of $F(ab')_2$ antibody fragments specific for L2C surface antigens on the binding of syngeneic L2C antibodies to Ia^+ L2C leukemia cells

$F(ab')_2$ Specificity	^{125}I-Protein A Bound (CPM)[a]	^{125}I-IgG1 Anti-L2C Bound (CPM)[b]
NRS Control[c]	4,987 (0)[d]	7,734 (0)[d]
Ia	4,710 (6)	7,324 (5)
B.1[e]	4,656 (7)	7,512 (3)
β_2 microglobulin	4,811 (4)	7,216 (7)
L2C λ id	3,542 (29)	5,331 (31)
L2C Fabμ id	2,969 (40)	4,089 (47)
λ id & Fabμ id	2,131 (57)	2,860 (63)

[a] L2C leukemia cells were incubated first with the respective $F(ab')_2$ reagent, then immune serum and afterwards with the ^{125}I-protein A reagent as described in Methods. The tumor cells were incubated with the reagents at 4°C in the presence of sodium azide. The values represent the mean radioactivity bound, in counts per minute (CPM), to the L2C tumor cells for four experiments.

[b] L2C leukemia cells were incubated first with the respective $F(ab')_2$ reagents and then ^{125}I-IgG1 purified from immune serum. The values represent the mean radioactivity bound, in counts per minute (CPM), to L2C tumor cells for two experiments, each performed in triplicate.

[c] Pooled normal rabbit serum (NRS) was used in place of $F(ab')_2$ reagents.

[d] The amount of radioactivity bound was considered the 100% level (zero inhibition) and the values were used in calculating the percentage of inhibition given in parentheses.

[e] B.1 alloantigen is the guinea pig homology to the murine K and D histocompatibility antigens.

appreciable inhibition of binding of L2C antibodies was achieved when the L2C tumor cells were preincubated with the xenogeneic anti-λ id or anti-Fabμ id reagents. The greatest inhibition was observed when the L2C tumor cells were pretreated with both anti-id reagents. Identical results were obtained with the indirect

(^{125}I-protein A) and direct (anti-L2C ^{125}I-IgG1) radiobinding assay. The IgG1 fraction of the syngeneic L2C immune serum was used because in 11 of the 12 sera fractionated by ion-exchange chromatography the anti-L2C reactivity was preferentially associated with the IgG1 pool (Fig. 1).

Reactivity of Splenocytes From L2C Protected Guinea Pigs With Normal And Malignant Guinea Pig Cells

Splenocytes obtained from L2C protected guinea pigs were assayed for the capacity to specifically lyse L2C tumor cells. The results given in Table 3 are representative of the cellular reactivity detected in the spleens of some of the L2C protected guinea pigs. Immune splenocytes that were stimulated in vitro with Ia$^+$ L2C tumor cells for 5 days selectively lysed either Ia$^+$ or Ia$^-$ L2C cells, but did not lyse normal guinea pig B cells or hepatocarcinoma L-1 and L-10 tumor cells, as assessed by a chromium-51 release assay. The cytotoxic activity was abrogated when the immune splenocytes were treated with antiguinea pig T cell serum and complement (Table 3). Furthermore, Ia$^-$ L2C tumor cells failed to elicit a secondary stimulation of L2C cytotoxic T cells in vitro.

Molecular Specificity Of The Syngeneic L2C Cytotoxic T Cells

Complementary binding competition experiments were performed using the same F(ab')$_2$ reagents as in the antibody studies in order

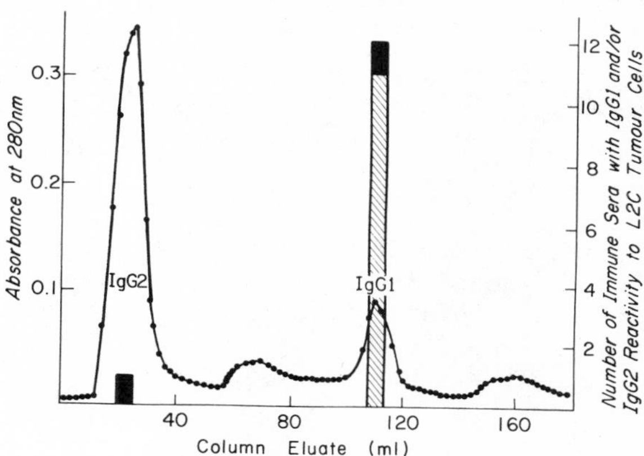

Fig. 1. Demonstration of the preferential binding of IgG1 (▧) to L2C tumor cells in 11 of 12 L2C immune sera fractionated on DE-cellulose. One immune serum (■) contained reactivity in the IgG1 and IgG2 fractions to the L2C leukemia cells. The relative position of IgG1 and IgG2 are indicated on the chromatographic profile. Fractionation was achieved employing a discontinuous gradient of sodium phosphate buffers (0.005M, pH 8.0; 0.04 M, pH 6.2; 0.06 M, pH 6.1).

Table 3. Secondary stimulation of cytotoxic immune splenocytes in vitro with Ia^+ L2C tumor cells[a]

Stimulator L2C	Target Cell	Chromium-51 Release (CPM)[b]
None	Ia^+ L2C	461 ± 26
Ia^+	Ia^+ L2C	1338 ± 73
Ia^+	Ia^- L2C	1261 ± 50
Ia^+	L-1	561 ± 30
Ia^+	L-10	503 ± 41
Ia^+	B cells	418 ± 33
Ia^-	Ia^+ L2C	532 ± 27
Ia^-	Ia^- L2C	610 ± 32
Ia^{+}[c]	Ia^+ L2C	463 ± 48

[a] Splenocytes were harvested from L2C protected guinea pigs and were stimulated in vitro with stimulator cells that were pretreated with mitomycin C as described in Methods.

[b] The values represent the mean radioactivity release in counts per minute (CPM). Standard error is given by ±.

[c] In these experiments, splenocytes were depleted of T cell before in vitro stimulation with Ia^+ L2C cells.

to assess the molecular specificity of the cytotoxic T cells. From the results presented in Table 4, it is apparent that the anti-id reagents failed to inhibit appreciably the cytotoxicity caused by the L2C immune splenocytes. Only the anti-B.1 $F(ab')_2$ reagent was capable of inhibiting the cytolysis to an appreciable extent.

DISCUSSION

Our results have provisionally identified anti-L2C antibodies in leukemia protected strain 2 guinea pigs. This suggests that the IgM idiotype on the L2C leukemia might function as a tumor-associated antigen (TAA) in antibody induction. This is further supported by the finding that the antibodies precipitated only IgM from extracts of L2C cells (data not shown). By contrast no evidence was obtained that supports recognition of the IgM idiotype in cell-

Table 4. Lysis of L2C tumor cells by anti-L2C splenocytes in the presence of $F(ab')_2$ antibody fragments specific for plasma membrane antigens on L2C tumor cells

$F(ab')_2$ Specificity	Percentage of Chromium-51 release[a]	Percentage of Inhibition
None	23 ± 2	0
Ia	24 ± 3	0
B.1	16 ± 3	30
β2 microglobulin	26 ± 4	0
L2C λ id	23 ± 3	0
L2C Fabμ id	22 ± 3	4
L2C λ id & Fabμ id	1 ± 2	9
NRS Control[b]	27 ± 2	0
NGPS Control[b]	25 ± 2	0

[a] The data represents 5 separate experiments each done in triplicate. Standard error of the mean is given by ±.

[b] Pooled normal rabbit serum (NRS) or normal guinea pig serum (NGPS) was used in place of $F(ab')_2$ reagents.

mediated immunity against the L2C tumor. It is conceivable, therefore, that the spectrum of antigenic determinents recognized by T lymphocytes may be somewhat different from that recognized by B lymphocytes and their antibody products as suggested previously (13). The partial inhibition of cellular immunity against the L2C tumor by anti-B.1 $F(ab')_2$ fragment supports the thought that L2C T effector cells recognize other biologically important TAAs other than the IgM idiotype. The B.1 alloantigen may form part of or is near one of the antigenic complexes recognized by the effector T cells. In addition, presumably other TAAs exist on the L2C tumor cell surface but do not elicit strong antibody or cellular responses in the syngeneic host. Relevant to this point is the observation that in many (>50%) of the L2C protected guinea pigs neither humoral or cellular immunity could be detected in vitro. With regard to the antibody response, however, it is possible that low concentrations of L2C antibodies were present in the circulation in the form of immune complexes and thus were not detected in the sera obtained from L2C protected guinea pigs. The lack of detectable L2C antibodies in these sera did not result from antigenic modulation because the binding assays were done at 4^oC in the presence of azide and immunofluorescence analysis did not show appreciable redistribution of the L2C surface IgM under these conditions.

The predominance of IgGl L2C antibodies in 11 of the 12 positive immune sera was an unexpected finding. The reason for this is not known. However, there might be a tight association, that is governed by DNA splicing dynamics, between heavy chain variable gene sequence specific for L2C determinants and the λ_1 constant region gene sequence. Another possibility could be that in the IgGl isotype compartment there is a larger repertoire of low affinity anti-L2C clones that are less effectively down-regulated by autoanti-idiotypic mechanisms compared to the IgG2 compartment. The more rapid dissociation of syngeneic antibodies from the L2C cell surface at acid pH as compared to xenogeneic L2C antibodies (data not shown) supports the view that the IgGl syngeneic antibodies are products of low affinity clones. It has been suggested that autoantiidiotypic antibodies develop during the course of tumor bearing, thus, leading to a fall in antitumor antibody levels and the failure of the host to control metastatic spread by antibody mediated mechanisms. The role humoral mechanisms play in L2C tumor protection in the syngeneic host remains unclear. However, on the basis of our results, we conclude that antibody probably affects a minimum level of L2C protection. In the guinea pig, IgGl does not bind complement by the classical pathway (14) and does not participate in K cell-mediated cytolysis (15), thereby, restricting its capacity to mediate tumor rejection by secondary immune mechanisms.

SUMMARY

Immunization of strain 2 guinea pigs with 10^7 syngeneic Ia^+ L2C leukemia cells in adjuvant leads to L2C tumor protection. After subsequent challenges with L2C tumor cells, the sera and spleens of the protected guinea pigs had detectable anti-L2C reactivity. The L2C antibody reactivity was preferentially associated with the IgGl isotype fraction and bound equally well to Ia^+ or Ia^- L2C cells but failed to bind to normal guinea pig lymphoid cells or hepatocarcinoma tumor cells. The binding was inhibited appreciably with $F(ab')_2$ fragments specific for the L2C surface IgM idiotypic determinants. By contrast, the same reagent failed to inhibit the specific cytolysis of L2C tumor cells by T lymphocytes present in the spleens of L2C protected guinea pigs. However, the T cell mediated cytolysis was inhibited to some extent by $F(ab')_2$ fragments specific for the B.1 alloantigen on the L2C tumor cells. These results indicate that the specificity of the L2C T effector cells appears to differ from that of the L2C antibodies and that in the elicitation of a humoral response the IgM idiotypic determinants may function as a tumor-associated antigen.

ACKNOWLEDGEMENT

This work was supported in part by United States Public Health Service grant CA-28253.

REFERENCES

1. Congdon, C. C., and E. Lorenz. 1954. Leukemia in guinea pigs. Am. J. Pathol. 30: 337-359.

2. Shevach, E. M., L. Ellman, J. M. Davie, and I Green. 1972. L2C guinea pig lymphatic leukemia: a "B" cell leukemia. Blood 39: 1-12.

3. Forni, G., E. M. Shevach, and I. Green. 1976. Mutant lines of guinea pig L2C leukemia. I Deletion of Ia alloantigens is associated with a loss in immunogenicity of tumor-associated transplantation antigens. J. Exp. Med. 143: 1067-1081.

4. Whang-Peng, J. 1977. Cytogenetic studies in L2C leukemia. Fed. Proc. 36: 2255-2259.

5. Gross, L. 1970. Specific, active intradermal immunization against leukemia in guinea pigs. Acta Haemat. 44: 1-10.

6. Hu, C. P., B. O. Schwartz, and I. Green. 1978. Identification of a tumor-associated antigen of the guinea pig L2C leukemia by using syngeneic antisera. J. Immunol. 120: 579-601.

7. Ricardo, M. J., Jr., and D. T. Grimm. 1982. Preferential expression of IgG1 antibodies specific for the L2C leukemia IgM idiotypic determinants in tumor-protected strain 2 guinea pigs. Immunol. (in press).

8. Ricardo, M. J., Jr., 1980. Heterogeneity of Fc-receptors on guinea pig T lymphocytes. J. Immunol. 123: 2009-2016.

9. Ricardo, M. J., Jr., 1981. Isotype specificity of Fcλ-receptors on guinea pig T lymphocytes and their modulation by homologous immune complexes. Immunol. 42: 459-467.

10. Shevach, E. M., W. E. Paul, and I. Green. 1972. Histocompatibility-linked immune response gene function in the guinea pigs. J. Exp. Med. 136: 1207-1221.

11. Schwartz, B. D., M. McMillan, E. Shevach, Y. Hohn, S. M. Rose, and L. Hood. 1980. Partial N-terminal amino acid sequences of guinea pig classic histocompatibility antigens. J. Immunol. 125: 1055-1059.

12. Stevenson, G. T., and F. K. Stevenson. 1975. Antibody to a molecularly-defined antigen to a tumor cell surface. Nature 254: 714-716.

13. Bradley, B. A., and H. Festenstein. 1978. Cellular typing. Br. Med. Bull. 34: 223-232.

14. Bloch, K. J., F. M. Kourilsky, Z. Ovary and B. Benacerraf. 1963. Properties of guinea pig 7S antibodies. III Identification of antibodies involved in complement fixation and hemolysis. J. Exp. Med. 117: 965-981.

15. Öhlander, C., A. Larson, and P. Perlmann. 1978. Specificity of Fc-receptors on lymphocytes and monocytes for guinea pig IgG1 and IgG2: Induction and inhibition of cytolysis or phagocytosis of erythrocytes. Scand. J. Immunol. 7: 285-296.

DIMINISHED SYNTHESIS OF IMMUNOGLOBULINS BY LYMPHOCYTES OF PATIENTS TREATED WITH THYMOSIN (TFX) AND CYCLOPHOSPHAMIDE

A. Gorski, Z. Rancewicz, M. Nowaczyk, M. Malejczyk and M. Waski

The Transplantation Institute, Warsaw Medical School
02006 Warsaw, Poland

INTRODUCTION

Thymosin fraction V, one of the most important hormonal-like peptides produced by the thymus, has been shown to be a useful agent in treating patients with primary and secondary immunodeficiency diseases (4). Thymus Factor X (TFX), an extract corresponding to thymosin fraction V prepared from calf thymus by Polfa Pharmaceuticals (Jelenia Góra, Poland) has been found to have similar immunomodulating properties (3). Thymic factors participate in the process of immune regulation by affecting the functions of various T lymphocyte subsets. Therefore, it may be anticipated that the final effect of their action depends on a number of factors including the immune status of a patient and the conditions of administration. This may explain why a thymic factor can cause opposing effects in vitro, and when administered in vivo, may lead to both amelioration and aggravation in the same clinical situation (15). We have recently shown that TFX is a potent inducer of helper T cells for antibody production in man. However, when TFX is added to lymphocytes generating high numbers of plasma cells in culture the resulting immunoglobulin synthesis is markedly reduced (7, 8). This data indicates that in some situations thymosin could have immunosuppressive properties. This further suggests the feasibility of combining TFX with immunosuppressive drugs which might be a more efficient immunosuppressive protocol to inhibit humoral responses.

METHODS

Immunoglobulin Synthesis In Vitro

An assay to detect intracellular deposits of immunoglobulins (Ic-Ig) in lymphocytes stimulated with pokeweed mitogen (PWM) has been described in detail elsewhere (8). Briefly, peripheral blood mononuclear cells were isolated on a Ficoll-Isopaque gradient, washed and cultured in a final volume of 10^6 cells/ml in medium RPMI 1640 (Seromed, FRG) with 20% AB serum, L-glutamine and gentamicin 25 μg/ml. The cultures were stimulated with 10 μl of PWM (Seromed, FRG). Following 7 days of culture in a fully humidified atmosphere with 5% CO_2, the cells were cytocentrifuged, washed, counted, fixed and stained with FITC-labelled antibodies to human gamma globulins (Behring). The slides were scored with an aid of fluorescence microscope (Biolar FL, PZO, Warsaw).

Immunomodulating Drugs

TFX, 4-hydroperoxycyclophosphamide (4HCy, an in vitro active metabolite of Cy, Asta Werke AG, FRG) as well as azathioprine (AZ, Imuran, Burroughs-Wellcome) were dissolved in tissue culture medium and added directly to lymphocyte cultures.

Detection of EA Rosettes

Detection of EA-mu and EA-gamma rosettes was performed similar to the technique described by Spiegelberg and Dainer (13). Ox red blood cells (ORBC) were coated with a subagglutinating dilution of IgM (purified from a rabbit anti-ORBC antiserum) by incubation for 90 min at 37° followed by 30 min at 4°. To obtain ORBC coated with IgG, ORBC were incubated with IgG for 30 min at 37° followed by 30 min at 4°. Freshly isolated lymphocytes were mixed with ORBC, centrifuged for 5 min at 200g at 4° and incubated for at least 30 min at 4°. The pellet was gently resuspended and rosettes scored in a hemocytometer.

ADCC Assay

This was performed as described previously (16) using L1210 mouse lymphoma target cells and rabbit anti-L1210 serum. Effector cells were mononuclears isolated from peripheral blood of normal donors.

Patients

Seven patients with aplastic anemia received TFX alone, injected intramuscularly at a daily dose of 2.5 milligrams. Two patients with IgA nephropathy and 10 renal allograft recipients received a brief course (3-10 days) of TFX followed by cyclophosphamide at 50-150 milligrams. In addition to TFX and Cy, the transplant patients were also receiving prednisone 15-30 mg daily. Finally, 10 patients with primary glomerulopathies receiving Cy alone were also studied.

RESULTS

Aplastic anemia provides a good model for studying TFX action since those patients have an inverted ratio of T-mu (helper) to T-gamma (suppressor) lymphocytes caused by a reduction of T cells (mu/gamma = 0.18 $\pm$ 0.04). Following 3 weeks of TFX therapy there was a marked increase of T-mu cells. Since the number of T-gamma cells remained unchanged, the mu/gamma ratio increased to 0.94 $\pm$ 0.04 (p <0.001 when compared to the pretreatment value) which was also significantly higher than the value we have found in normals (0.39 $\pm$ 0.02) (5, 13).

Figure 1 shows the dual effect of TFX on PWM-driven humoral responses in vitro. The primary effect of TFX is to enhance T cell dependent antibody synthesis, which is in accord with the above finding suggesting that TFX increases the number of T helper cells. Similar effects are observed when thymosin is added at the beginning of culture or up to day 5, as shown in the figure. However, when TFX-activated cultures receive a second dose of thymosin on day 5, the resulting immunoglobulin production is not enhanced. Such a phenomenon is frequently seen with lymphocytes of normal blood donors. Of particular note, a more striking reduction of immunoglobulin synthesis is seen when lymphocytes of patients treated with TFX are cultured with PWM and TFX. Moreover, similar lowering of Ic-Ig formation is observed when TFX is added to lymphocytes generating markedly elevated humoral responses in vitro, for example lymphocytes from renal allograft recipients undergoing acute rejection (data not shown).

Figure 2 demonstrates that lymphocytes of patients treated with TFX are more susceptible to the inhibitory action of Cy than the normal cells. Thus, a given concentration of 4HCy causes in most cases a more pronounced inhibition of antibody synthesis in vitro of cells derived from patients than normal donors. The 5 μg/ml dose completely abrogates immunoglobulin synthesis of TFX-lymphocytes while normal cells still produce some immunoglobulins. Interestingly, TFX treatment does not appear to change the sensitivity to azathioprine.

Two patients with IgA nephropathy and 10 allograft recipients with deteriorating renal function due to biopsy-proven humoral rejection entered a study to determine the efficacy of TFX with Cy as a modality for treatment of immunologic disorders with increased B cell reactivity. The effects of such treatment (2-6 weeks) in

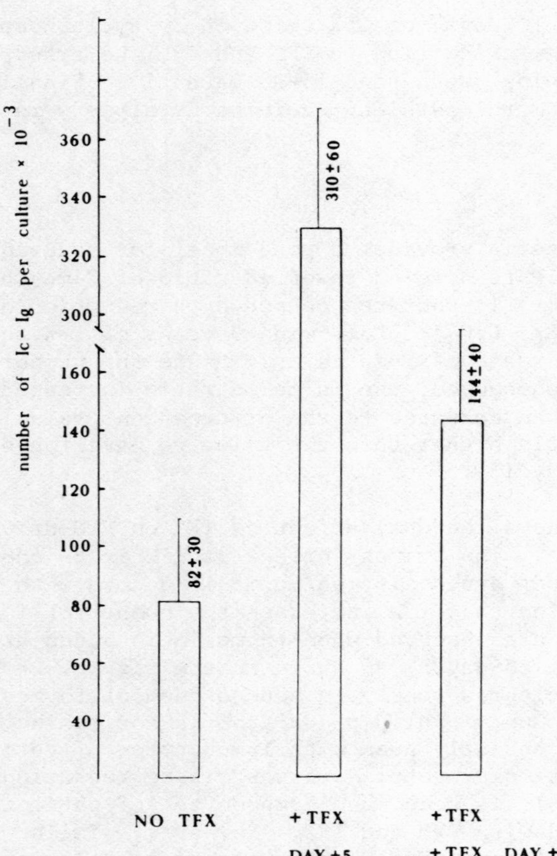

Fig. 1. The effect of TFX added on either day 5 (second bar) or on days 0 and 5 (third bar). Standard deviations are shown. The difference between the first and third bars is not significant, while differences between first and second and second and third are significant ($p < 0.01$).

terms of the ability of patient lymphocytes to synthesize antibodies in vitro in response to PWM are shown in Figure 3. It may be seen that this immunomodulating protocol causes a marked inhibition of the ability of the patient lymphocytes to mount humoral responses in vitro. On the other hand, lymphocytes of patients treated with Cy alone or in association with steroids have a normal ability to produce immunoglobulins, while TFX alone (given to patients with nephropathy prior to Cy and patients with aplastic anemia) causes a marked enhancement of humoral responses.

Figure 4 shows that TFX does not alter significantly the ADCC activity, while at higher doses inhibits the activity of effector

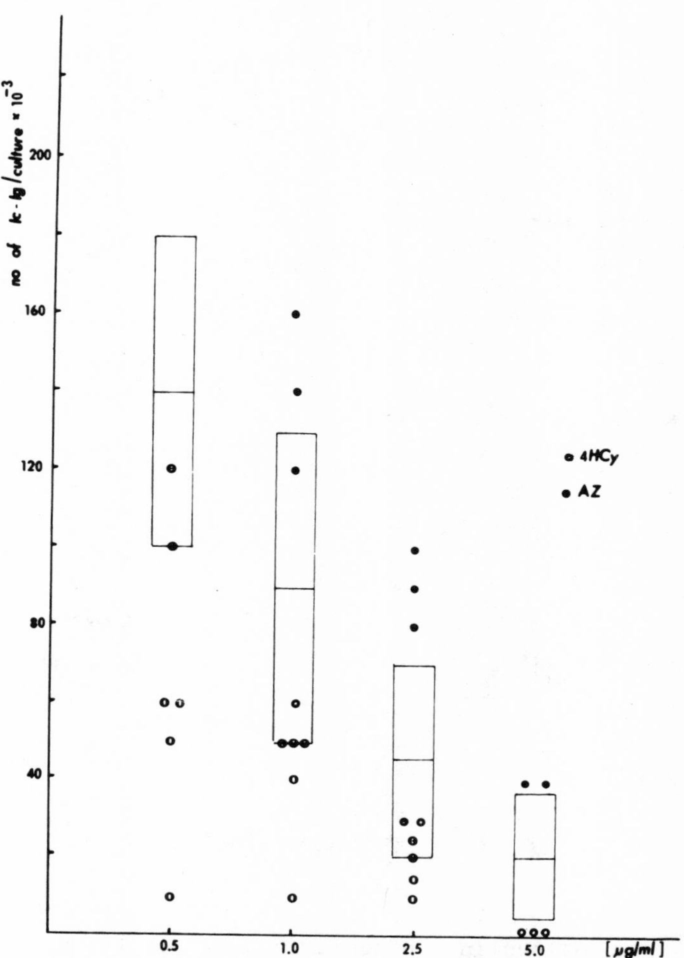

Fig 2. 4HCy- and AZ-dependent inhibition of immunoglobulin synthesis of lymphocytes from patients treated with TFX. The boxes represent the 4HCy-induced inhibition of immunoglobulin synthesis of normal lymphocytes for each concentration of the drug (mean ± SD).

cells. Also, culturing effector cells for 3 days in the presence of TFX prior to the assay does not change their activity (data not shown).

DISCUSSION

Recent advances in the search for new biological response modifiers have included the identification of remarkable immunosup-

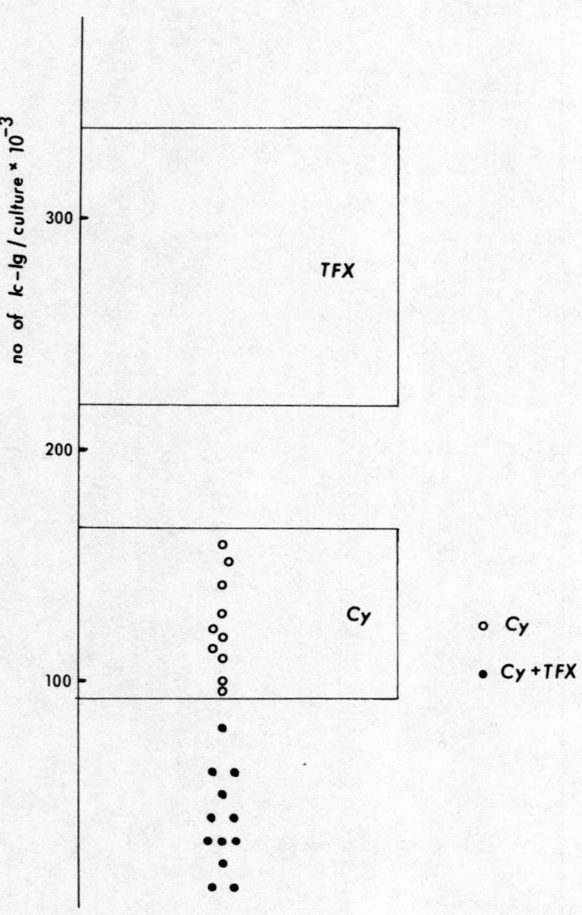

Fig. 3. Immunoglobulin synthesis in vitro of lymphocytes from patients treated with TFX, Cy and TFX + Cy. Mean ± SD is shown for TFX and Cy group.

pressive agents such as cyclosporin A and monoclonals. Clinical testing of those agents indicates, however, that they are not free of serious side effects. On the other hand, the use of monoclonals may be limited by their immunogenicity. It has been shown (1) that the administration of monoclonals to renal allograft recipients causes antibody formation that blocks their effect. These results indicate that the classical immunomodulating drugs continue to have an important role and their combining with new agents may lead to synergistic effects (14).

Evidence has accumulated to indicate that the major effect of thymosin is to induce T cell differentiation and enhance immunologic

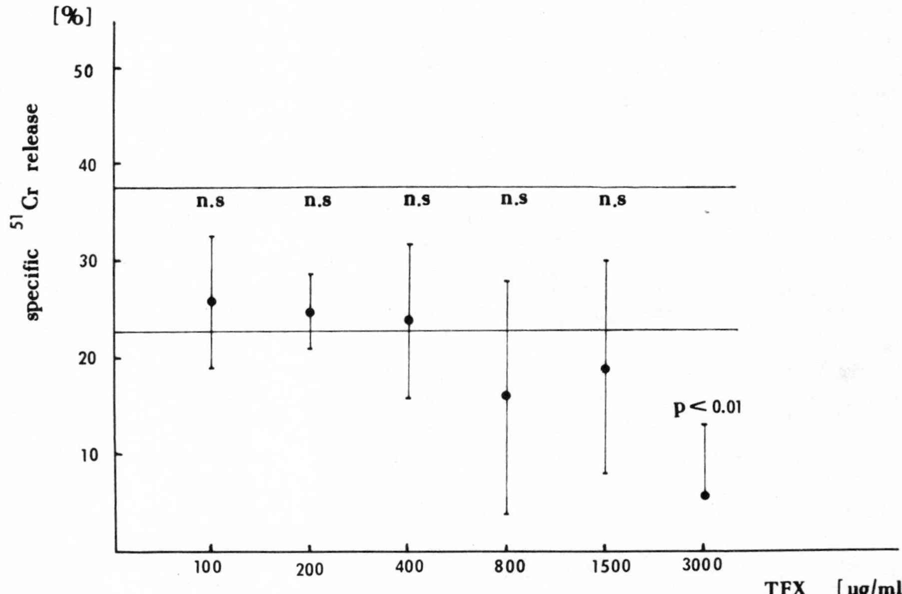

Fig. 4. The effect of TFX on ADCC assay. The horizontal lines represent the mean and standard deviation for cultures minus TFX.

functions in vivo and in vitro (4). However, it appears that the final effect of thymosin action depends, at least to some extent, upon the immune status of the patient (6). Our data seems to confirm this assumption. The primary effect of TFX is to enhance T cell dependent humoral responses, however, the agent is also capable of decreasing antibody synthesis to a normal level in cultures of lymphocytes rendered hyperactive by their prior exposure to TFX or unknown activators in vivo. Of particular note, TFX frequently completely abrogated immunoglobulin synthesis suggesting that it might be a useful agent in diseases with hyperactivity of the B cell system, especially caused by dysfunctions of T helper and suppressor cells. Furthermore, because the ADCC assay is believed to be an in vitro correlate of allograft rejection (16) the fact that TFX may be inhibitory to the effector cells suggests that TFX can be also useful in clinical transplantation.

Our data indicate that thymosin administration enhances the inhibitory effect of Cy on immunoglobulin-synthesizing B cells. In fact, a regimen involving both agents has been shown to cause a marked inhibition of antibody synthesis. This data is especially interesting in view of our previous observations showing that TFX alone enhances T cell dependent antibody synthesis, while the treatment with standard doses of Cy does not affect immunoglobulin production of peripheral blood lymphocytes (9). Interestingly, thymosin with chemotherapy (including Cy as its major component) has been shown to be superior to chemotherapy alone in the treatment of cancer (11). One could hypothesize that TFX recruits lymphocytes into the cell cycle rendering them more susceptible to chemotherapeutic agents. In fact, Dabrowski and Goldstein (2) have shown that thymosin accelerates the S + G phase of lymphocytes of thymectomized rats. That thymic hormones and immunosuppressive agents may have a synergistic effect is also supported by the observation of Bach et al (1) who put forward a hypothesis that the thymus liberates a humoral factor rendering lymphocytes sensitive to azathioprine. Although in our experiments Cy was clearly superior to AZ in inhibiting immunoglobulin synthesis, this finding is in agreement with the concept that Cy is more effective than AZ in inhibiting B cell functions (12).

Our data suggest that in some circumstances thymosin alone may have immunosuppressive properties and the concomitent use of TFX and Cy may be of potential value in clinical transplantation. Such therapy should provide an effective management of diseases with hyperactivity of the B cell system. Furthermore, as TFX is moderatel[y] inhibitory to ADCC, such a treatment should not precipitate rejection episodes.

ACKNOWLEDGEMENTS

This work was supported by grants IV/A/437 from Polfa Pharmaceuticals, Jelenia Gora and 10.5.1.4 from Polish Academy of Sciences. We are indebted to J. Gahr and M. Friedrich of Seromed, Munich, FRG for their generous gift of tissue culture media and reagents as well as Hoechst AG-Behring/FRG/for FITC-labelled antibodies. We also thank Dr. H. Brukert of Asta Werke AG, FRG for 4HCy and J. Pelkey of Burroughs-Wellcome, USA for Imuran.

REFERENCES

1. Bach, J. F., M. Dardanne, and A. J. S. Davies. 1971. Early effect of adult thymectomy. Nature 231: 110.

2. Dabrowski, M. P., and A. L. Goldstein. 1976. Thymosin induced changes in the cell cycle of lymphocytes from aging neonatally thymectomized rats. Immunol. Commun. 5: 695.

3. Dabrowski, M. P., B. K. Dabrowska-Bernstein, W. J. Brzosko, L. Babiuch, and B. Kassur. 1980. Maturation of human T lymphocytes under the influence of calf thymus hormone. Clin. Immun. Immunopath. 16: 297.

4. Goldstein, A. L., T. L. K. Low, G. B. Thurman, M. M. Zatz, N. Hall, J. Chen, S. K. Hu, P. B. Naylor, and J. E. McClure. 1981. Current status of thymosin and other hormones of the thymus gland. Recent Prog. Horm. Res. 37: 369.

5. Golightly, M. G., and S. H. Golub. 1980. The in vitro culture characteristic and requirements for expression of receptors for IgM on human peripheral blood lymphocytes. Clin. Exp. Immunol. 39: 227.

6. Gorski, A., A. B. Skotnicki, Z. Gaciong, and G. Korczak. 1981. The effect of calf thymus extract (TFX) on human and mouse hematopoiesis. Thymus 3: 129.

7. Górski, A., G. Korczak-Kowalska, Z. Gaciong and L. Paczek. 1982. Transient hypogammaglobulinemia of infancy. New Engl. J. Med. 306: 939.

8. Górski, A., G. Korczak-Kowalska, M. Nowaczyk, Z. Gaciong, and E. Skopinska-Rozewska. 1982. Thymosin (TFX): an immunomodulator of antibody production in man. Immunology 47: (in press).

9. Górski, A., M. Nowaczyk, G. Korczak-Kowalska, M. Wasik, I. Podobińska, M. Malejczyk, Z. Gaciong and L. Paczek. 1983. Mode of action of cyclophosphamide as assessed by in vitro activity of its active metabolite. Transplant. Proc. (in press).

10. Jaffers, G., R. B. Colvin, A. B. Cosimi, J. V. Giorgi, T. C. Fuller, C. Lillehei, and P. S. Russell. 1983. The human immune response to murine OKT3 monoclonal antibody. Transplant. Proc. (in press).

11. Lipson, S. D., P. B. Chretien, R. Maluch, D. E. Kenady, and M. K. Cohen. 1979. Thymosin immunotherapy in patients with small cell carcinoma of the lung. Cancer 43: 863.

12. Otterness, I. G., and Y. H. Chang. 1976. Comparative study of cyclophosphamide, 6-mercaptopurine, azathioprine and methotrexate. Clin. Exp. Immunol. 26: 346.

13. Spiegelberg, H. L., and P. M. Dainer. 1979. Fc receptors for IgG, IgM and IgE on human leukaemic lymphocytes. Clin. Exp. Immunol. 35: 286.

14. Squifflet, J. P., D. E. R. Sutherland, J. Field, J. Rynasiewicz, and J. Keil. 1982. Synergistic immunosuppressive effect of cyclosporin A and azathioprine. IX International Congress of the Transplantation Society, Brighton. (abstract).

15. Touraine, J. L., and R. A. Good. 1982. Therapy communication session on thymic hormones. Thymus 4: 57.

16. Wasik, M., L. Gradowska, D. Rowinska, M. Lao, and T. Orlowski. 1981. Diagnostic and prognostic value of ADCC and lectin-induced cellular cytotoxicity tests for renal allograft rejection. Transplantation 32: 217.

PROTECTIVE ACTIVITY OF THYMOSIN α_1 AGAINST TUMOR PROGRESSION IN IMMUNOSUPPRESSED MICE

Hideo Ishitsuka, Yukio Umeda, Atsuko Sakamoto, and Yasuo Yagi.

Nippon Roche Research Center, 200 Kajiwara, Kamakura City, Kanagawa Pref. 247, Japan

INTRODUCTION

Thymus gland has been shown to play an important role in the development, growth and function of lymphoid systems through a hormonal mechanism. One of the thymic hormones, thymosin (1), stimulates T cell development and corrects some immunodeficiency diseases resulting from lack of thymus functions. Considering the importance of T cells in immunoregulatory systems, thymosin is expected to be useful as a pharmaceutical agent for a variety of diseases which are caused by or which accompany the aberration of these systems.

Clinical efficacy of thymosin hormones has been shown in patients with some types of primary immunodeficiency (2). However, the efficacy of thymic hormones in patients with secondary immunodeficiency diseases has not been fully investigated. Patients with secondary immunodeficiency diseases such as cancer patients receiving intensive cancer therapies are faced with serious problems such as opportunisitic infections and recurrence of tumors presumably due to therapies with immunosuppressive side effects. One would expect that biological response modifiers like thymosin which can restore immunodeficient status would be effective in prevention of the diseases caused by immunosuppressive cancer therapies. Therefore, we have explored animal model systems which are relevant to such clinical situations.

In this report we describe animal model systems utilizing mice immunosuppressed by cytostatics or x-ray irradiation, where thymosin α_1(3), one of the thymosin peptides, was shown to be effective against the tumor progression. In addition, we describe studies on the mode of action of thymosin α_1 in immunosuppressed mice, which suggests that thymosin α_1 serves to maintain the natural killer (NK) cell activity and the barrier systems for the spread of tumor cells in circulation.

METHODS

Animals

Male mice (6 weeks old) of DBA/2, C57Bl/6 and CDF_1 (DBA/2 x BALB/c)F_1 strains were purchased from Shizuoka Agricultural Cooperative Association for Laboratory Animals, Hamamatsu, Japan.

Tumors

L1210 leukemic cells resistant to 5-FU (5-fluorouacil) were kindly supplied by Dr. A. Hoshino, Aichi Cancer Center. B16 melanoma was obtained from Cancer Institute, Japanese Foundation for Cancer Research, Tokyo. L1210 and B16 were maintained by continuous passage in DBA/2 mice and in tissue culture, respectively.

Treatment With Immunosuppressive Agents and Thymosin α_1

Immunosuppressed mice were obtained by treatment with cytostatic agents or X-ray irradiation as follows. Mice were treated with 5-FU (25 mg/kg, i.p.) daily for 7 to 10 days or with cyclophosphamide (CY, 100 mg/kg, i.p.) three times at 5, 3 and 1 days before inoculation of tumors. Alternatively, mice received 600 rad of X-ray once at 5 days before inoculation of tumor. Thymosin α_1 (40 μg/kg, i.p.) was given daily for 7 to 10 days concomitantly with the cytostatic agents or after X-ray.

Preparation of Radioactively Labeled Cells

^{125}IUdR-labeled L1210 and B16 cells were prepared by a previously described method (4).

YAC-1 lymphoma cells for cytotoxicity testing, and lymph node cells and bone marrow cells for lymphocyte homing were labeled by ^{51}Cr as described elsewhere (5).

Cytotoxicity Assay

Cytolytic reactivity of spleen cells was assayed by using a 4 hr ^{51}Cr-release test with ^{51}Cr-YAC-1 cell target as described (6). Cytolytic activity was quantified by using the equation: Percent specific release = (Experimental release - Spontaneous release)/(Maximum release - Spontaneous release) x 100.

Compounds

Thymosin $\alpha 1$ synthesized chemically was obtained from Dr. J. Neienhofer, Hoffmann-La Roche Inc., New Jersey, USA. Mouse monoclonal anti-Thy 1.2 and Lyt 5.1 sera were purchased from Flow Laboratory and New England Nuclear Co., respectively. Rabbit anti-asialo GM1 serum was obtained from Wako Pure Chemical Co.

Statistical Analyses

Statistical significance was analyzed using Student's t-test for paired data. Differences were considered to be significant when probability values $p < 0.05$. were obtained

RESULTS

High Incidence of Pulmonary Metastasis Caused By Immunosuppressive Agents and Preventive Effect of Thymosin $\alpha 1$

Impairment of the immune system against tumor growth by treatment with cytostatic agents or X-ray irradiation was demonstrated in mice. As shown in Figure 1, in normal mice, inoculation of B16 melanoma (10^4 cells) intravenously did not cause any pulmonary metastasis for two weeks, whereas in mice pretreated with cyclophosphamide (CY), it caused a high incidence of tumor metastasis in

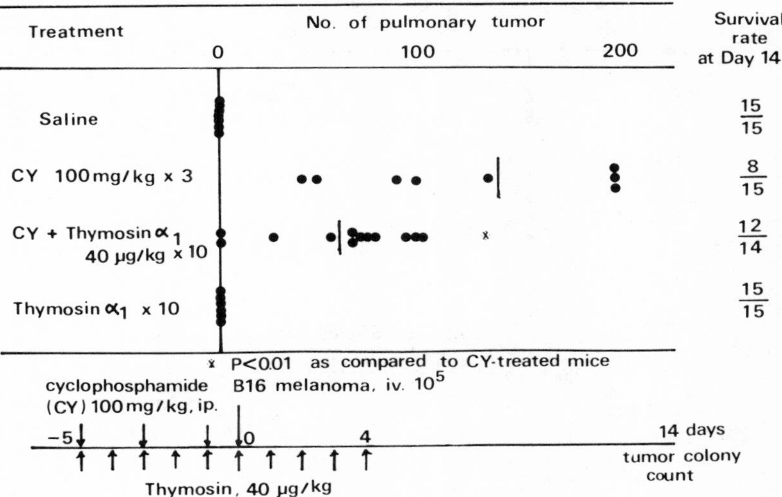

Fig. 1. Protective activity of thymosin $\alpha 1$ against pulmonary metastasis caused by inoculation of B16 melanoma in C57BL/6 mice treated with cyclophosphamide.

lungs. The treatment with CY also increased the mortality, i.e. 7 out of 15 mice died with tumor within two weeks. On the other hand, thymosin α_1 given with CY reduced the number of tumor colonies in lungs and mortality, i.e. only 2 out of 14 mice died.

Similar phenomena were observed in mice treated with 5-fluoroacil (5-FU) (Figure 2) and X-ray (Figure 3). These agents also increased the incidence of the pulmonary metastasis, although the number of tumor colonies metastasized was fewer probably because of less immunosuppressive activity of both agents than that of CY in these experiments. In these systems thymosin α_1 given concomitantly with 5-FU or after X-ray irradiation again suppressed the pulmonary metastasis.

Rapid Death Caused By Tumor Inoculation In Immunosuppressed Mice And Its Prevention By Thymosin α_1

Protective activity was also demonstrated following inoculation of L1210 leukemia. As shown in Figure 4, when mice were pretreated with 5-FU and then inoculated with the leukemic cells, the mice died very rapidly within a few days (rapid death). In this system, thymosin α_1 given concomitantly with 5-FU again protected the mice from the rapid death, although the mice eventually died with leukemia as in the case of normal mice inoculated with the same dose of the tumor cells (Figure 4).

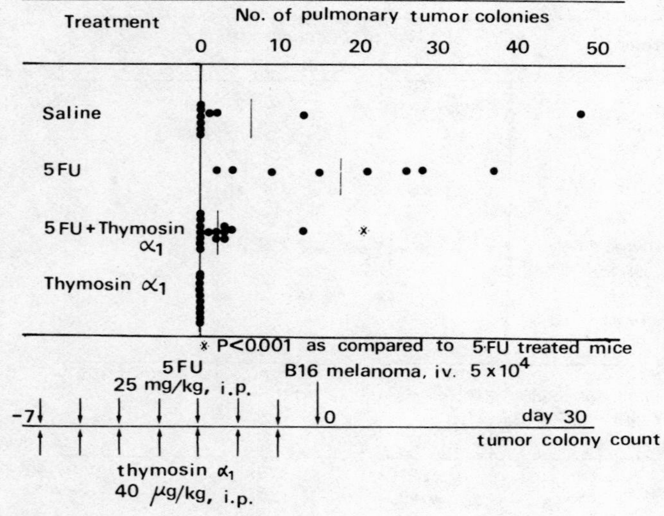

Fig. 2. Protective activity of thymosin α_1 against B16 pulmonary metastasis in C57BL/6 mice treated with 5-fluoruracil (5-FU).

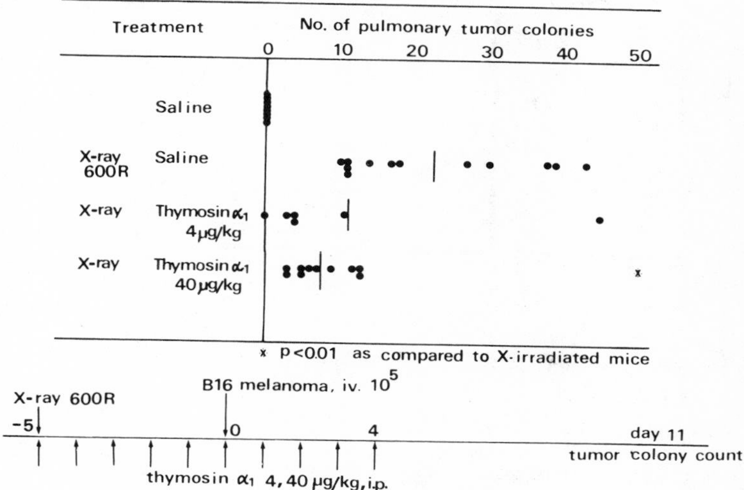

Fig. 3. Protective activity of thymosin α_1 against B16 pulmonary metastasis in C57BL/6 mice irradiated with x-ray.

In order to have some insight into the mechanism of this rapid death in these mice, the adoptive transfer of spleen cells was performed. As shown in Figure 5, when spleen cells from the donor mice treated with thymosin α_1 and 5-FU were transferred into the mice immunosuppressed with 5-FU and then L1210 leukemic cells were inoculated into the recipient mice, the rapid death did not occur, whereas spleen cells from donor mice treated with 5-FU alone did not show such activity.

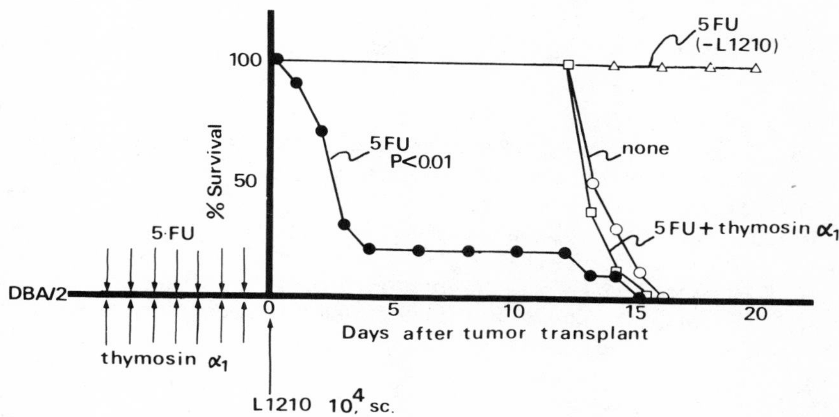

Fig. 4. Protective activity of thymosin α_1 against rapid death caused by inoculation of L1210 leukemic cells in DBA/2 mice treated with 5-FU.

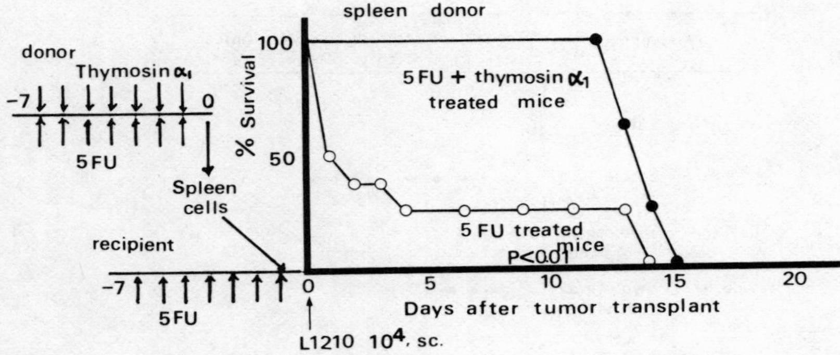

Fig. 5. Prevention of rapid death in DBA/2 recipient mice by adoptive transfer of spleen cells from donor mice treated with 5-FU and thymosin α_1 but not treated with 5-FU alone.

In separate experiments (7), treatment with anti-asialo GM1 or anti-Lyt5 serum of the donor cells from 5-FU + thymosin α_1-treated mice abrogated their activity to prevent the rapid death. These results suggest that the damage to NK cells by the 5-FU-treatment seems to be at least a part of the cause of the rapid death, and that thymosin α_1 affects NK cells or their progenitor cells in the 5-FU-treated mice. This possibility was suggested by the fact that the 5-FU treatment reduced the NK activity in spleen, but the combined treatment with thymosin α_1 prevented such reduction (Figure 6) However, the thymosin α_1 activity preventing the rapid death was not abrogated by injection with anti-asialo GM1 serum before the inoculation of the tumor cells, although NK cell activity in spleen was abolished. Some mechanism other than the damage to the NK cells may be involved in causing the rapid death in immunosuppressed mice.

Aberration Of The Barrier System For Spread Of Tumor Cells In Circulation And Its Prevention By Thymosin α1

The mechanisms leading to the rapid death and causing the high incidence of the pulmonary metastasis was investigated by examining the tissue distribution of tumor cells inoculated in immunosuppressed mice. In Figure 7, the tissue distribution of the radioactivity after inoculation of ^{125}I-labeled L1210 leukemic cells was compared between normal and the 5-FU-treated mice. The level of radioactivity in the 5-FU-treated mice was higher in blood and lung, but lower in liver and spleen. On the other hand, when thymosin α_1 was given concomitantly with 5-FU, the distribution pattern was almost the same as that in normal mice. These phenomena were also observed when ^{125}I-B16 melanoma (Figure 8), ^{51}Cr-lymph node (Figure 9) and bone marrow cells (Figure 10) were inoculated. The barrier system for spread of tumor cells and the trapping system for lymphocytes may be damaged by the 5-FU-treatment, but thymosin α_1 may maintain the function.

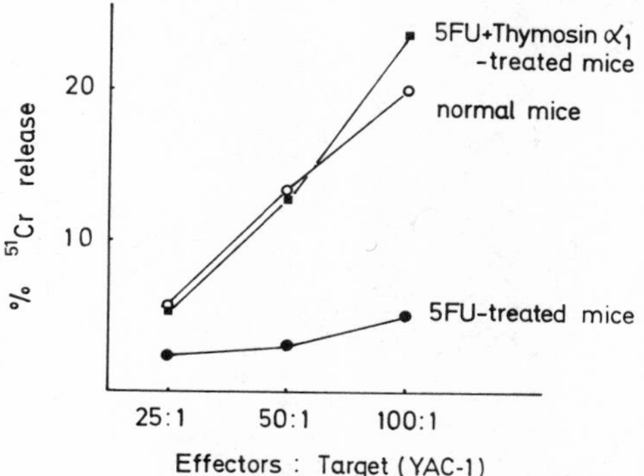

Fig. 6. Maintenance of NK activity by treatment with thymosin α_1 in 5-FU-treated mice. C57BL/6 mice were injected daily for 7 days with 5-FU (25 mg/kg, i.p.) and thymosin α_1 (40 μg/kg, i.p.).

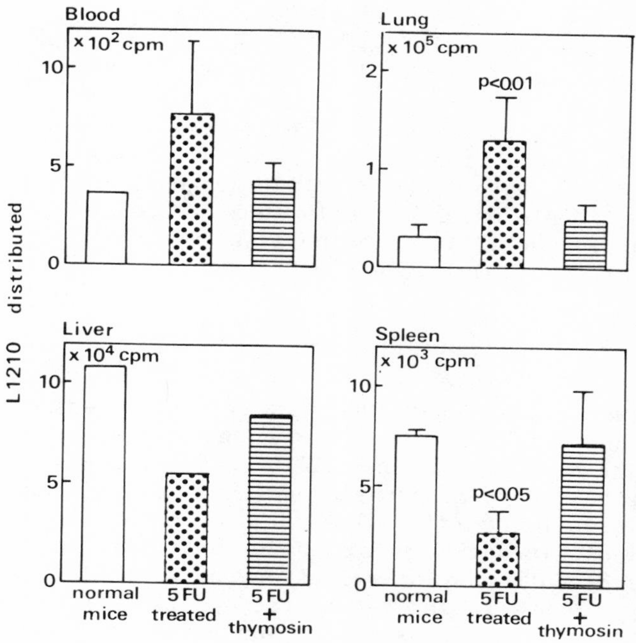

Fig. 7. Tissue distribution of ^{125}IUdR-labeled L1210 leukemic cells. DBA/2 mice treated daily for 7 days with or without 5-FU (25 mg/kg, i.p.) and thymosin α_1 (40 μg/kg, i.p.) were inoculated intravenously with ^{125}IUdR-labeled L1210 leukemic cells (10^6 cells/5.7 x 10^5 cpm). The radioactivity in each tissue was measured at 22 hr after the inoculation.

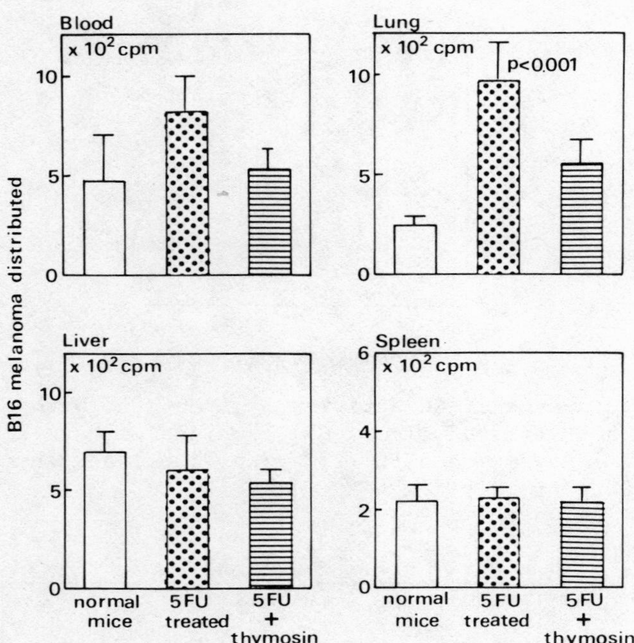

Fig. 8. Tissue distribution of ^{125}IUdR-labeled B16 melanoma cells. C57BL/6 mice treated with 5-FU and thymosin as described in Fig. 7 were inoculated intravenously with ^{125}IUdR-labeled B16 melanoma cells (6×10^5 cells/3.5×10^4 cpm). The radioactivity in each tissue was measured at 24 hr after the inoculation.

DISCUSSION

The present study showed that in immunosuppressed mice such as those which had received cytostatic agents or X-ray irradiation, inoculation of B16 melanoma and L1210 leukemic cells caused a high incidence of pulmonary metastasis and rapid death, respectively, to the host animals. These animal model systems are rather analogous to the clinical situation, where cancer patients are immunosuppressed by intensive chemotherapy or radiation therapy. In these systems, thymosin α_1, given with the cytostatic agents or after X-ray before the inoculation of the tumor cells, suppressed the metastasis and prevented the accelerated death. The mice consequently survived as long as the control mice inoculated with the same tumor cells.

Since NK cells are reported to participate in the suppression of pulmonary metastasis (8), the mechanism causing the high incidence of the metastasis was expected to be due to the damage to the NK cells by the immunosuppressive agents. The adoptive transfer

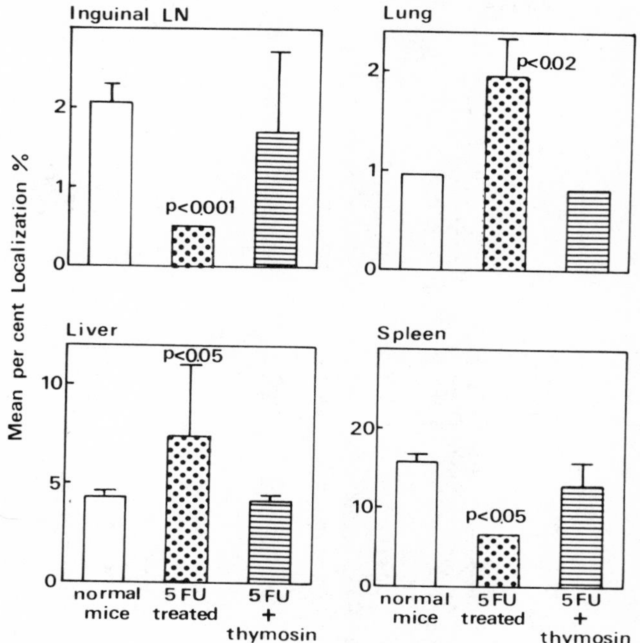

Fig. 9. Homing of ^{51}Cr-lymph node cells. DBA/2 mice treated with 5-FU and thymosin α_1 as described in Fig. 7 were inoculated with ^{51}Cr-inguinal lymph node cells (10^6 cells/1.97 x 10^5 cpm, i.v.). The radioactivity of each tissue was measured at 30 hr after the inoculation and expressed as % of total radioactivity inoculation.

of spleen cells with antisera against surface antigens of NK and T cells indicated that one of the effector cells preventing the rapid death was the NK cells. In addition, the NK activity was damaged by the 5-FU treatment, but thymosin α_1 served to maintain it at the normal level. On the other hand, treatment with anti-asialo GM1 serum (which should react with NK cells) before inoculation of L1210 failed to abolish the activity of thymosin α_1 to prevent the rapid death. This negative finding suggests that some mechanism other than the damage to NK cells may be involved in causing the rapid death in immunosuppressed mice.

Another possible mechanism causing the rapid death and increasing the metastasis is the damage to the barrier system for spread of tumor cells in blood circulation. In the 5-FU-treated mice, the trapping system against the tumor cells in tissues such as spleen and liver did not appear to function smoothly, resulting in poor clearance of the tumor cells from the blood and an accumulation into lung. In such mice, the tumor cells could migrate into some specific sites, where growth of the tumor cells may be lethal.

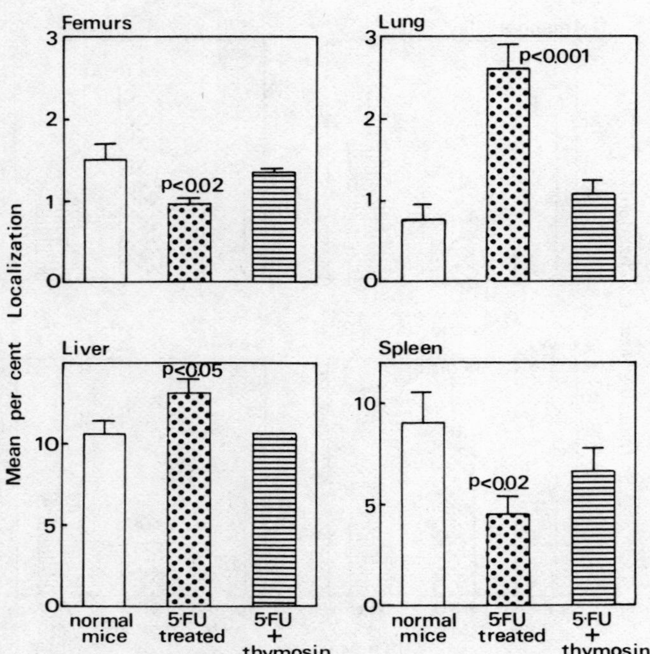

Fig. 10. Homing of ^{51}Cr-bone marrow cells. DBA/2 mice treated with 5-FU and thymosin as described in Fig. 7 were inoculated with ^{51}Cr-bone marrow cells (femurs) (5×10^6 cells/1.46×10^5 cpm, i.v.). The radioactivity of each tissue was measured at 24 hr after the inoculation and expressed as % of total radioactivity inoculated.

Abnormal homing of lymph node and bone marrow cells also suggests that an ability of lymphoid tissues to recognize surface marker of lymphocytes as well as tumor cells is reduced in the 5-FU-treated mice, and that it is restored by thymosin α_1. Thymosin α_1 seems to affect various cell populations. In separate experiments, thymosin α_1 was shown to prevent opportunistic infections in immunosuppressed mice probably through affecting not only T cells but also macrophages, neutrophils or their progenitor cells (9).

Thymosin has been shown to have beneficial effects in animal tumors (10) and human neoplasm (11) as an adjuvant. The present study gives some insight into the mode of action of thymosin. Although thymosin α_1 itself did not show any activity against tumors inoculated into normal mice (data were not shown), it could prevent the tumor progression through restoration or maintenance of immune functions in mice pretreated with therapeutic agents for cancer therapies. The present study also indicates that chemotherapy with a cytostatic agent, particularly when the agent is not effective against the tumor, may be quite deleterious. In combination with thymosin α_1 undesirable effects of cytostatics may be avoided and extensive chemotherapy for a longer duration may be possible.

SUMMARY

The effect of thymosin α_1 was examined in mice immunosuppressed by cytostatics or X-ray irradiation. Inoculation of B16 melanoma or L1210 leukemic cells into these immunosuppressed mice caused a high incidence of pulmonary metastasis or rapid death, respectively. Thymosin α_1 given concomitantly with cytostatics or after X-ray prevented such deleterious effects of these agents. One of possible mechanisms causing the rapid death and increasing the metastasis is the damage to NK cells. Thymosin α_1 prevented the reduction of NK cell activity caused by these agents. The preventive activity could be transferred to immunosuppressed recipients by spleen cells and those deprived of T cells, but not by those deprived of NK cells. Another possible mechanism is the aberration of the barrier system for spread of tumor cells in blood circulation, which may allow the tumor cells to migrate to various sites in the host. In 5-FU-treated mice, distribution of ^{125}I-L1210 cells upon inoculation was higher in blood and lung, but lower in liver and spleen as compared with that in normal mice. On the other hand, when thymosin α_1 was given with 5-FU, the pattern of the tissue distribution was almost the same as that in normal mice. Thus, thymosin α_1 protected mice which received immunosuppressive agents from undesirable effects of the agents on surveillance systems against tumor. Thymosin α_1 may be useful as an adjuvant in cancer therapies.

REFERENCES

1. Hooper, J. A., M. C. McDaniel, G. B. Thurman, G. H. Cohen, R. S. Schulof, and A. L. Goldstein. 1975. Purification and properties of bovine thymosin. Ann. N. Y. Acad. Sci. 249: 125.

2. Wara, D. W., A. L. Goldstein, W. Doyle, and A. J. Ammann. 1975. Thymosin activity in patients with cellular immunodeficiency. New Engl. J. Med. 292: 70.

3. Goldstein, A. L., T. L. K. Low, M. McAdoo, J. McClure, G. B. Thurman, J. Rossio, C-Y. Lai, D. Chang, S-S. Wang, C. Harvey, A. H. Ramel, and J. Meienhofer. 1977. Thymosin α_1 : Isolation and sequence analysis of an immunologically active thymic polypeptide. Proc. Natl. Acad. Sci. U.S.A. 74: 725.

4. Fidler, I. J. 1970. Metastasis: Quantitative analysis of distribution and fate of tumor emboli labeled with ^{125}I-5-iodo-2'-deoxyuridine. J. Natl. Cancer Inst. 45: 775.

5. Kasai, M., M. Iwamori, Y. Nagai, K. Okumura, and T. Tada. 1980. A glycolipid on the surface of mouse natural killer cells. Eur. J. Immunol. 10: 175.

6. Zatz, M. M., E. M. Lance. 1971. The distribution of ^{51}Cr-labeled lymphocytes into antigen stimulated mice. J. Exp. Med. 134: 224.

7. Umeda, Y., J. Nakamura, H. Ishitsuka, and Y. Yagi. Protective activity of thymosin α_1 against tumor progression in immunosuppressed mice through affecting NK cells (in preparation).

8. Hanna, N., and C. R. Burton. 1981. Definitive evidence that natural killer (NK) cells inhibit experimental tumor metastasis *in vivo*. J. Immunol. 127: 1754.

9. Ishitsuka, H., Y. Umeda, J. Nakamura and Y. Yagi. Protective activity of thymosin α_1 against opportunistic infection in immunosuppressed mice (submitted).

10. Chirigos, M. A. 1978. *In vitro* and *in vivo* studies with thymosin, p. 305. *In* M. A. Chirigos (ed.), Immune modulation and control of neoplasia by adjuvant therapy. Raven Press, New York.

11. Lipson, S. D., P. B. Chretien, R. Makuch, D. E. Kenady, and M. H. Cohen. 1973. Thymosin immunotherapy in patients with small cell carcinoma of the lung: Correlation of *in vitro* studies with clinical course. Cancer 43: 863.

EFFECT OF THYMOSTIMULIN ON HUMAN LYMPHOCYTE ADENOSINE DEAMINASE AND PURINE NUCLEOSIDE PHOSPHORYLASE ACTIVITIES: PHYSIOLOGICAL AND THERAPEUTIC EFFECTS

F. Ambrogi, M. Petrini, F. Caracciolo, A. Azzara, and G. Carulli

I Clinica Medica, Università di Pisa, Ospedali S. Chiara Pisa, Italy

INTRODUCTION

Thymostimulin (TP1 - Serono), which has several immunobiological activities in vivo and in vitro, is a pool of thermostable polypeptides extracted from calf thymus and has been used in the treatment of primary and secondary immunodeficiencies (1, 2). However, the immunobiological properties and the mechanism of action of this cellular extract is still not completely understood. For this reason, we have studied the activity of thymostimulin on the intracellular levels of adenosine deaminase (ADA) and purine nucleoside phosphorylase (PNP) enzymes in peripheral blood lymphocytes of patients with hematological malignancies. We also hoped to reveal the effects of thymostimulin on lymphocytes from cord blood and from elderly patients. In fact, these enzymes have important roles in both lymphocyte ontogenesis (3, 4) and in the maintenance of immunological functions (5, 6).

METHODS

The lymphocytes from 22 consenting control subjects were assayed to evaluate the normal levels of intralymphocyte ADA and PNP. Nineteen patients with Hodgkin's lymphoma (H.D.), 16 patients with non Hodgkin's (N.H.L.) lymphoma, 40 patients with chronic lymphocytic leukaemia (CLL) and 17 healthy, elderly subjects were evaluated. Cord blood lymphocytes taken from 7 babies, immediately after birth, were included in our study. Lymphocyte purification, mitogenic response to PHA and enzymatic evaluation of ADA and PNP have already been described in previous reports (4-9). To evaluate thymostimulin activity in vivo, 100 mg was administered daily for 7 days to individual human subjects. To evaluate activity in vitro, lymphocytes were incubated with 10 mg of thymostimulin for 1 hour at 37°C, and then washed twice. Statistical analysis was determined using the Student's t test unless otherwise indicated.

RESULTS

ADA and PNP activities evaluated in lymphocytes from the consenting healthy donors were 6.9 ± 1.1 and 32.0 ± 6.8 respectively. Lymphocyte ADA levels of 19 patients with H.D. (6.6 ± 1.2) and 16 NHL (6.2 ± 3.0) fell within normal values. The Tpl treatment was carried out in 7 of these patients with widely varying results (Table 1). In 40 cases of CLL, we found a significantly reduced ADA level (2.4 ± 2.1; $p < 0.001$). In 5 cases, treated with Tpl, we found a significant increase of enzymatic activity, from 2.4 ± 1.5 to 5.3 ± 3.4 ($p < 0.01$).

Incubation of lymphocytes from elderly subjects with Tpl significantly increased the mitogenic response to PHA (data not shown). This occurred after both cell preincubation (for 1 hr at 37°) and maintaining Tpl in the culture medium throughout the experiment. However, cell preincubation with Tpl produced no effects on PNP and ADA activities. ADA and PNP activities were respectively 11.5 ± 4.3 and 41.7 ± 14.3 before and 10.8 ± 5.8 and 41.3 ± 8.2 after Tpl preincubation. In cord blood lymphocytes, the basic ADA activity (12.9 ± 2.3) was found statistically unchanged after incubation with Tpl (14.9 ± 2.0) but PNP activity that was initially 38.8 ± 14.3 was significantly ($p < 0.05$) increased to 50.2 ± 19.0 as evaluated on the basis of the Wilcoxon's test.

DISCUSSION

In some hematological malignancies, such as CLL, we found low ADA activity. In a few cases, Tpl was found to increase this activity. Variable results were found in patients with HD and NHL. Restoration of immunological function by Tpl in elderly subjects, was assessed by testing in vitro the modification of the PHA response after Tpl addition. The drug demonstrated mitogenic activity alone and also significantly increased the PHA response (10). However, it produced no effects on PNP and ADA levels in these elderly patients. Lymphocytes from human cord blood were evaluated to assess the ability of Tpl to induce lymphocyte maturation. These cells have shown high levels of ADA (4-9). We found a significant PNP increase but no ADA modification as expected following the initial cell differentiation.

In conclusion, this preliminary data seems to indicate that

Table 1. Adenosine deaminase activity in peripheral blood lymphocytes from patients with lymphomas before and after Tpl administration

Lymphoma*	Adenosine deaminase activity	
	Before Treatment	After Treatment
NHL	12.3	8.5
NHL	15.8	15.0
NHL	49.7	11.0
NHL	4.3	9.5
NHL	4.4	17.1
NHL	4.7	10.7
HD	8.9	6.9

* NHL, non Hodgkin's lymphoma; HD, Hodgkin's lymphoma.

the evaluation of intralymphocytic enzymes of purine catabolism may be a useful methodological approach in assessing immunomodulator agents. By this approach we can confirm some effect of Tpl on lymphocyte differentiation. The treatment with Tpl may be useful in CLL.

REFERENCES

1. Fiorilli, M., R. Ammirati, M. C. Sirianni, R. D'Amelio, I. Quinti, M. C. Voci, and F. Aiuti. 1980. In Thymus, thymic hormones and T lymphocytes. F. Aiuti and H. Wigzell (eds.), Academic Press, London.

2. Falchetti, R., G. Bergesi, A. Esvol, C. Cafiero, L. Adorini, and L. Caprino. 1977. Drugs Exp. Clin. Res. 3: 39.

3. Barton, R., F. Martiniuk, P. Hirschnorn, and I. Goldschneider. 1980. Cell. Immunol. 49: 208.

4. Petrini, M., R. Testi, N. Capelli, F. Caracciolo, S. Ronca-Testoni, and F. Ambrogi. 1980. In F. Gasosto, G. P. Bagnara, M. A. Brunelli, and C. Castaldini (eds.), Editrice Esculapio, Bologna.

5. Giblett, E., E. Anderson, E. Cohen, B. Pollara, and H. J. Meuwissen. 1972. Lancet 2: 1067.

6. Giblett, E., A. T. Amman, D. W. Wara, R. Sandman, and L. K. Diamon. 1975. Lancet 1: 1010.

7. Ambrogi, F., B. Grassi, S. Ronca-Testoni, and G. Ronca. 1977. Clin. Exp. Immunol. 28: 80.

8. Petrini, M., A. Azzara, R. Polidori, Maria L. Vatteroni, F. Caracciolo, G. Carulli, and F. Ambrogi. 1982. Clin. Immunol. Immunopathol. 23: 124

9. Ambrogi, F. 1982. Cell. Immunol. (in press).

10. Petrini, M., R. Polidori, A. Azzara, Maria L. Vatteroni, and F. Ambrogi. 1981. Curr. Therap. Res. 30: 367.

INTERLEUKINS IN EXPERIMENTAL AUTOIMMUNE DISEASE

Norman Talal and Michael Fischbach

The University of Texas Health Science Center Department of Medicine, Division of Clinical Immunology and the Veterans Administration, San Antonio, Texas (USA)

INTRODUCTION

In autoimmune disorders, the organism's ability to discriminate self from foreign antigens is disturbed, leading to tissue destruction due to a variety of immunopathologic mechanisms. Autoantibodies and immune complexes may be present in the serum, and target organs may undergo vasculitic destruction or become infiltrated with lymphocytes and plasma cells. Recognition of histocompatibility antigens and Ia antigens on lymphocyte and macrophage membranes is an important regulatory mechanism allowing the immune system to react against viral and other foreign antigens. The immune system is exquisitely regulated. In part, this regulation is dependent upon specific immune response genes which are located within the major histocompatibility complex. Genetic factors influence specialized subpopulations of T-lymphocytes, which function either to suppress or enhance immune responses. Recognition of idiotypic receptors on lymphocyte membranes by antibody or by other lymphocytes can also result in either suppression or priming of an immune response. Since these regulatory mechanisms play an important role in immunologic control, one must look to some derangement in their function to explain the existence of autoimmunity and autoimmune disorders.

Interleukin-2 (IL-2), or T cell growth factor, is a protein essential for T cell proliferation and for the development of appropriate pathways of immunologic control. IL-2 is produced by Lyt $1^{+}23^{-}$ cells and interacts with specific receptors on Lyt $1^{+}23^{+}$ cells to promote the development of T effector cells (1). Since autoimmune diseases can be viewed as problems of disordered immunologic regulation, we undertook a study of immunoregulatory factors which might be qualitatively or quantitatively abnormal in autoimmune states. We argued that deficiency in an immunoregulatory factor might be particularly important since replacement of such a material could have therapeutic potential. Our studies focused on IL-2 because its chemistry and biology were relatively well defined.

For over twenty years the NZB mouse and its variants were the only murine models for systemic lupus erythematosus available for examination. In recent years, a second model has been introduced called MRL/lpr which differs from the NZB in developing a very fulminant form of disease with early death (2). A cardinal feature in this disease is the marked proliferation of an unusual T lymphocyte which is weakly expressive of the Lyt $1^{+}23^{-}$ phenotype (3). Disease in this strain is related to the presence of the lpr gene since a congenic MRL mouse lacking this gene, MRL/++, develops only very mild disease. The lpr gene has also been introduced into C57Bl/6, C3H and AKR mice. Although the time of disease onset may vary, all of these lpr mice develop hypergammaglobulinemia, autoantibodies, immune complex glomerulonephritis and massive lymphoproliferation.

We find that IL-2 deficiency is a common feature in several autoimmune susceptible strains of mice, suggesting that defective IL-2 may contribute to their immunoregulatory disorder. We have utilized an antigen presentation system to study IL-2 dependent T cell proliferation in MRL/lpr, C57Bl6/lpr and C3H/He/lpr mice and their normal congenic counterparts. The normal mice proliferate well whereas there is little proliferation in the lpr variants. Mixing experiments demonstrate that the defects reside with the lpr responding T cells and not with the lpr macrophages.

An IL-2 defect is also present in patients with systemic lupus erythematosus and rheumatoid arthritis. In this respect, there is a parallel between the human disease and the animal model. We are currently investigating the mechanism responsible for the IL-2 defect in these patients.

METHODS

MRL/Mp-lpr/lpr (MRL/lpr), MRL/Mp-+/+, C57Bl/6J-lpr/lpr (57/lpr), C3H/HeJ-lpr/lpr (C3H/lpr), and NZB/NZW F_1 mice were obtained from our breeding colonies at The University of Texas Health Science Center at San Antonio. The normal congenic partners, C57Bl/6J and C3H/HeJ were obtained from Jackson Laboratory, Bar Harbor, ME.

The following methods have been described previously (4).

IL-2 Production

Briefly, spleen cells were suspended at a density of 1 x 10^7/ml in culture medium supplemented with 10 μg/ml Concanavalin A. The cells were incubated in multiwell tissue culture plates for 36 hours at 37°C in a humidified atmosphere containing 5% CO_2. Cells were removed from the culture supernatants by centrifugation at 1500g for 10 minutes. Cell-free supernatants were subsequently passed through 0.22 μm filters and stored at -20°C.

IL-2 Assay

Normal spleen cells were cultured for 48 hours with Con A (2 μg/ml) and subsequently washed three times in 10 mg/ml α-methyl-D-mannoside. The cells were then incubated in microtiter plates with serial dilutions of the culture supernatant being tested for IL-2 activity. Each well contained 5 x 10^3 cells in a volume of 200 μl. Cultures were supplemented with 10 mg/ml α-methyl-D-mannoside to block the possible mitogenic effects of Con A in the test samples. One μCi of (^{3}H)thymidine added during the last 24 hours of a 72-hour incubation yield optimal thymidine incorporation. The cultures were then harvested onto glass fiber filter strips, and retained radioactivity was measured in a Packard liquid scintillation counter.

IL-2 Response

The assay described above was also used to determine IL-2 response. Spleen cells from the strains to be tested were substituted for the normal spleen cells and known amounts of purified human IL-2 from Associated Biomedic Systems, Inc., was added in place of supernatants.

IL-2 Production In Humans

Two million peripheral blood mononuclear cells were stimulated with 1 μg/ml PHA for 24 hours. Supernatants were collected and assayed for IL-2 activity.

IL-2 Assay

Spleen cells from C57Bl/6J mice (2-3 month old) are stimulated with 5 μg/ml of Con A for 36 hours. Cells are harvested and washed with media containing 10 mg/ml of α-methyl-D-mannoside. Various dilutions of culture supernatants are added to the cells (5 x 10^4/well) and ^{3}H-Tdr incorporation is measured after 48 hours.

IL-2 Response

Five million peripheral blood mononuclear cells were activated by 10 μg/ml Con A. Excess Con A was removed by treatment with α-methyl-D-mannoside. Exogeneous IL-2 was added to 10 thousand cells and incorporation of tritiated thymidine determined after 72 hours in culture.

Antigen Presentation

This was studied by using the method of Alkan (5). Mice were immunized at the base of the tail with 10 μg $TNP_{25}KLH$ emulsified in complete Freund's adjuvant. Seven days later, draining lymph nodes were removed and the T cells purified by nylon wool chromatography. Non-immune spleen cells, 1×10^7, were incubated with TNP-KLH in the presence of Mitomycin C for one hour at 37°C. After extensive washing, 2×10^5 antigen pulsed spleen cells were incubated with 4×10^5 immune T cells for 5 days in culture. The incorporation of tritiated thymidine was used to measure the degree of antigen stimulation.

In some experiments, purified human IL-2 was added to the cultures or IL-2 was administered daily *in vivo* at the base of the tail during the initial antigen priming.

RESULTS

IL-2 Production

An age related decline in IL-2 production was noted in autoimmune mice. The exact time course varied from strain to strain, for example, in MRL/*lpr* and C57/*lpr*, the decreased IL-2 production preceded the development of autoimmune disease manifestations occurring as early as six weeks of age. In the B/W mice, there was a gradual decline in IL-2 production, paralleling the development of autoimmunity (6).

The macrophage factor Interleukin-1 or the compound phorbol myristic acetate stimulate IL-2 production. Neither of these substances was capable of inducing IL-2 when added to *in vitro* cultures of autoimmune mice (4).

A search for suppressor cells or factors as an explanation for the decreased production of IL-2 was undertaken. Lymphocytes from *lpr* strains were mixed with their normal congenic partners during Con A stimulation. No decrease in IL-2 production was observed (4).

IL-2 Response

Lymphocytes from autoimmune strains failed to respond to exogeneous IL-2. In the MRL/*lpr*, the IL-2 response was reduced by 50%

at 2 months of age, and decreased to 5% of that of age-matched controls (MRL/++) by 5 months of age (5).

The failure of autoimmune spleen cells to respond normally to IL-2 suggested that they might be unable to bind the lymphokine. To investigate this possibility, exogeneous IL-2 was incubated with Con A stimulated cells. Lymphocytes from normal strains were able to remove most of the IL-2 activity, in contrast to MRL/lpr cells which hardly removed any. This suggests an actual or functional defect in surface receptors for IL-2.

Human Studies

To determine the relevance of these findings to human autoimmune disease, lymphocytes from patients with SLE, rheumatoid arthritis (RA) and Sjogren's syndrome (SS) were examined for their ability to produce and respond to IL-2. The results given in Table 1 show a statistically significant reduction in IL-2 production by peripheral blood lymphocytes from patients with SLE and RA. However, unlike the situation in autoimmune mice, IL-2 response was not uniformally low.

The data presented in Table 2 demonstrates that only lymphocytes from patients with RA failed to respond to IL-2.

Antigen Presentation

In order to better define and hopefully elucidate the cellular nature of the IL-2 defect, the interaction between macrophages and T cells during the important activity of presenting antigen was studied.

Table 1. Production of IL-2 by peripheral blood lymphocytes from patients with systemic lupus erythematosus (SLE), rheumatoid arthritis (RA), and Sjogren's syndrome (SS).

SLE (n=22)	0.40 ±0.05*
RA (n=17)	0.32 ± 0.03**
SS (n=10)	0.52 ± 0.19
Controls (n=19)	0.67 ± 0.07

*p <0.012; Data in units of activity
**p <0.001

Table 2. Proliferative responsiveness to IL-2 of blood lymphocytes from patients with systemic lupus erythematosus (SLE), rheumatoid arthritis (RA), and Sjogren's syndrome (SS).

SLE (n=22)	20,821 ± 1585
RA (n=17)	14,613 ± 1315*
SS (n=10)	23,734 ± 3443
Controls (n=19)	24,945 ± 2628

*p <0.02; Data in counts per minute

Not surprisingly, all the mice possessing the lpr gene did not respond normally to antigen. A representative study employing C57/lpr and its normal C57/B6 partner is shown in Table 3. The lpr mouse failed to respond whereas the normal congenic mouse gave a brisk response. To determine the cell responsible for this defect, normal antigen presenting cells were mixed with lpr T cells and vice versa. As can be seen in Table 3, the lpr spleen cells can present antigen to normal T cells. However, lpr T cells are unable to respond to antigen when presented by normal spleen cells.

Table 3. Lymphoproliferation in response to antigen employing co-culture combinations of normal and lpr lymphoid cells.

Cells	Incorporation Tritiated Thymidine (cpm)
1. Normal antigen presenting cells + normal T cells	41,300 ± 4322
2. lpr antigen presenting cells + lpr T cells	322 ± 165
3. Normal antigen presenting cells + lpr T cells	1,402 ± 629
4. lpr antigen presenting cells + normal T cells	38,039 ± 4147

Controls: Primed T cells, antigen presenting cells, unprimed T cells or antigen presenting cells alone or in any combination gave less than 900 cpm.

This finding held true for three strains possessing the *lpr* gene, and demonstrates that the *lpr* macrophage can perform normally in this assay. These results imply that there is enough Interleukin-1 produced by *lpr* macrophages to initiate a normal proliferative response.

A pharmacologic attempt to stimulate the defective *lpr* T cell was undertaken (Table 4). Purified IL-2 was added *in vitro* to the antigen presentation cultures. Cells from normal mice increased their antigen induced proliferation by 48%. The *lpr* cells did not change. IL-2 was given *in vivo* at the time of initial immunization and daily thereafter. Again in the normal mouse, antigen induced proliferation increased by the same amount, 48%, but *lpr* mice remained unresponsive. Finally, IL-2 was administered both *in vivo* and *in vitro*. Normal mice increased by approximately 75%, but *lpr* mice could not be stimulated.

DISCUSSION

Autoimmune disorders are complex and multifactorial in etiology. Genetic, immunologic, hormonal, environmental and possible viral factors may all play a role in pathogenesis. Studies performed in inbred strains of mice that are genetically predisposed to lupus-like illness likewise indicate a variety of immunologic abnormalities associated or predisposing to disease.

Our laboratory has utilized several autoimmune-susceptible mouse strains as models for human lupus. Our strategy has been to define immunologic defects that are also present in patients and that might be corrected by specific immunologic means. Our recent interest has focused on IL-2 or T cell growth factor. Murine IL-2 is a 30,000 m.w. protein produced by Lyt $1^{+}23^{-}$ T cells in response to

Table 4. Failure to modify antigen-induced lymphoproliferative response of *lpr* cells by IL-2 treatment.

Strain	IL-2	Net Percent Increase
C3H	in vitro	48%
C3H/lpr	in vitro	0%
C3H	in vivo	48%
C3H/lpr	in vivo	0%
C3H	in vivo and vitro	75%
C3H/lpr	in vivo and vitro	0%

antigen or mitogen stimulation (7-9). IL-2 has diverse effects on lymphocytes *in vitro*, including 1) augmentation of antibody synthesis by splenocytes from nude mice (7, 10, 11), 2) long-term maintenance of specific alloreactive cytotoxic and helper-T cells (7, 10, 12-16), and 3) enhancement of thymocyte proliferation after mitogen stimulation (7, 17-20). Receptors for IL-2 are present on activated T cells (21-27), which are then stimulated to undergo clonal expansion. IL-2 is also active *in vivo* (21, 22) and is an important mediator of immune function and regulation.

The several laboratory models for SLE offer an opportunity to identify common immunopathologic features that contribute to immune dysregulation, such as the deficiency of IL-2. This defect arises within the first two months of life in the MRL/*lpr* and C57Bl/6/*lpr* strains. We have not yet defined mechanisms responsible for the IL-2 defect although we have defined the cell responsible for their abnormality. The antigen presentation studies employing TNP-KLH have localized the defect to the responding T cells rather than to the antigen presenting macrophages. In every instance, T cells from *lpr* lymph nodes remain unresponsive even when exposed to antigen presented with normal macrophages. Conversely, *lpr* macrophages can present antigen well to normal T cells.

The response to IL-2 is also defective in addition to the impaired production. Thus, at least two T cell subpopulations are implicated (IL-2 producers as well as IL-2 responders), presumably the Lyt 1^+23^- and Lyt 123^+ subsets. This inability to respond to IL-2 probably explains the relative ineffectiveness of IL-2 added *in vivo* or *in vitro* to augment the proliferative response to TNP-KLH.

The lymphoid enlargement present in *lpr* mice in the face of IL-2 deficiency suggests an IL-2 independent lymphoproliferation. The proliferating cells are weakly Lyt 1^+ (3). We hypothesize that these cells are arrested in a developmental phase characterized by deficient expression of the Lyt 1^+ phenotype and by defective production of IL-2. These two features may not necessarily be related, although perhaps the Lyt 1^+ marker contributes to a cell surface receptor normally responsive to signals stimulating IL-2 production. This would be analogous to the involvement of the Lyt 2^+ antigen in recognition events leading to cellular cytotoxicity.

The defective production of IL-2 in patients with SLE and rheumatoid arthritis demonstrate that the animal model can provide information relevant to human disease. The diseases of immunologic dysregulation, which include SLE, may be susceptible to specific forms of immunoregulatory molecules. Much progress has been made recently due to our understanding of the immunobiology of the interleukins and interferon. Hopefully, better definition of immunoregulatory abnormalities in animal models and patients will one day yield appropriate drugs or biologicals that can restore immune control in these diseases.

SUMMARY

New mouse models of SLE have been developed recently including strains bearing the *lpr* gene. The presence of this gene results in antibodies to nucleoproteins and DNA, immune complex glomerulonephritis, and proliferation of Lyt 1^+23^- T cells. A defect in Interleukin-2 (IL-2) production is a common abnormality in these autoimmune mice. We have utilized an antigen presentation system to study T cell proliferation in MRL/*lpr*, C57B16/*lpr* and C3H/He/*lpr* mice and their normal congenic counterparts. The normal mice proliferate well whereas there is little proliferation in the *lpr* variants. Mixing experiments demonstrate that the defect resides with the *lpr* responding T cells and not with the *lpr* macrophages. This abnormality could be due to defective IL-2 production by Lyt 1^+23^- T cells.

REFERENCES

1. Smith, K. A. and F. W. Ruscetti. 1981. T cell growth factor and the culture of cloned functional T cells. Adv. Immunol. *31*: 137-175.

2. Andrews, B. S., R. A. Eisenberg, A. N. Theofilopoulos, S. Izui, C. B. Wilson, P. J. McConahey, E. D. Murphy, J. B. Roths and F. J. Dixon. 1978. Spontaneous murine lupus-like syndromes. Clinical and immunopathological manifestations in several strains. J. Exp. Med. *148*: 1198-1215.

3. Wofsy, D., J. R. Roubinian, J. A. Ledbetter, W. C. Seaman and N. Talal. Thymic influences on autoimmunity in MRL/lpr mice. Scand. J. Immunol. (in press)

4. Wofsy, D., E. D. Murphy, J. B. Roths, M. J. Dauphinee, S. B. Kipper and N. Talal. 1981. Deficient interleukin-2 activity in MRL/Mp and C57Bl/6J mice bearing the *lpr* gene. J. Exp. Med. *154*: 1671-1680.

5. Alkan, S. S. 1978. Antigen-induced proliferation assay for mouse T lymphocytes. Response to a monovalent antigen. Eur. J. Immunol. *8*: 112-118.

6. Dauphinee, M. J., S. B. Kipper, D. Wofsy and N. Talal. 1981. Interleukin-2 deficiency is a common feature of autoimmune mice. J. Immunol. 127: 2483-2487.

7. Watson, J., S. Gillis, J. Marbrook, D. Mochizuki and K. A. Smith 1979. Biochemical and biological characterization of lymphocyte regulatory molecules. I. Purification of a class of murine lymphokines. J. Exp. Med. 150: 840.

8. Watson, J. and D. Mochizuki. 1980. Interleukin-2: A class of T cell growth factors. Immunol. Rev. 51: 257.

9. Smith, K. A. 1980. T cell growth factor. Immunol. Rev. 51: 337.

10. Farrar, J. J., P. L. Simon, W. J. Koopman and J. Fuller-Bonar. 1978. Biochemical relationship of thymocyte mitogenic factor a factors enhancing humoral and cell-mediated immune responses. J. Immunol. 121: 1353.

11. Stotter, H., E. Rude and H. Wagner. 1980. T cell factor (Interleukin-2) allows *in vivo* induction of T helper cells against heterologous erythrocytes in athymic (nu/nu) mice. Eur. J. Immunol. 10: 719.

12. Gillis, S and K. A. Smith. 1977. Long-term culture of tumor-specific cytotoxic T cells. Nature 268: 154.

13. Rosenberg, S. A., P. J. Spiess and S. Schwarz. 1978. *In vitro* growth of murine T cells. I. Production of factors necessary for T cell growth. J. Immunol. 121: 1946.

14. Rosenberg, S. A., S. Schwarz and P. J. Spiess. 1978. *In vitro* growth of murine T cells. II. Growth of *in vitro* sensitized cells cytotoxic for alloantigens. J. Immunol. 121: 1951.

15. Ruscetti, F. A., D. A. Morgan and R. C. Gallo. 1977. Functional and morphologic characterization of human T cells continuously grown *in vitro*. J. Immunol. 119: 131.

16. Gillis, S., P. E. Baker, R. W. Ruscetti and K. A. Smith. 1978. Long-term culture of human antigen-specific cytotoxic T cell lines. J. Exp. Med. 148: 1093.

17. Shaw, J., V. Monticone, G. Mills and V. Paetkau. 1978. Effects of costimulator on immune responses *in vitro*. J. Immunol. 120: 1974.

18. Koopman, W. J., J. J. Farrar, J. J. Oppenheim, J. Fuller-Bonar and S. Dougherty. 1977. Association of a low molecular weight helper factor(s) with thymocyte proliferative activity. J. Immunol. 119: 55.

19. Draber, P. and P. Kisielow. 1981. Identification and characterization of immature thymocytes responsive to T cell growth factor. Eur. J. Immunol. 11: 1.

20. Wagner, H. and M. Rollinghoff. 1978. T-T cell interactions during *in vitro* cytotoxic allograft responses. I. Soluble products from activated $Ly1^+$ cells trigger autonomously antigen-primed Ly2, 3^+ T cells to cell proliferation and cytolytic activity. J. Exp. Med. 148: 1523.

21. Wagner, H., C. Hardt, K. Heeg, M. Rollinghoff and K. Pfizenmaier. 1980. T-cell-derived helper factor allows *in vivo* induction of cytotoxic T cells in nu/nu mice. Nature 284: 278.

22. Baker, P. E. and K. A. Smith. 1980. The potential therapeutic utility of T cell growth factor. Fed. Proc. 39: 803.

23. Bonnard, G. D., K. Yasaka and D. Jacobson. 1979. Ligand-activated T cell growth factor-induced proliferation: Absorption of T cell growth factor by activated T cells. J. Immunol. 123: 2704.

24. Beller, D. K. and E. R. Unanue. 1979. Evidence that thymocytes require at least two distinct signals to proliferate. J. Immunol. 123: 2890.

25. Larsson, E. 1981. Mechanism of T cell activation. II. Antigen- and lectin-dependent acquisition of responsiveness to TCGF is nonmitogenic, active response of resting T cells. J. Immunol. 126: 1323.

26. Larsson, E., A. Coutinho and C. Martinez-A. 1980. A suggested mechanism for lymphocyte activation: Implications on the acquisition of functional reactivities. Immunol. Rev. 51: 61.

27. Smith, K. A., S. Gillis, F. W. Ruscetti, P. E. Baker and D. McKenzie. 1979. T cell growth factor: the second signal in the T cell immune response. N. Y. Acad. Sci. 332.

MURAMYL DIPEPTIDES: PROSPECT FOR CANCER TREATMENTS AND IMMUNO-STIMULATION

Shozo Kotani[1], Ichiro Azuma[2], Haruhiko Takada[1], Masachika Tsujimoto[1], and Yuichi Yamamura[3]

Department of Microbiology[1], Osaka University Dental School, Kita-ku, Osaka 530; Institute of Immunological Science[2], Hokkaido University, Kita-15, Nishi-7, Kita-ku Sapporo 060; Osaka University[3], Yamadagami, Suita 565 Japan

INTRODUCTION

It has been well established that bacterial cell walls, especially their peptidoglycan portions, exhibit a number of biological activities capable of modulating host defense mechanisms in various ways. Table 1 summarizes the activities detected by in vivo assays. The in vivo activities include the modulation (mainly potentiation) of antibody- and cell-mediated immune responses and the stimulation of reticuloendothelial system. These activities possibly relate to the other effects such as antigen-specific and nonspecific enhancement of host resistance to microbial infections and tumor development, and the induction of autoimmune diseases such as an experimental allergic encephalomyelitis with encephalitogenic antigens and "adjuvant" arthritis with or without foreign antigens. Other reported activities are concerned with the induction of a transient leukopenia, the following leukocytosis and the lasting monocytosis, the pyrogenicity, the induction of acute inflammatory reaction, epitheloid granulomas and recurrent multinodular lesions, the provocation of necrotic inflammation at the site prepared with tubercle bacilli, a transient decrease and the following increase of serum complement component levels, the promotion and inhibition of sleep, and others.

The immunopharmacological activities shown by in vitro assays are presented in Table 2. Corresponding to the in vivo immunomodulating activities described above, cell walls and their peptidoglycan portions are shown to stimulate macrophages/monocytes,

Table 1. Biological activities of bacterial cell walls and muramyl peptides (in vivo)[a]

I. Modulation of immune responses.

A. Potentiation of antibody-mediated immune responses (1-4, 208) including an increase in serum IgG (guinea pigs) (2, 5), IgG_1 (mice) (6, 7) and IgE (mice) (8, 9) levels, and activation of helper T cells (10-12).

B. Potentiation of cell-mediated immune responses (1-4, 13, 208) and induction of cytotoxic effector T cells (14-19).

C. Inhibition of antibody-mediated immune responses (20-22) including suppression of the IgE response (23), and induction of suppressor T cells (24).

D. Modulation of vaccination (25-37, 56, 197) including induction of transplantation tolerance (38), and preparation of totally synthetic vaccines (35-37, 56).

II. Stimulation of reticuloendothelial system (39-42).

III. Induction of transient leukopenia and subsequent leukocytosis (43, 44), monocytosis (44, 45), and stimulation of proliferation of bone-marrow progenitor cells (44).

IV. Increase of interferon production (46, 47).

V. Increase of natural resistance against microbial infections (49-67, 116, 206, 209, 210) and tumor development (16-18, 68-76) including the induction of activated macrophages (19, 76-78) and natural killer cells (79).

VI. Induction of experimental allergic encephalomyelitis with exogenous antigens (80-84) and adjuvant polyarthiritis with or without exogenous antigens (85, 91).

VII. Pyrogenicity (15, 16, 43, 52, 55, 56, 92-95, 188, 197).

VIII. Promotion (96) or inhibition (94) of sleep.

IX. Induction of acute inflammatory reaction (97), epitheloid granuloma (64, 89, 98-100), recurrent multinodular lesions (97, 182) and increased vascular permeability (101).

(con't)

Table 1 continued

X. Provocation of necrotic inflammation at the site prepared with tubercle bacilli (102, 206).

XI. Increase and suppression of complement levels in serum (103, 104).

XII. Immunogenicity (105-107) and the induction of delayed-type hypersensitivity-like skin reaction (109), and lung granuloma (110, 111).

XIII. Acute and chronic toxicity (112) involving the degradation and excretion (113-117).

---

[a] As a rule, the literature cited is limited to articles using synthetic muramyl peptides except in cases where given activities have not been detected with synthetic compounds. References are only representative.

B and T lymphocytes, natural killer cells, neutrophils, basophils and mast cells, in a word, many cells playing important roles in natural and acquired host-defense mechanisms. Furthermore, cell walls exert stimulating or injurious effects on thrombocytes, fibroblasts, osteoclasts, and other cells. They also activate the complement system via the alternative (and classical) pathways, cause the contraction (or relaxation) of ileal strips, and induce the gelation of an amoebocyte lysate of the horse-shoe crab.

Some of the activities listed above may be beneficial to the host, while others are more detrimental, though it is indeed not easy to make a clear distinction between beneficial and detrimental effects. It may be added here that there is little definite information on the primary target cells or mechanisms bringing about these extremely versatile immunomodulating activities.

The minimum effective structure responsible for the majority of the immunomodulating activities listed in Tables 1 and 2 has been shown to be _N_-acetylmuramyl-_L_-alanyl-_D_-isoglutamine (MDP), a key structure common to peptidoglycans of essentially all bacterial species parasitic to mammals. It should be pointed out, however, that some biological activities distinctly exhibited by the cell walls and peptidoglycans are not manifested, at least in terms of comparable efficiency, by synthetic MDP. On the other hand, it is becoming apparent that by appropriate chemical modifications of MDP, some activities of the molecule can be increased and the others can be abolished or significantly decreased.

Table 2. Biological activities of bacterial cell walls and muramyl peptides (in vitro)[a]

I. Modulation of cells involved in natural and acquired immunity.

A. Monocyte and macrophage functions including chemotactic activity (118, 119), stimulation of differentiation (140, 141), inhibition of DNA synthesis (125), enhancement of adherence and spreading on surfaces (120-122), inhibition of migration (142-145), increase of glucosamine uptake (123, 124), stimulation of lysosomal enzyme release (126), increase of ornithine decarboxylase levels (127), increase of superoxide release (122, 128), increase of glucose oxidation (124), stimulation (129-131) or inhibition (132) of phagocytosis, increase of candidacidal activity (59, 133), induction of cytotoxicity or cytostasis of tumor cells (19, 134-138, 148) or fibroblasts (139), production of collagenase (146), enhancement of proliferation of dengue virus (155), stimulation of monokine production such as endogenous pyrogen (52, 93), fibroblast proliferating factor (146, 153), chemoattractant for fibroblasts (150), plasminogen activator (151,152), lymphocyte activating factor (147, 154), thymocyte mitogenic protein (148), T cell activating factor (149) and colony-stimulating factor (183).

B. B lymphocyte functions including mitogenesis (156-162), polyclonal activation (163-169) and inhibition of mitogen-induced polyclonal activation (170), enhancement (163-166, 168, 171, 172) or inhibition (22, 172) of antigen-specific antibody formation and helper T cell replacing activity (166, 173).

C. T lymphocyte functions including mitogenesis (160, 174-177), stimulation of differentiation (178), enhancement of helper function (171), induction of cytotoxic effector cells (19, 156) and stimulation of mixed lymphocyte reaction (19).

D. Natural killer cell stimulation (79).

E. Neutrophil functions including stimulation (179) or inhibition (180, 181) of phagocytosis, inhibition of chemotaxis (181, 182), stimulation of release of leukocyte pyrogen (52, 93).

F. Basophil increase of histidine uptake (184).

G. Enhancement of mast cell histamine release (185).

Table 2 continued

H. Enhancement of cell viability (120, 165).

II. Modulation of cells other than those listed in item I.

A. Thrombocyte lysis and serotonin release (186-189).

B. Fibroblast stimulation and proliferation (146).

C. Osteoclast stimulation and bone resorption (190).

C. Kidney cell inhibition of proliferation (180).

III. Activation of complement system through alternative (and classical) pathway (191-197).

IV. Gelation of amoebocyte lysate of horse-shoe crab (92).

V. Contraction (or relaxation) of ileal strips (198).

VI. Binding with cytoplasmic membranes of mammalian cells and stabilization of artificial cell membranes (199).

VII. Antigenicity in vitro (105, 108).

VIII. Degradation in vitro (115).

---

[a] As a rule, the literature cited is limited to articles using synthetic muramyl peptides except in cases where given activities have not been detected with synthetic compounds.

ATTEMPTS TO UTILIZE IMMUNOSTIMULATING ACTIVITIES OF MURAMYL PEPTIDES AND THEIR ANALOGUES FOR ANTITUMOR IMMUNOTHERAPY.

The immunostimulating activities of bacterial cell walls, and especially of muramyl peptides synthesized as a part of the peptidoglycan, are attracting the attention of many research workers with the object of making use of the activities in clinical and preventive medicine. One of the most fascinating possibilities is for coping with human malignant tumors.

There seems to be three possible approaches for this purpose. The first approach is the nonspecific enhancement of natural host defense mechanisms against tumor cells by the induction of cytotoxic or cytostatic effector T cells, natural killers or activated macrophages. The second approach is the increase of nonspecific resistance to microbial infections, stubbornly resistant to antimicrobial chemotherapy alone, which are frequently encountered in the advance stage of tumor patients whose defense mechanisms were unfavorably affected by tumor. The third approach is the stimulation of specific immune responses, either humoral or cell-mediated, against tumor-specific or tumor-associated antigens if they were available.

As delivered by Yamamura in the keynote address of this Symposium, purified cell wall preparations (CWS) of *Mycobacterium bovis* (BCG) and *Nocardia rubra* were shown to exhibit a limited, but definite antitumor activity in animal tumor model systems and human tumor patients. It is important to investigate whether or not the antitumor activity of BCG-CWS and *Nocarida*-CWS can be reproduced by MDP or related synthetic compounds, with the aim to find out chemically well-defined compounds which are both superior to CWS and without side effects.

The first study on the antitumor activity of MDP was made by Juy and Chedid in 1975 (134). They demonstrated by in vitro assay that MDP activated murine peritoneal macrophages of F_1 hybrid mice (DBA/2 X C57BL) inhibited the growth of mastocytoma cells derived from DBA/2 mice. However, the peritonal macrophages from the F_1 mice previously injected intraperitoneally with MDP did not show any cytostatic activity against mastocytoma cells. On the other hand, in similar studies wherein mice received either water-soluble adjuvants extracted from *Mycobacterium smegmatis* cell wall or interphase materials prepared from the whole cells, the macrophages showed a definite activity.

Subsequent studies have failed to demonstrate a significant antitumor activity of MDP in transplantable, synergistic or autochthonous animal tumor model systems until a recent study of Fidler and his colleagues. They have shown that MDP encapsulated in multilamellar liposomes activates rat alveolar macrophages to exhibit cytocidal effects against syngeneic as well as xenogeneic or allogeneic tumor cells (137). Based on this finding, they proceeded to examine the antitumor effects of liposome-encapsulated MDP against spontaneous B16 - BL-6 melanoma metastases in C57BL/6 mice, and demonstrated that liposome-encapsulated MDP effectively reduced the incidence of metastases, especially of those of lungs (76). They have further shown in a succeeding study (77), using three lines of T cell deficient mice, that the antitumor activity induced by liposome-MDP is dependent upon macrophage activation by thymus-independent mechanisms. The finding of Fidler's group indicates the importance of vehicles for the administration of MDP in tumor immunotherapy.

McLaughlin and his coworkers (74), on the other hand, reported that combined intratumor injection of some analogues of MDP, namely, N-acetylmuramyl-L-seryl-D-isoglutamine and N-acetyldes-methylmuramyl-L-valyl- (or L-alanyl-) D-isoglutamine with trehalose dimycolate in mineral oil-in-water emulsion caused a significant regression of primary and metastic line 10 hepatocellular carcinomata in strain 2 guinea pigs. They also showed that acylated compounds such as N-acetyldesmethyl-L-α-aminobutyryl-D-isoglutamine were more active than parent compounds. No curative effects were observed in tumor-bearing animals treated with the muramyl peptides described above in the absence of trehalose dimycolate. At almost the same time, Yarkoni, Lederer and Rapp (75) reported synergistic antitumor effects of the combined use of muramyl peptides and trehalose dimycolate. They further showed that mineral oil and squalane served as an effective vehicle for intralesional injection, but neither squalene nor hexadecane did. This finding again indicates the importance of selection of appropriate vehicles for administration of MDP related compounds in tumor immunotherapy.

6-O-MYCOLOYL-MURAMYL DIPEPTIDES AND QUINONYL-MDP-66 AS USEFUL ANTITUMOR MDP ANALOGUES

Along a different line of approach from that described above research groups of Azuma and Yamamura have carried out extensive studies on the antitumor activity of a variety of lipophilic derivatives of muramyl dipeptides. The first study was made on 6-O-mycoloyl-muramyl dipeptides (200-201). Test compounds were prepared by introduction of either natural mycolic acids extracted from mycobacteria and nocardia or mycolic acid-like synthetic fatty acids into 6-O-position of the muramic acid residue by ester linkage. These 6-O-mycoloyl MDP analogues showed the potent adjuvant activity in the induction of allogeneic cell-mediated cytotoxicity in vivo and the antitumor activity in transplantable tumor systems in mice and guinea pigs, under the assay conditions where MDP and its non-lipophilic analogues were ineffective (14-16, 68-72). Among test 6-O-acyl-MDPs, 6-O-(3-hydroxy-2-tetradecyloctadecanoyl)- and 6-O-(3-hydroxy-2-docosylhexacosanoyl)-N-acetylmuramyl-L-valyl-D-isoglutamines were shown to have a limited, but significant, regressive activity on line 10 hepatoma in strain 2 guinea pigs when administrated intralesionally with squalene.

Studies have been continued to pursue MDP derivatives having stronger antitumor activity than 6-O-mycoloyl-MDP. After all, Azuma and his colleagues (17, 18) have chosen quinonyl-MDP-66 (Figure 1) as a provisional leading compound which might be worthy of human trial. This new compound, a benzoquinonyl derivative of N-acetyl-muramyl-L-valyl-D-isoglutamine methyl ester, was synthesized in consideration of the fact that ubiquinone and related compounds had manifold biological activities such as the activation of reticulo-endothelial system, the enhancement of humoral immune responses and so on (202-204).

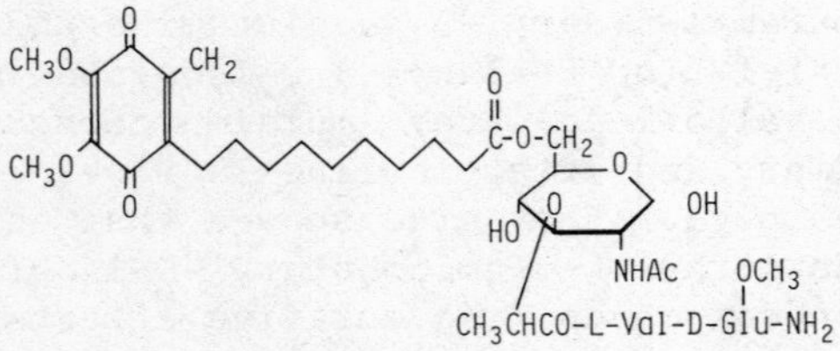

Fig. 1. Chemical structure of quinonyl-MDP-66, methyl 2-(acetamido-2-deoxy-6-O-[10-(2,3-dimethoxy-5-methyl-1,4-benzoquinon-6-yl)-decanoyl]-D-glucopyranos-3-O-yl)-D-propionyl-L-valyl-D-isoglutaminate.

The results of comparison of the antitumor activity of quinonyl-MDP-66 with that of 6-O-mycoloyl (natural or synthetic)-MDP are summarized in Table 3. Quinonyl-MDP-66 has been proved to be more effective than 6-O-mycoloyl-MDP forms in both the regression of the original tumor and the suppression of lymph node metastases under the assay conditions described in the legend.

The immunoadjuvant activity of quinonyl-MDP-66 and parent compounds was examined in guinea pigs and mice. As shown in Table 4, all four test compounds were equally active for the development of delayed-type hypersensitivity to ABA-N-acetyl-L-tyrosine in guinea pigs. Quinonyl-MDP-66 (compound D) was shown to be active as an adjuvant on the induction of cytotoxic effector T cells in allogeneic mice by Brunner's method (205), while its demethyl derivative (C), N-acetylmuramyl-L-valyl-D-isoglutamine (A) and its methyl ester (B) were found inactive. Regarding the suppressive activity against Meth-A sarcoma growth in synergistic BALB/c mice, quinonyl-MDP-66 was the sole effective compound, that is, the development of systemic tumor immunity in the mice, whose tumor growth was suppressed by the intralesional injection of quinonyl-MDP-66, was demonstrated by re-inoculation of Meth-A cells (10^5). The results described above suggest that both benzoquinonyl group and methyl ester play roles in the manifestation of antitumor activity and the induction of allogeneic cell-mediated cytotoxicity by quinonyl-MDP-66 molecule.

The antitumor activity of quinonyl-MDP-66 was further studied with the line 10 hepatoma in strain 2 guinea pigs (Table 5). Tumor cells (10^6) were inoculated intradermally into the guinea pigs, and 10% squalene-treated quinonyl-MDP-66 (400 or 100 μg) as well as 400 of 10% squalene-treated quinonyl-MDP-66) (100 μg as well as 400 μg per animal) completely regressed the tumor growth and prevented the metastases to the lymph nodes. Twice injection of 400 μg was partially effective.

The effect of quinonyl-MDP-66 to induce cell-mediated cyto-

Table 3. Comparison of antitumor activity against line 10 hepatoma in strain 2 guinea pigs of quinonyl-MDP-66 and 6-O-mycoloyl-MDPs[a]

Test Material[b]	Tumor-free / Treated	Metastases in regional lymph node
6-O-QS-10-MurNAc-L-Val-D-Glu(OCH)-NH (Quinonyl-MDP-66)	4/7	2/7
6-O-Nocardomycoloyl-MurNAc-L-Ser-D-isoGln	1/7	6/7
6-O-BH32-MurNAc-L-Ser-D-isoGln	2/7	5/7
6-O-BH48-MurNAc-L-Ser-D-isoGln	3/6	3/6
6-O-BH32-MurNAc-L-Val-D-isoGln	2/6	4/6
6-O-BH48-MurNAc-L-Val-D-isoGln	1/6	5/6
Control (10% Squalene)	0/6	6/6

[a] A group of 6 to 7 strain 2 guinea pigs were inoculated intradermally with line 10 hepatoma cells (10^6). 10% Squalene-treated adjuvant (400 μg each) or 10% Squalene alone was injected intralesionally on days 2 and 5.

[b] BH means α-branched and β-hydroxylated fatty acid and the figure means total number of carbon atoms in fatty acid. Therefore BH32- and BH48- mean 3-hydroxy-2-tetradecyloctadecanoyl- and 3-hydroxy-2-docosylhexacosanoyl-, respectively.

toxicity in tumor-bearing mice was recently examined (unpublished study). As shown in Table 6, the cell-mediated cytotoxic activity of the spleen cells obtained from 3LL-bearing mice on allogeneic P815 tumor was markedly decreased by tumor bearing, and this impaired cell-mediated cytotoxic activity could be restored to a normal level, when the mice were treated by intraperitoneal, intravenous or intralesional injection of a suspension of quinonyl-MDP-66 in phosphate buffered saline.

ENHANCEMENT OF HOST RESISTANCE TO EXPERIMENTAL MICROBIAL INFECTIONS WITH LIPOPHILIC DERIVATIVES OF MURAMYL PEPTIDES

Chedid's group took the initiative in this field (48-56, 66,

Table 4. Adjuvant and antitumor activities of MurNAc-L-Val-D-isoGln derivatives

Test material	Dose (μg)	Delayed-type hypersensitivity[a]: Skin reaction with ABA-BαA at 24 h (mm)	Cytotoxicity[b]: Specific target cell lysis (%) (25 h)	Suppression of Meth-A growth in BALB/C mice[c]
(A) MurNAc-L-Val-D-Glu(OH)-NH_2	100	23.6	ND	0/10
(B) MurNAc-L-Val-D-Glu(OCH_3)-NH_2	100	24.1	ND	0/10
(C) QS-10-MurNAc-L-Val-D-Glu(OH)-NH_2	100	21.9	24.9	0/10
(D) QS-10-MurNAC-L-Val-D-Glu(OCH_3)-NH_2 (quinonyl-MDP-66)	100	24.4	84.2	8/10
Control		0	26.9	0/10

[a] Five Hartley guinea pigs immunized in four footpads with 50 μg of ABA-N-acetyl-L-tyrosine with synthetic adjuvant in Freund's incomplete adjuvant. Control group was immunized with ABA-N-acetyl-L-tyrosine alone in Freund's incomplete adjuvant. Skin tests were carried out after 2 weeks with 100 μg of ABA-bacterial α-amylase (ABA-BαA) and skin reactions were measured 24 hr after intradermal injection of the test antigens.

[b] Four C57BL/6J mice in each group were immunized intraperitoneally with a mixture of mastocytoma P815-X2 (1×10^4) cells and synthetic adjuvant suspended in phosphate-buffered saline. After 11 days, cell mediated cytotoxicity was determined by the incubation of spleen cells (1×10^7) and [^{51}Cr]-labeled mastocytoma P815-X2 cells (1×10^5) for 20 h. Control group was immunized with mastocytoma P815-X2 cells alone.

[c] A mixture of tumor cells (Meth-A, 1×10^5) and 100 μg of synthetic adjuvant suspended in phosphate-buffered saline was inoculated intradermally in BALB/c female mice. Results 4 weeks after inoculation. Values give No. of tumor-free mice/No. of mice tested.

Table 5. Regression of line 10 hepatoma by repeated intralesional injections of quinonyl-MDP-66 in strain 2 guinea pigs[a]

Dose (μg)	Injection (on day)	Tumor-free/treated (on day 60)
400 x 4	2, 5, 8, 15	7/7
100 x 4	2, 5, 8, 15	7/7
400 x 2	2, 5	4/7
None x 4	2, 5, 8, 15	1/7
None x 2	2, 5	0/10

[a] Groups of 7 to 10 strain 2 guinea pigs were inoculated intradermally with line 10 hepatoma cells (10^6), and injected intralesionally with 10% Squalene-treated quinonyl-MDP-66 (test groups) or 10% Squalene alone (control groups).

116), and accomplished very productive achievements. The recent studies (61-63, 206) of Japanese colleagues Ogawa, Matsumoto and their coworkers are briefly summarized here. In the study shown in Table 7, male 5-week-old STD:ddY mice were subcutaneously injected with 0.2 μmole, namely a dose equivalent to 100 μg of MDP, of 6-O-linear, α-branched or α-branched and β-hydroxylated fatty acid derivatives of MDP. Twenty-four hours later, the treated mice and non-treated control animals were challenged by subcutaneous injection of 1×10^7 or 5×10^6 cells of a highly virulent E77156(06) strain of *Escherichia coli*. Lipophilic derivatives of MDP having linear fatty acids of 16 to 20 total carbon atoms, namely L16- to L20-MDP, protected mice more effectively than MDP against the sepsis type of *E. coli* infection. On the contrary, substitution of C6 hydroxy group on the muramic acid residue with either α-branched or α-branched and β-hydroxylated higher fatty acid group resulted in marked decrease or disappearance of the antiinfectious activity of the MDP molecule. No data are available on the nonspecific antiinfectious activity of quinonyl-MDP-66 in this experimental system for the present moment.

Table 8 shows the results of a similar study done with lipophilic MDP derivatives having substituted groups at the γ-carboxyl position of D-isoglutamine residue of MDP: namely 1) γ-alkyl amides, 2) γ-esters and 3) γ-(N^{α}-MDP-N^{α}-acyllysyl) derivatives. The results obtained by this and other (206, 209, 210) experiments led us to a tentative conclusion that γ-(N^{α}-MDP-N^{α}-stearoyl lysyl) derivative of MDP, MDP-Lys(L18) (Figure 2) is a compound of choice.

Table 6. Effect of quinonyl-MDP-66 on depressed cell-mediated cytotoxicity and pulmonary metastases in 3LL-bearing mice

Group	C57BL/6 mice inoculated with	Treatment with quinonyl-MDP-66	Allo-antigen (4×10^5)	Weight (g) of Primary tumor mean ± S.E.	Lysis (%) mean ± S.E.	No. of lung nodules/mouse	
	Day 0	Day 2, 5	Day 7	Day 18		Individual	Median
1	-	-	P815	-	69.3 2.2	-	-
2	3LL	(PBS, *i.p.*)	P815	2.01 ± 0.05	3.1 ± 4.6	29, 34, 40, 61	37
3	3LL	400 μg x 2, *i.p.*	P815	1.65 ± 0.34	67.0 ± 1.5	32, 33, 33, 37, 52	33
4	3LL	400 μg x 2, *i.v.*	P815	1.73 ± 0.22	53.2 ± 6.3	17, 37, 51, 58, 100	51
5	3LL	400 μg x 2, *i.t.*	P815	1.89 ± 0.36	61.1 ± 2.7	9, 21, 31, 42, 70	31

Table 7. Stimulation of nonspecific resistance to *Escherichia coli* infection induced by 6-*O*-acyl muramyl dipeptides in mice[a]

Test material[b]	Protective activity with: 5 x 10^6 cells[c]	1 x 10^7 cells[d]
MDP	+[e]	+[e]
MDP(L-Val)	+[e]	±[f]
MDP (L-Ser)	+[e]	–
S. mycol-MDP	–[g]	–
S. mycol-MDP(L-Ser)	–	–
N. mycol-MDP(L-Ser)	–	–
B30-MDP	–	–
BH32-MDP	–	–
B46-MDP	–	–
BH48-MDP	–	–
Iso.15-MDP	++[e]	++[e]
L2-MDP	+[e]	+[e]
L4-MDP	+[e]	+[e]
L8-MDP	+[e]	+[e]
L10-MDP	+[e]	+[e]
L12-MDP	+[e]	+[e]
L14-MDP	+[e]	+[e]
L16-MDP	++[e]	++[e]
L17-MDP	++[e]	++[e]
L18-MDP	++[e]	++[e]
L19-MDP	++[e]	++[e]
L20-MDP	++[e]	++[e]
L24-MDP	++[e]	+[e]
L30-MDP	+[e]	+[e]
L18-MDP(L-Val)	++[e]	++[e]
L18-MDP(L-Ser)	++[e]	++[e]
L18-MDP(L-isoGln)	–	–
α-Bzl-MDP	–	–

Table 7 continued

α-Bzl-Iso.15-MDP	+[e]	±[e]
α-Bzl-MDP-OBzl	–	–
α-Bzl-MDP(L-Val)-OBzl	–	–
α-Bzl-MDP(L-Ser-Bzl)-OBzl	–	–
Isopentadecanoic acid	–	–
Stearic acid	–	–
N-acetyl muramic acid	–	–

[a] Groups of more than 20 outbred STD:ddY mice (5 week old, male) were subcutaneously injected with a test material at a dose of 0.2 μmol/ mouse (equivalent to 100 μg of MDP) 24 h before infection with *Escherichia coli* E77156(06).

[b] MDP, MurNAc-L-Ala-D-isoGln; MDP(L-Val), MurNAc-L-Val-D-isoGln; MDP(L-Ser), MurNAc-L-Ser-D-isoGln; MDP(L-isoGln), MurNAc-L-Ala-L-isoGln); S.mycol, mycolic acid from *Mycobacterium smegmatis*; N.mycol, mycolic acid from *Nocardia rubra*; B, BH, L and figures α-branched, α-branched and β-hydroxyl, lineal fatty acids, and a total carbon number in fatty acid, respectively; Iso.15, Iso-pentadecanoic acid; α-Bzl-MDP, 1-α-O-bezyl-MDP; α-Bzl-MDP(L-Ser-Bzl)-OBzl, 1-α-O-bezyl-MurNAc-O-benzyl-L-Ser-D-isoGln-benzyl-ester.

[c] Percent survival 7 days after infection with 5 x 10^6 *E. coli* cells per mouse: –, <30%; ±, 31 to 45%; +, 46 to 75%; ++, >75%.

[d] Percent survival 7 days after infection with 1 x 10^7 *E. coli* cells per mouse; –, <10%; ±, 11 to 20%; +, 21 to 44%; ++. >45%.

[e, f, g] Significantly different from control as determined by the adjusted Chi-square method: e P <0.001, f P <0.01, and g P <0.05.

Quoted from the report (62) by K. Matsumoto et al. and partially modified.

Table 8. Stimulation of nonspecific resistance to *Escherichia coli* infection induced by MDP derivatives[a]

Test material[b]	Protective activity	
	5×10^{6} [c]	1×10^{7} [d]
MDP	+	+
MDP(L-Val)	+	+
MDP(L-Ser)	+	−
MurNAc-L-Ala-D-Glu[NH$(CH_2)_7CH_3$]-NH_2	−	−
MurNAc-L-Ala-D-Glu[NH$(CH_2)_{11}CH_3$]-NH_2	−	−
MurNAc-L-Ala-D-Glu[NH$(CH_2)_{17}CH_3$]-NH_2	−	−
MurNAc-L-Ala-D-Glu(OCH_3)-NH_2	±	−
MurNAc-L-Ala-D-Glu[O$(CH_2)_7CH_3$]-NH_2	+	+
MurNAc-L-Ala-D-Glu[O$(CH_2)_{17}CH_3$]-NH_2	+	+
L18-MurNAc-L-Ala-D-Glu(OCH_3)-NH_2	++	+
L18-MurNAc-L-Ala-D-Glu[O$(CH_2)_7CH_3$]-NH_2	±	−
L18-MurNAc-L-Ala-D-Glu[O$(CH_2)_{17}CH_3$]-NH_2	±	−
MurNAc-L-Ala-D-Glu(L-Lys-OH)-NH_2	+	+
MDP-Lys(L8)[e]	+	+
MDP-Lys(L12)[e]	++	++
MDP-Lys(L18)[e]	++	++
MDP-Lys(L30)[e]	+	+
MDP(L-Val)-Lys(L18)[e]	++	+
MDP(L-Ser)-Lys(L18)[e]	++	+
MDP-Lys(Iso.15)[e]	++	++
MurNAc(L-Val)-Lys(N.mycol)[e]	±	±
MurNAc(L-Ser)-Lys(N.mycol)[e]	±	±
MurNAc-L-Ala-D-Glu[L-Lys(CO$(CH_2)_{17}CH_3$)-OCH_3]-NH_2	++	+
MurNAc-L-Val-D-Glu[L-Lys(CO$(CH_2)_{17}CH_3$)-NH$(CH_2)_{17}CH_3$]-NH_2	±	±

[a-d] Same as the footnotes in Table 7.

[e] γ-(N^{α}-MDP-N^{α}-actyllysyl) derivatives of MDP (See Figure 2). Quoted from the report (209) by Matsumoto et al. and partially modified.

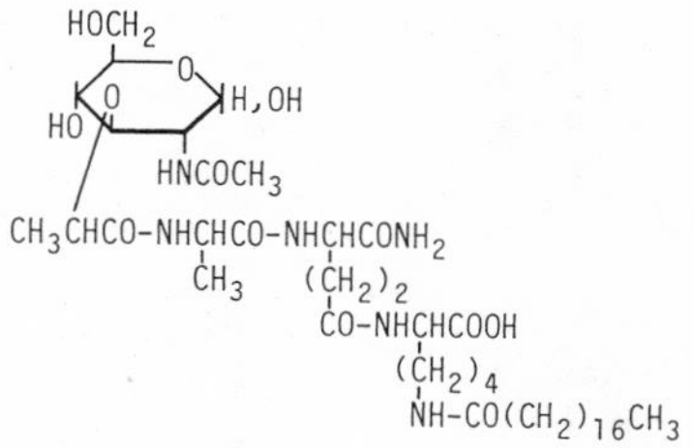

HOCH$_2$
O
O H,OH
HO
HNCOCH$_3$
CH$_3$CHCO-NHCHCO-NHCHCONH$_2$
CH$_3$ (CH$_2$)$_2$
CO-NHCHCOOH
(CH$_2$)$_4$
NH-CO(CH$_2$)$_{16}$CH$_3$

Fig. 2. Chemical structure of N^{α}-(N-acetylmuramyl-L-alanyl-D-isoglutamine)-N^{ε}-stearoyl-L-Lys, MDP-Lys(L18).

The antiinfectious activity of MDP-Lys(L18) in mice immunocompromised by cyclophosphamide pretreatment was studied as presented in Figure 3. The reduced resistance against *E. coli* infection of STD:ddY mice which had received intraperitoneal injection of cyclophosphamide was restored to the normal resistance level by subcutaneous injection of MDP-Lys(L18) 22 h prior to the infection.

ATTEMPTS TO INCREASE TUMOR-SPECIFIC IMMUNITY BY MURAMYL PEPTIDES

This approach has so far failed to obtain successful results. The failure seems to be mainly due to the fact that the very poor immunogenicity of syngeneic and autochtonous tumor cells makes it difficult to utilize the antigen-specific immunopotentiating activity of MDP and its derivatives.

In this respect, a recent study of Binz, Dukor and their colleagues(38) to increase the immunogenicity of MLC T-lymphoblasts by covalently coupling of muramyl peptides to their membranes is noteworthy. Their results suggest that there might be a good possibility to increase the tumor-specific immune responses by use of membrane constituents of tumor cells modified by suitable treatments and then coupled with appropriate MDP analogues or derivatives.

If there would be no need for covalent coupling, 6-O-(2-tetradecylhexadacanoyl)-MDP, B30-MDP, is provisionally the most favorable candidate for human trials to potentiate tumor-specific or tumor-associated immune responses. This is because of the low effective dose, the high extent of specific immunopotentiation, the limited accompanying detrimental side effects, and the adaptability to a wide range of vehicles for administration (197, 207) associated with this compound. Although so far we have no data on specific or systemic stimulation of antitumor immunity by B30-MDP, the proved usefulness of this compound for the enhancement of the potency of highly purified influenza HA-NA (hemagglutinin and neuraminidase) vaccine (206) and the enhanced potency of the *Plasmodium falciparum* vaccine prepared from a long-term culture of the parasite (206), suggests that B30-MDP might be effective in the augmentation of

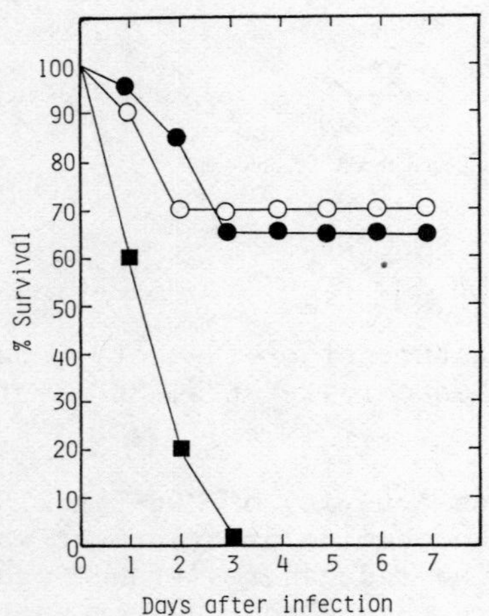

Fig. 3. Effect of MDP-Lys-(L18) on resistance of mice immunocompromised by cyclophosphamide treatment to infection with <u>Escerichia coli</u> E77156. Two groups of 20 ddY male mice were treated intraperitoneally with 100 mg/kg of cyclophosphamide. One group (●) was treated subcutaneously 24 h later with 1.5 x 10^6 cells/mouse (1/4 MLD for a normal, untreated mouse) and MDP-Lys(L18) 22 h prior to infection. The other immunocompromised group (■) receiving no MDP-Lys(L18) treatment was similarly infected. A group of 20 mice not treated with either cyclophosphamide or MDP-Lys(L18) was submitted to the similar infection (○).

specific antitumor immune responses, especially if poor immunogenicity of tumor cells could be raised by sophisticated methods.

DISCUSSION (PROSPECT)

Available evidence suggests that the use of derivatives or analogues of muramyl peptides for antitumor immunotherapy may be promising. But the fruits harvested to date do not seem to be satisfactory. For example, the results obtained with quinonyl-MDP-66 have been favorable. However, we must point out that although quinonyl-MDP-66 has significant antitumor activity by intralesional injection, it is hardly effective by other administration routes, indicating that this compound is not fully effective in the potentiation of systemic antitumor immune mechanisms. Much remains to be studied, particularly in the restoration and enhancement of specific antitumor host immune mechanisms by combined use of appropriate derivatives of muramyl peptides and suitable methods to increase the immunogenicity of tumor antigens. The prerequisite for this approach should be the decrease of tumor loading by surgery and other means.

We must realize that biological response modifiers such as muramyl peptides which mainly exert their biological effects through modulation of host defense mechanisms, either natural or acquired, may primarily act as a double-edged sword. Over-stimulation of defense mechanisms sometimes brings about more deleterious than beneficial effects in the host. So, we must be cautious about the possible occurrence of adverse side effects in clinical applications of MDP-related compounds, especially in the case where repeated injections of larger dosage are needed.

SUMMARY

The immunopharmacological activities of bacterial cell walls and muramyl peptides were collected in table form with a comprehensive literature. The past and present studies emphasizing the host-defense enhancing activities of muramyl peptides for antitumor immunotherapy were surveyed along three possible approaches: 1) the nonspecific enhancement of natural defense ability of host against tumor cells themselves; 2) the enhancement of nonspecific resistance of host to microbial infections which are frequently encountered and difficult to treat in the advanced stage of tumor patients; and 3) the stimulation of immunity against tumor-specific or tumor-associated immunogens. Finally, the prospects of successful antitumor immunotherapy with muramyl peptides and their derivatives was discussed.

REFERENCES

1. Ellouz, F., A. Adam, R. Ciorbaru, and E. Lederer. 1974. Minimal structural requirements for adjuvant activity of bacterial peptidoglycan derivatives. Biochem. Biophys. Res. Commun. 59: 1317-1325.

2. Kotani, S., Y. Watanabe, F. Kinoshita, T. Shimono, I. Morisaki, T. Shiba, S. Kusumoto, Y. Tarumi, and K. Ikenaka. 1975. Immunoadjuvant activities of synthetic N-acetylmuramyl-peptides or -amino acids. Biken J. 18: 105-111.

3. Azuma, I., K. Sugimura, T. Taniyama, M. Yamawaki, Y. Yamamura, S. Kusumoto, S. Okada, and T. Shiba. 1976. Adjuvant activity of mycobacterial fractions: adjuvant activity of synthetic N-acetylmuramyl-dipeptide and the related compounds. Infect. Immun. 14: 18-27.

4. Tanaka, A., R. Saito, K. Sugimura, I. Morisaki, S. Kotani, S. Kusumoto, and T. Shiba. 1977. Adjuvant activity of synthetic N-acetylmuramyl peptides in rats. Infect. Immun. 15: 131-136.

5. Souvannavong, V., A. Adam, and E. Lederer. 1978. Kinetics of the humoral and cellular immune response of guinea pigs after injection of the synthetic adjuvant N-acetylmuramyl L-alanyl-D-isoglutamine: comparison with Freund complete adjuvant. Infect. Immun. 19: 966-971.

6. Heymer, B., H. Finger, and C.-H. Wirsing. 1978. Immunoadjuvant effects of the synthetic muramyl-dipeptide (MDP) N-acetylmuramyo-L-alanyl-D-isoglutamine. Z. Immunitaetsforsch. 155: 87-92.

7. Leclerc, C., F. Audibert, and L. Chedid. 1978. Influence of a synthetic adjuvant (MDP) on qualitative and quantitative changes of serum globulins. Immunology 35: 963-970.

8. Ohkuni, H., Y. Norose, M. Hayama, Y. Kimura, S. Kotani, T. Shiba, S. Kusumoto, K. Yokogawa, and S. Kawata. 1977. Adjuvant activities in production of reaginic antibody in mice of bacterial cell wall peptidoglycans or peptidoglycan subunits and of synthetic N-acetylmuramyl dipeptides. Biken J. 20: 131-136.

9. Ohkuni, H., Y. Norose, M. Ohta, M. Hayama, Y. Kimura, M. Tsujimoto, S. Kotani, T. Shiba, S. Kusumoto, K. Yokogawa, and S. Kawata. 1979. Adjuvant activities in production of reaginic antibody by bacterial cell wall peptidoglycan or synthetic N-acetylmuramyl-L-alanyl-D-isoglutamine. Infect. Immun. 24: 313-318.

10. Löwy, I., C. Bona, and L. Chedid. 1977. Target cells for the activity of a synthetic adjuvant: muramyl dipeptide. Cell. Immunol. 29: 195-199.

11. Sugimoto, M., R. N. Germain, L. Chedid, and B. Benecerraf. 1978. Enhancement of carrier-specific helper T cell function by the synthetic adjuvant, N-acetyl muramyl-L-alanyl-D-isoglutamine (MDP). J. Immunol. 120: 980-982.

12. Löwy, I., J. Theze, and L. Chedid. 1980. Stimulation of the *in vivo* dinitrophanyl antibody response to the DNP conjugate of L-glutamic acid^{60}-L-ananine^{30}-L-tyrosine^{10} (GAT) polymer by a synthetic adjuvant, muramyl dipeptide (MDP): target cells for adjuvant activity and isotypic pattern of MDP-stimulated response. J. Immunol. 124: 100-104.

13. Masek, K., M. Zaoral, J. Jezek, and R. Straka. 1978. Immunoadjuvant activity of synthetic N-acetyl muramyl dipeptide. Experientia 34: 1363-1365.

14. Yamamura, Y., I. Azuma, K. Sugimura, M. Yamawaki, M. Uemiya, S. Okada, S. Okada, T. Shiba, and Y. Yamamura. 1978. Adjuvant activity of 6-O-mycoloyl derivatives of N-acetyl-muramyl-L-alanyl-D-isoglutamine. Gann 67: 867-877.

15. Azuma, I., K. Sugimura, M. Yamawaki, M. Uemiya, S. Kusumoto, S. Okada, S. Okada, T. Shiba, and Y. Yamamura. 1978. Adjuvant activity of synthetic 6-O-"mycoloyl"-N-acetylmuramyl-L-alanyl-D-isoglutamine and related compounds. Infect. Immun. 20: 600-607.

16. Uemiya, M., K. Sugimura, T. Kusama, I. Saiki, M. Yamawaki, I. Azuma, and Y. Yamamura. 1979. Adjuvant activity of 6-O--mycoloyl derivatives of M-acetyl-muramyl-L-alanyl-D-isoglutamine and related compounds in mice and guinea pigs. Infect. Immun. 24: 83-89.

17. Azuma, I., M. Yamawaki, M. Uemiya, I. Saiki, Y. Tanio, S. Kobayashi, T. Fukuda, I. Imada, and Y. Yamamura. 1979. Adjuvant and antitumor activities of quinonyl-N-acetyl muramyl dipeptides. Gann 70: 847-848.

18. Saiki, I., Y. Tanio, M. Yamawaki, M. Uemiya, S. Kobayashi, T. Fukuda, H. Yukimasa, Y. Yamamura, and I. Azuma. 1981. Adjuvant activities of quinonyl-N-acetyl muramyl dipeptides in mice and quinea pigs. Infect. Immun. 31: 114-121.

19. Matter, A. 1979. The effects of muramyldipeptide (MDP) in cell-mediated immunity. A comparison between in vitro and in vivo systems. Cancer Immunol. Immunother. 6: 201-210.

20. Chedid, L., F. Audibert, P. Lefrancier, J. Choay, and E. Lederer. 1976. Modulation of the immune response by a synthetic adjuvant and analogs. Proc. Natl. Acad. Sci. USA 73: 2472-2475.

21. Leclerc, C., D. Juy, E. Bourgeois, and L. Chedid. 1979. In vivo regulation of humoral and cellular immune responses of mice by a synthetic adjuvant, N-acetyl-muramyl-L-alanyl-D-isoglutamine, muramyl dipeptide for MDP. Cell. Immunol. 45: 199-206.

22. Souvannavong, V., and A. Adam. 1980. Opposite effects of the synthetic adjuvant N-acetyl-muramyl-L-alanyl-D-isoglutamine on the immune response in mice depending on experimental conditions. Eur. J. Immunol. 10: 654-656.

23. Kishimoto, T., Y. Hirai, K. Nakanishi, I. Azuma, A. Nagamatsu, and Y. Yamamura. 1979. Regulation of antibody response in different immunoglobulin classes. VI. Selective suppression of IgE response by administration of antigen-conjugated muramylpeptides. J. Immunol. 123: 2709-2715.

24. Leclerc, C., E. Bouregois, and L. Chedid. 1982. Demonstration of muramyl dipeptide (MDP)-induced T suppressor cells responsible for MDP immunosuppressive activity. Eur. J. Immunol. 12: 249-252.

25. Siddiqui, W. A., D. W. Taylor, S. Kan, K. Kramer, S. M. Richmond-Crum, S. Kotani, T. Shiba, and S. Kusumoto. 1978. Vaccination of experimental monkeys against *Plasmodium falciparum*: a possible safe adjuvant. Science 201: 1237-1338.

26. Reese, R. T., W. Trager, J. B. Jensen, D. A. Miller, and R. Tantravehi. 1978. Immunization against malaria with antigen from *Plasmodium falciparum* cultivated *in vitro*. Proc. Natl. Acad. Sci. USA 75: 5665-5668.

27. Mitchell, W. H., G. Richards, A. Voller, F. M. Dietrich, and P. Dukor. 1979. Nor-MDP, saponin, corynebacteria, and pertussis organisms as immunological adjuvants in experimental malaria vaccination of macaques. Bull. W. H. O. 57(Suppl.1): 189-197.

28. Siddiqui, W. A. 1982. Synthetic adjuvants and experimental human malaria vaccine, p. 245-249. *In* Y. Yamamura, S. Kotani, I. Azuma, A. Koda and T. Shiba (eds.), Immunomodulation by microbial products and related synthetic compounds. Excerpta Medica, Amsterdam.

29. Webster, R. G., W. P. Glezen, C. Hannoun, and W. G. Laver. 1977. Potentiation of the immune response to influenza virus subunit vaccines. J. Immunol. 119: 2073-2077.

30. Okunaga, T. 1980. Potentiation of immune responses to influenza split virus vaccine by synthetic 6-*O*-acyl-muramylpeptides. J. Osaka Univ. Dent. Soc. 25: 29-52. (In Japanese with English summary).

31. Woodard, L. F., N. M. Toone, and C. A. McLaughlin. 1980. Immunogenic properties of soluble antigens or whole cells of *Brucella abortus* strain 45/20 associated with immunoadjuvants. I. Soluble antigens. Can. J. Comp. Med. 44: 453-455.

32. Woodard, L. F., N. M. Toone, and C. A. McLaughlin. 1980. Immunogenic properties of soluble antigens or whole cells of *Brucella abortus* strain 45/20 associated with immunoadjuvants. II. Whole cells. Can. J. Comp. Med. 44: 456-458.

33. Woodard, L. F., N. M. Toone, and C. A. McLaughlin. 1980. Comparison of muramyl dipeptide, trehalose dimycolate, and dimethyl dioctadecyl ammonium bromide as adjuvants in *Brucella abortus* 45/20 vaccines. Infect. Immun. 30: 409-412.

34. Langbeheim, H., R. Arnon, and M. Sela. 1978. Adjuvant effect of a peptidoglycan attached covalently to a synthetic antigen provoking anti-phage antibodies. Immunology 35: 573-579.

35. Audibert, F., M. Jolivet, L. Chedid, J. E. Alouf, P. Boquet, P. Rivaille, and O. Siffert. 1981. Active antitoxic immunization by a diphtheria toxin synthetic oligopeptide. Nature 289: 593-594.

36. Audibert, F., and M. Jolivet. 1982. Immunization by a diphtheria toxin olibopeptide and MDP, a model for synthetic vaccines, p. 241-244. *In* Y. Yamamura, S. Kotani, I. Azuma, A. Koda and T. Shiba (eds.), Immunomodulation by microbial products and related synthetic compounds. Excerpta Medica, Amsterdam.

37. Chedid, L., and F. Audibert. 1982. Utilization of muramyl dipeptide derivatives as adjuvants of synthetic vaccines, p. 48-59. *In* Y. Yamamura, S. Kotani, I. Azuma, A. Koda and T. Shiba (eds.), Immunomodulation by microbial products and related synthetic compounds. Excerpta Medica, Amsterdam.

38. Binz, H., L. Tarcsay, H. Wigzell, and P. Dukor. 1981. Specific impaired alloreactivity of mice immunized with synthetic MLC T-lymphoblasts using muramylpeptides as adjuvant. Transplant. Proc. 13: 566-573.

39. Tanaka, A., S. Nagao, R. Saito, S. Kotani, S. Kusumoto, and T. Shiba. 1977. Correlation of sterochemically specific structure in muramyl dipeptide between macrophage activation and adjuvant activity. Biochem. Biophys. Res. Commun. 77: 621-627.

40. Tanaka, A., S. Nagao, R. Saito, S. Kotani, S. Kusumoto, and T. Shiba. 1979. Stimulation of the reticuloendothelial system of mice by muramyl dipeptide. Infect. Immun. 24: 302-307.

41. Waters, R. V., and R. W. Ferraresi. 1980. Muramyl dipeptide stimulation of particle clearance in several animal species. J. Reticuloendothel. Soc. 28: 457-471.

42. Fraser-Smith, E. B., R. V. Waters, and T. R. Matthews. 1982. Correlation between in vivo anti-Pseudomonas and anti-Candida activities and clearance of carbon by the reticuloendothelial system for various muramyl dipeptide analogs, using normal and immunosuppressed mice. Infect. Immun. 35: 105-110.

43. Kotani, S., Y. Watanabe, T. Shimono, K. Harada, T. Shiba, S. Kusumoto, K. Yokogawa, and M. Taniguchi. 1976. Correlation between the immunoadjuvant activities and pyrogenicities of synthetic N-acetylmuramyl-peptides or -amino acids. Biken J. 19: 9-13.

44. Wuest, B., and E. D. Wachsmuth. 1982. Stimulatory effect of N-acetyl muramyl dipeptide in vivo: proliferation of bone marrow progenitor cells in mice. Infect. Immun. 37: 452-462.

45. Kato, K., S. Kotani, K. Kawano, T. Monodane, H. Kitamura, S. Kusumoto, and T. Shiba. 1982. Monocytosis-inducing activity of L. monocytogenes cell wall and muramyl dipeptides, p. 181-184. In Y, Yamamura, S. Kotani, I. Azuma, A. Koda and T. Shiba (eds.), Immunomodulation by microbial products and related synthetic compounds. Excerpta Medica, Amsterdam.

46. Barot-Ciorbaru, R., J. Wietzerbin, J.-F. Petit, L. Chedid, E. Falcoff, and E. Lederer. 1978. Induction of interferon synthesis in mice by fractions from Nocardia. Infect. Immun. 19: 353-356.

47. Barot-Ciorbaru, R., L. Catinot, J. Wietzerbin, J.-F Petit, L. Chedid, and E. Falcoff. 1981. Involvement of a radioresistant cell in the production of circulating interferon induced by Nocardia fractions in mice. J. Reticuloendothel. Soc. 30: 247-257.

48. Chedid, L., M. Parant, F. Parant, P. Lefrancier, J. Choay, and E. Lederer. 1977. Enhancement of nonspecific immunity to Klebsiella pneumoniae infection by a synthetic immunoadjuvant (N-acetylmuramyl-L-alanyl-D-isoglutamine) and several analogs. Proc. Natl. Acad. Sci. USA 74: 2089-2093.

49. Parant, M., F. Parant, and L. Chedid. 1978. Enhancement of the neonate's nonspecific immunity to Klebsiella infection by muramyl dipeptide, a synthetic immunoadjuvant. Proc. Natl. Acad. Sci. USA 75: 3395-3399.

50. Parant, M., C. Damais, F. Audibert, F. Parant, L. Chedid, E. Sache, P. Lefrancier, J. Choay, and E. Lederer. 1978. In vivo and in vitro stimulation of nonspecific immunity by the β-D-p-aminophenyl glycoside of N-acetylmuramyl-L-alanyl-D-isoglutamine and an oligomer prepared by cross-linking with glutaraldehyde. J. Infect. Dis. 138: 378-386.

51. Chedid, L., M. Parant, F. Parant, F. Audibert, F. Lefrancier, J. Choay, and M. Sela. 1979. Enhancement of certain biological activities of muramyl dipeptide derivatives after conjugation to a multi-poly (DL-alanine)--poly-(L-lysine) carrier. Proc. Natl. Acad. Sci. USA 76: 6557-6561.

52. Parant, M., G. Riveau, F. Parant, C. A. Dinarello, S. M. Wolff, and L. Chedid. 1980. Effect of indomethacin on increased resistance to bacterial infection and on febrile responses induced by muramyl dipeptide. J. Infect. Dis. 142: 708-715.

53. Parant, M. A., F. M. Audibert, L. A. Chedid, M. R. Level, P. L. Lefrancier, J. P. Choay, and E. Lederer. 1980. Immunostimulant activities of a lipophilic muramyl dipeptide derivative and of desmuramyl peptidolipid analogs. Infect. Immun. 27: 826-831.

54. Audibert, F., M. Parant, C. Damais, P. Lefrancier, M. Derrien, J. Choay, and L. Chedid. 1980. Dissociation of immunostimulant activities of muramyl dipeptide (MDP) by linking amino-acids or peptides to the glutaminil residue. Biochem. Biophys. Res. Commun. 96: 915-923.

55. Lefrancier, P., M. Derrien, X. Jamet, J. Choay, E. Lederer, F. Audibert, M. Parant, F. Parant, and L. Chedid. Apyrogenic, adjuvant-active N-acetyl-muramyl-dipeptides. J. Med. Chem. 25: 87-90.

56. Chedid, L. A., M. A. Parant, F. M. Audibert, G. J. Riveau, F. J. Parant, E. Lederer, J. P. Choay, and P. L. Lefrancier. 1982. Biological activity of a new synthetic muramyl peptide adjuvant devoid of pyrogenicity. Infect. Immun. 35: 417-424.

57. Finger, H., and C.-H Wirsing von Konig. 1980. Failure of synthetic muramyl dipeptide to increase antibacterial resistance. Infect. Immun. 27: 288-291.

58. Humphres, R. C., P. R. Henika, R. W. Ferraresti, and J. L. Krhenbuhl. 1980. Effects of treatment with muramyl dipeptide and certain of its analogs on resistance to Listeria monocytogenes in mice. Infect. Immun. 30: 462-466.

59. Cummings, N. P., M. J. Pabst, and R. B. Johnston, Jr. 1980. Activation of macrophages for enhanced release of superoxide anion and greater killing of Candida albicans by injection of muramyl dipeptide. J. Exp. Med. 152: 1659-1669.

60. Fraser-Smith, E. B., and T. R. Matthews. 1981. Protective effect of muramyl dipeptide analogs against infections of Pseudomonas aeruginosa or Candida albicans in mice. Infect. Immun. 34: 676-683.

61. Matsumoto, K., H. Ogawa, O. Nagase, T. Kusama, and I. Azuma. 1981. Stimulation of nonspecific host resistance to infection induced by muramyl-dipeptides. Microbiol. Immunol. 24: 1047-1058.

62. Matsumoto, K., H. Ogawa, T. Kusama, O. Nagase, N. Sawaki, M. Inage, S. Kusumoto, T. Shiba, and I. Azuma. 1981. Stimulation of nonspecific resistance to infection induced by 6-O-acyl muramyl dipeptide analogs in mice. Infect. Immun. 32: 746-758.

63. Osada, Y., M. Mitsuyama, T. Une, K. Matsumoto, T. Otani, M. Satoh, H. Ogawa, and K. Nomoto. 1982. Effect of L18-MDP(Ala), a synthetic derivative of muramyl dipeptide, on nonspecific resistance of mice to microbial infections. Infect. Immun. 37: 292-300.

64. Tanaka, A. 1982. Macrophage activation by muramyl dipeptide (MDP), p. 72-83. In Y. Yamamura, S. Kotani, I. Azuma, A. Koda and T. Shiba (eds.), Immunomodulation by microbial products and related synthetic compounds. Excerpta Medica, Amsterdam.

65. Kierszenbaum, and R. W. Ferraresi. 1979. Enhancement of host resistance against Trypanosoma cruzi infection by the immunoregulatory agent muramyl dipeptide. Infect. Immun. 25: 273-278.

66. Olds, G. R., L. Chedid, E. Lederer, and A. A. F. Mahmoud. 1980. Induction of resistance to Schistosoma mansoni by natural cord factor and synthetic lower homologues. J. Infect. Dis. 141: 473-478.

67. Krahenbuhl, J. L., S. D. Sharma, R. W. Ferraresi, and J. S. Remington. 1981. Effects of muramyl dipeptide treatment on resistance to infection with Toxoplasma gondii in mice. Infect. Immun. 31: 716-722.

68. Azuma, I., and Y. Yamamura. 1979. Immunotherapy of cancer with BCG cell-wall skeleton and related materials. Gann Monograph Cancer Res. 24: 121-141.

69. Azuma, I., M. Uemiya, I. Saiki, M. Yamawaki, Y. Tanio, S. Kusumoto, T. Shiba, T. Kusama, K. Tobe, H. Ogawa, and Y. Yamamura. 1979. Synthetic immunoadjuvants--new immunotherapeutic agents. Dev. Immunol. 6: 311-330.

70. Yamamura, Y., K. Yasumoto, T. Ogura, and I. Azuma. 1981. Nocardia rubra-cell wall skeleton in the therapy of animal and human cancer, p. 71-90. In E. M. Hersh, M. A. Chirigos, and M. J. Mastrangelo (eds.), Augmentating agents in cancer immunity. Raven Press, New York.

71. Yamamura, Y., and I. Azuma. 1982. Cancer immunotherapy with cell-wall skeletons of BCG and Nocardia rubra and related synthetic compounds, p. 17-36. In Y. Yamamura, S. Kotani, I. Azuma, A. Koda and T. Shiba (eds.), Immunomodulation by microbial products and related synthetic compounds. Excerpta Medica, Amsterdam.

72. Ribi, E., C. A. McLaughlin, J. L. Cantrell, W. Brehmer, I. Azuma, Y. Yamamura, S. M. Strain, K. M. Hwang, and R. Toubiana. 1978. Immunotherapy for tumors with microbial constituents or their synthetic analogues, p. 131-154. In Staff of the University of Texas System Cancer Center (eds.), Immunotherapy of human cancer. Raven Press, New York.

73. Ribi, E., J. Cantrell, S. Schwartzman, and R. Parker. 1981. BCG cell wall skeleton, P3, MDP and other microbial components-structure activity studies in animal models, p. 15-31. In E. M. Hersh, M. A. Chirigos and M. J. Mastrangelo (eds.), Augmentating agents in cancer therapy. Raven Press, New York.

74. McLaughlin, S. M. Schwartzman, B. L. Horner, G. H. Jones, J. G. Moffatt, J. J. Nestor, Jr., and D. Tedd. 1980. Regression of tumors in guinea pigs after treatment with synthetic muramyl dipeptides and trehalose dimycolate. Science 208: 415-416.

75. Yarkoni, E., E. Lederer, and H. J. Rapp. 1981. Immunotherapy of experimental cancer with a mixture of synthetic muramyl dipeptide and trehalose dimycolate. Infect. Immun. 32: 273-276.

76. Fidler, I. J., S. Sone, W. E. Fogler, and Z. L. Barnes. 1981. Eradication of spontaneous metastases and activation of alveolar macrophages by intravenous injection of liposomes containing muramyl dipeptide. Proc. Natl. Acad. Sci. USA 78: 1680-1684.

77. Fidler, I. J. 1981. The in situ induction of tumoricidal activity in alveolar macrophages by liposomes containing muramyl dipeptide is a thymus-independent process. J. Immunol. 127: 1719-1720.

78. Bruley-Rosset, M., I. Florentin, and G. Mathe. 1981. Macrophage activation by tufsin and muramyl-dipeptide. Mol. Cell. Biochem. 41: 113-118.

79. Sharma, S. D., V. Tsai, J. L. Krahenbuhl, and J. S. Remington. 1981. Augmentation of mouse natural killer cell activity by muramyl dipeptide and its analogs. Cell. Immunol. 62: 101-109.

80. Nagai, Y., K. Akiyama, K. Suzuki, S. Kotani, Y. Watanabe, T. Shimono, T. Shiba, S. Kusumoto, F. Ikuta, and S. Takeda. 1978. Minimum structural requirements for encephalitogen and for adjuvant in the induction of experimental allergic encephalomyelitis. Cell. Immunol. 35: 158-167.

81. Nagai, Y., K. Akiyama, S. Kotani, Y. Watanabe, T. Shimono, T. Shiba, and S. Kusumoto. 1978. Structural specificity of synthetic peptide adjuvant for induction of experimental allergic encephalomyelitis. Cell. Immunol. 35: 168-172.

82. Koga, T., K. Maeda, K. Onoue, K. Kato, and S. Kotani. 1979. Chemical structure required for immunoadjuvant and arthritogenic activities of cell wall peptidoglycans. Mol. Immunol. 16: 153-162.

83. Maeda, K., T. Koga, S. Sakamoto, K. Onoue, S. Kotani, S. Kusumoto, T. Shiba, and A. Sumiyoshi. 1980. Structural requirement of synthetic N-acetyl-muramyl dipeptides for induction of experimental allergic encephalomyelitis in the rat. Microbiol. Immunol. 24: 771-776.

84. Mitsuzawa, E., T. Yasuda, N. Tamura, and S. Ohtani. 1981. Experimental allergic encephalomyelitis induced by basic protein with synthetic adjuvant in comparison with Freund's adjuvant. J. Neurol. Sci. 52: 133-145.

85. Kohashi, O., S. Kotani, T. Shiba, and A. Ozawa. 1979. Synergistic effect of polyriboinosinic acid:polyribocytidylic acid and either bacterial peptidoglycans or synthetic N-acetylmuramyl peptides on production of adjuvant-induced arthritis in rats. Infect. Immun. 26: 690-697.

86. Koga, T., S. Sakamoto, K. Onoue, S. Kotani, and A. Sumiyoshi. 1980. Efficient induction of collagen arthritis by the use of a synthetic muramyl dipeptide. Arthritis Rheumat. 23: 993-997.

87. Nagao, S., and A. Tanaka. 1980. Muramyl dipeptide-induced adjuvant arthritis. Infect. Immun. 28: 624-626.

88. Kohashi, O., A. Tanaka, S. Kotani, T. Shiba, S. Kusumoto, K. Yokogawa, S. Kawata, and A. Ozawa. 1980. Arthritis-inducing ability of a synthetic adjuvant, N-acetylmuramyl peptides, and bacterial disaccharide peptides related to different oil vehicles and their composition. Infect. Immun. 29: 70-75.

89. Kohashi, O., C. M. Pearson, N. Tamaoki, A. Tanaka, K. Shimamura, A. Ozawa, S. Kotani, M. Saito, and K. Hioki. 1981. Role of thymus for N-acetyl muramyl-L-alanyl-D-isoglutamine-induced polyarhtritis and granuloma formation in euthymic and athymic nude rats or in neonatally thymectomized rats. Infect. Immun. 31: 758-766.

90. Kohashi, O., Y. Kohashi, S. Kotani, and A. Ozawa. 1981. A new model of experimental arthritis induced by an aqueous form of synthetic adjuvant in immunodeficient rats (SHR and nude rats). Ryumachi 21(Suppl.): 149-156.

91. Zidek, Z., K. Masek, and Z. Jiricka. 1982. Arthritogenic activity of a synthetic immunoadjuvant, muramyl dipeptide. Infect. Immun. 35: 674-679.

92. Kotani, S., Y. Watanabe, F. Kinoshita, K. Kato, K. Harada, T. Shiba, S. Kusumoto, Y. Tarumi, K. Ikenaka, S. Okada, S. Kawata, and K. Yokogawa. 1977. Gelation of the amoebocyte lysate of Tachypleus tridentatus by cell wall digest of several gram-positive bacteria and synthetic peptidoglycan subunits of natural and unnatural configurations. Biken J. 20: 5-10.

93. Dinarello, C. A., R. J. Elin, L. Chedid, and S. M. Wolff. 1978. The pyrogenicity of the synthetic muramyl dipeptide and two structural analogues. J. Infect. Dis. 138: 760-767.

94. Masek, K., O. Kadlecova, and P. Petrovicky. 1978. Pharmacological activity of bacterial peptidoglycan: the effect on temperature and sleep in the rat, p. 991-1003. In P. Rosenberd (ed.), Toxins: animal, plant and microbial. (Proceedings of the fifth international symposium). Pergamon Press, Oxford and New York.

95. Riveau, G., K. Masek. M. Parant, and L. Chedid. 1980. Central pyrogenic activity of muramyl peptide. J. Exp. Med. 152: 869-877.

96. Krueger, J. M., J. R. Pappenheimer, and M. L. Karnovsky. 1982. The composition of sleep-promoting factor isolated from human urine. J. Biol. Chem. 257: 1664-1669.

97. Schwab, J. H. 1979. Acute and chronic inflammation induced by bacterial cell wall structures, p. 209-214. In D. Schlessinger (ed.), Microbiology 1979. American Society for Microbiology, Washington, D. C.

98. Emori, K., and A. Tanaka. 1978. Granuloma formation by synthetic bacterial cell wall fragment: muramyl dipeptide. Infect. Immun. 19: 613-620.

99. Nagao, S., F. Ota, K. Emori, K. Inoue, and A. Tanaka. 1981. Epitheloid granuloma induced by muramyl dipeptide in immunologically deficient rats. Infect. Immun. 34: 993-999.

100. Tanaka, A., K. Emori, S. Nagao, K. Koshima, O. Kohashi, M. Saitoh, and T. Kataoka. 1982. Epitheloid granuloma formation requiring no T-cell function. Am. J. Pathol. 106: 165-170.

101. Ohkuni, H., and Y. Kimura. 1976. Increased capillary permeability in guinea pigs and rats by peptidoglycan fraction extracted from group A streptococcal cell walls. Exp. Cell. Biol. 44: 83-94.

102. Nagao, S., Y. Iwata, and A. Tanaka. 1982. Extensive necrosis caused by the injection of MDP, p. 189-192. In Y. Yamamura, S. Kotani, I. Azuma, A. Koda and T. Shiba (eds.), Immunomodulation by microbial products and related synthetic compounds. Excerpta Medica, Amsterdam.

103. Lambris, J. S., J. B. Allen, and J. H. Schwab. 1982. In vivo changes in complement induced with peptidoglycan-polysaccharide polymers from streptococcal cell walls. Infect. Immun. 35: 377-380.

104. Schwab, J. H., J. B. Allen, S. K. Anderle, F. Dalldorf, R. Eisenberg and W. J. Cromartie. 1982. Relationship of complement to experimental arthritis induced in rats with streptococcal cell walls. Immunology 46: 83-88.

105. Audibert, F., B. Heymer, C. Gros, K. H. Schleifer, P. H. Seidl, and L. Chedid. 1978. Absence of binding of MDP, a synthetic immunoadjuvant to antipeptidoglycan antibodies. J. Immunol. 121: 1219-1222.

106. Reichert, C. M., C. Carelli, M. Jolivet, F. Audibert, P. Lefrancier, and L. Chedid. Synthesis of conjugates containing N-acetylmuramyl-L-alanyl-D-isoglutaminyl (MDP). Their use as hapten-carrier systems. Mol. Immunol. 17: 357-363.

107. Bahr, G. M., F. Z. Modabber, G. A. W. Rook, M. L. Mehrotra, J. L. Stanford, and L. Chedid. 1982. Absence of antibodies to muramyl dipeptide in patients with tuberculosis or leprosy. Clin. Exp. Immunol. 47: 53-58.

108. Bahr, G. M., C. Carelli, F. Audibert, F. Modabber, and L. Chedid. 1982. Analysis of the antigenic relationship of various derivatives of N-acetyl-muramyl-L-ala-D-isoglutamine (MDP), using anti-MDP antibodies. Mol. Immunol. 19: 737-745.

109. Maeda, K., T. Koga, K. Onoue, S. Kotani, and A. Suumiyoshi. 1980. Induction of delayed type hypersensitivity-like skin reaction by peptidoglycans of bacterial cell walls. Microbiol. Immunol. 24: 335-348.

110. Yamamota, K., M. Kakinuma, K. Kato, H. Okuyama, and I. Azuma. 1980. Relationship of anti-tuberculous protection to lung granuloma produced by intravenous injection of synthetic 6-O-mycoloyl-N-acetylmuramyl-L-alanyl-D-isoglutamine with or without specific antigens. Immunology 40: 557-564.

111. Hamamoto, Y., Y. Kobara, A. Kojima, Y. Kumazawa, and K. Yasuhira. 1981. Experimental production of pulmonary granulomas. I. Immune granulomas induced by chemically modified cell walls and their constituents. Br. J. Pathol. 62: 259-269.

112. Wachsmuth, E. D., and P. Dukor. 1982. Immunopathology of muramyl peptides, p. 60-71. In Y. Yamamura, S. Kotani, I. Azuma, A. Koda and T. Shiba (eds.), Immunomodulation by microbial products and related synthetic compounds. Excerpta Medica, Amsterdam.

113. Parant, M., F. Parant, L. Chedid, A. Yapo, J. F. Petit, and E. Lederer. 1979. Fate of the synthetic immunoadjuvant, muramyl dipeptide (^{14}C-labelled) in the mouse. Int. J. Immunopharmacol. 1: 35-41.

114. Tomasic, J., B. Ladesic, Z. Valinger, and I. Hrsak. 1980. The metabolic fate of ^{14}C-labeled peptidoglycan monomer in mice. I. Identification of the monomer and the corresponding pentapeptide in urine. Biochim. Biophys. Acta 629: 77-82.

115. Ladesic, B., J. Tomasic, S. Kveder, I. Hrsak. 1981. The metabolic fate of ^{14}C-labeled immunoadjuvant peptidoglycan monomer. II. In vitro studies. Biochim. Biophys. Acta 678: 12-17.

116. Yapo, A., J. F. Petit, E. Lederer, M. Parant, F. Parant, and L. Chedid. 1982. Fate of two ^{14}C labelled muramyl peptides: Ac-Mur-L-Ala-γ-D-Glu-meso-A_2pm and Ac-Mur-L-Ala-γ-D-Glu-meso-A_2pm-D-Ala in mice. Evaluation of their ability to increase nonspecific resistance to Klebsiella infection. Int. J. Immunopharmacol. 4: 143-149.

117. Valinger, Z., B. Ladesic, and J. Tomasic. 1982. Partial purification and characterization of N-acetylmuramyl-L-alanine amidase from human and mouse serum. Biochim. Biophys. Acta 701: 63-71.

118. Ogawa, T., S. Kotani, K. Fukuda, Y. Tsukamoto, M. Mori, S. Kusumoto, and T. Shiba. Stimulation of migration of human monocytes by bacterial cell walls and muramylpeptides. Infect. Immun. (submitted).

119. Ogawa, T., S. Kotani, S. Kusumoto, and T. Shiba. Possible chemotaxis of human monocyte by N-acetylmuramyl-L-alanyl-D-isoglutamine, MDP. Infect. Immun. (submitted).

120. Tanaka, A., S. Nagao, K. Imai, and R. Mori. 1980. Macrophage activation by muramyl dipeptide as measured by macrophage spreading and attachment. Microbiol. Immunol. 24: 547-557.

121. Nagao, S., T. Miki, and A. Tanaka. 1981. Macrophage activation by muramyl dipeptide (MDP) without lymphocyte participation. Microbiol. Immunol. 24: 41-50.

122. Pabst, M. J., and R. B. Johnson, Jr. 1980. Increased production of superoxide anion by macrophages exposed in vitro to muramyl dipeptide or lipopolysaccharide. J. Exp. Med. 151: 101-114.

123. Takada, H., M. Tsujimoto, K. Kao, S. Kotani, S. Kusumoto, M. Inage, T. Shiba, I. Yano, S. Kawata, and K. Yokogawa. 1979. Macrophage activation by bacterial cell walls and related synthetic compounds. Infect. Immun. 25: 48-52.

124. Imai, K., M. Tomioka, S. Nagao, K. Kushima, and A. Tanaka. 1980. Biochemical evidence for activation of guinea pig macrophages by muramyl dipeptide. Biochem. Res. 25: 51-62.

125. Tanaka, A., S. Nagao, S. Ikegami, T. Shiba, and S. Kotani. 1982. The suppression of macrophage DNA synthesis by MDP, a possible correlate of macrophage activation, p. 201-204. In Y. Yamamura, S. Kotani, I. Azuma, A. Koda and T. Shiba (eds.), Immunomodulation by microbial products and related synthetic compounds. Excerpta Medica, Amsterdam.

126. Imai, K., and A. Tanaka. 1981. Effect of muramyldipeptide, a synthetic bacterial adjuvant, on enzyme release from cultured mouse macrophages. Microbiol. Immunol. 25: 51-62

127. Nichols, W. K., and F. H. Prosser. 1980. Induction of ornithine decarboxylase in macrophages by bacterial lipopolysaccharide (LPS) and mycobacterial cell wall material. Life Sci. 27: 913-920.

128. Pabst, M. J., N. P. Cummings, T. Shiba, S. Kusumoto, and S. Kotani. 1980. Lipophilic derivative of muramyl dipeptide is more active than muramyl dipeptide in priming macrophages to release superoxide anion. Infect. Immun. 29: 617-622.

129. Hadden, J. W. 1978. Effects of isoprinosine, levamisole, muramyl dipeptide and SM1213 on lymphocyte and macrophage function *in vitro*. Can. Treat. Res. 62: 1981-1985.

130. Hadden, J. W., A. England, J. R. Sadlik, and E. M. Hadden. 1979. The comparative effects of isoprinosine, levamisole, muramyl dipeptide and SM1213 on lymphocyte and macrophage proliferation and activation *in vitro*. Int. J. Immunopharmacol. 1: 17-27.

131. Takada, H., Y. Ishihara, S. Kotani, S. Kusumoto, T. Shiba, S. Kawata, and Y. Yokogawa. Macrophage activation by bacterial cell walls and related synthetic compounds. II. Phagocytosis stimulation. Microbiol. Immunol. (submitted).

132. Smialowicz, R. J., and J. H. Schwab. 1978. Inhibition of macrophage phagocytic activity by group A streptococcal cell walls. Infect. Immun. 20: 258-261.

133. Nozawa, R. T., R. Sekiguchi, and T. Yokota. 1980. Stimulation by conditioned medium of L-929 fibroblasts, *E. coli* lipopolysaccharide, and muramyl dipeptide of candidacidal activity of mouse macrophages. Cell. Immunol. 53: 116-124.

134. Juy, D., and L. Chedid. 1975. Comparison between macrophage activation and enhancement of nonspecific resistance to tumors by mycobacterial immunoadjuvants. Proc. Natl. Acad. Sci. USA 72: 4105-4109.

135. Taniyama, T., and H. T. Holden. 1979. Direct augmentation of cytolytic activity of tumor-derived macrophages and macrophage cell lines by muramyl dipeptide. Cell. Immunol. 48: 369-374.

136. Galelli, A., Y. L. Garrec, L. Chedid, P. Lefrancier, M. Derrien, and M. Level. 1980. Macrophage stimulation in vitro by an inactive muramyl dipeptide derivative after conjugation to multi-poly (DL alanyl)-poly(L-lysine) carrier. Infect. Immun. 28: 1-5.

137. Sone, S., and I. J. Fidler. 1980. Synergistic activation by lymphokines and muramyl dipeptide of tumoricidal properties in rat alveolar macrophages. J. Immunol. 125: 2454-2460.

138. Schroit, A. J., and I. J. Fidler. 1982. Effects of liposome structure and lipid composition on the activation of tumoricidal properties of macrophages by liposomes containing muramyl dipeptide. Cancer Res. 42: 161-167.

139. Smialowicz, R. J., and J. H. Schwab. 1977. Cytotoxicity of rat macrophages activated by persistent or biodegradable bacterial cell walls. Infect. Immun. 17: 599-606.

140. Akagawa, K. S., and T. Tokunaga. 1980. Effect of synthetic muramyl dipeptide (MDP) on differentiation of myeloid leukemic cells. Microbiol. Immunol. 24: 1005-1011.

141. Yamamoto, Y., M. Tomida, M. Hozumi, and I. Azuma. 1981. Enhancement by immunostimulants of the production of mouse spleen cells of factor(s) stimulating differentiation of mouse myeloid leukemic cells. Gann 72: 828-833.

142. Yamamoto, Y., S. Nagao, A. Tanaka, T. Koga, and K. Onoue. 1978. Inhibition of macrophage migration by synthetic muramyl dipeptide. Biochem. Biophys. Res. Commun. 80: 923-928.

143. Adam, A., V. Souvannavong, and E. Lederer. 1978. Nonspecific MIF-like activity induced by the synthetic immunoadjuvant: N-acetyl muramyl-L-alanyl-D-isoglutamine (MDP). Biochim. Biophys. Res. Commun. 85: 684-690.

144. Nagao, S., A. Tanaka, Y. Yamamoto, T. Koga, K. Onoue, T. Shiba, K. Kusumoto, and S. Kotani. 1979. Inhibition of macrophage migration by muramyl peptides. Infect. Immun. 24: 308-312.

145. Homma, Y., K. Onozaki, T. Hashimoto, K. Miura, S. Nagao, and A. Tanaka. 1981. Different effect of (L)-fucose binding lectin on macrophage migration inhibition caused by guinea pig migration inhibitory factor and synthetic muramyl dipeptide. Int. Arch. Aller. Appl. Immunol. 65: 27-33.

146. Wahl, S. M., L. M. Wahl, J. B. McCarthy, L. Chedid, and S. M. Mergenhagen. 1979. Macrophage activation by mycobacterial water soluble components and synthetic muramyl dipeptide. J. Immunol. 122: 2226-2231.

147. Oppenheim, J. J., A. Togawa, L. Chedid, and S. Mizel. 1980. Components of mycobacteria and muramyl dipeptide with adjuvant activity induce lymphocyte activating factor. Cell. Immunol. 50: 71-81.

148. Tenu, J.-P., E. Lederer, and J.-F Petit. 1980. Stimulation of thymocyte mitogenic protein secretion and of cytostatic activity of mouse peritoneal macrophages by trehalose dimycolate and muramyl-dipeptide. Eur. J. Immunol. 10: 647-653.

149. Iribe, H., T. Koga, K. Onoue, S. Kotani, S. Kusumoto, and T. Shiba. 1981. Macrophage-stimulating effect of a synthetic muramyl dipeptide and its adjuvant-active and -inactive analogs for the production of T-cell activating monokines. Cell. Immunol. 64: 73-83.

150. Tsukamoto, Y., W. Helsel, and S. M. Wahl. 1981. Macrophage production of fibronectin, a chemoattractant for fibroblasts. J. Immunol. 127: 673-678.

151. Drapier, J.-C., G. Lemaire, and J.-F. Petit. 1982. Regulation of plasminogen activator secretion in mouse peritoneal macrophages. II. Inhibition by immunomodulators of bacterial origin. Int. J. Immunopharmacol. 4: 21-34.

152. Hamilton, J. A., J. B. Zabriskie, L. B. Laghman, and Y.-S. Chen. 1982. Streptococcal cell walls and synovial cell activation. Stimulation of synovial fibroblasts plasminogen activator activity by monocytes treated with group A streptococcal cell wall sonicates and muramyl dipeptide. J. Exp. Med. 155: 1702-1818.

153. Rutherford, B., K. Steffin, and J. Sexton. 1982. Activated human mononuclear phagocytes release a substance(s) that induced replication of quiescent human fibroblasts. J. Reticuloendothel. Soc. 31: 281-293.

154. Damais, C., G. Riveau, M. Parant, J. Gerota, and L. Chedid. 1982. Production of lymphocyte activating factor in the absence of endogenous pyrogen by rabbit or human leukocytes stimulated by a muramyl dipeptide derivative. Int. J. Immunopharmacol. 4: 451-462.

155. Hotta, H., S. Hotta, H. Takada, and S. Kotani. Enhancement of Dengue-2 virus multiplication in cultured mouse peritoneal macrophages by bacterial cell walls and their related structural components. Infect. Immun. (submitted).

156. Igarashi, T., M. Okada, I. Azuma, and Y. Yamamura. 1977. Adjuvant activity of synthetic N-acetylmuramyl-L-alanyl-D-isoglutamine and related compounds on cell-mediated cytotoxicity in syngeneic mice. Cell. Immunol. 34: 270-278.

157. Takada, H., S. Kotani, S. Kusumoto, Y. Tarumi, K. Ikenaka, and T. Shiba. 1977. Mitogenic activity of adjuvant-active N-acetylmuramyl-L-alanyl-D-isoglutamine and its analogues. Biken J. 20: 81-85.

158. Damais, C., M. Parant, and L. Chedid. 1977. Nonspecific activation of murine spleen cells in vitro by a synthetic immunoadjuvant (N-acetylmuramyl-L-alanyl-D-isoglutamine). Cell. Immunol. 34: 49-56.

159. Damais, C., M. Parant, L. Chedid, P. Lefrancier, and J. Choay. 1978. In vitro spleen cells responsiveness to various analogs of MDP (N-acetylmuramyl-L-alanyl-D-isoglutamine), a synthetic immunoadjuvant, in MDP high-responder mice. Cell. Immunol. 35: 173-179.

160. Takada, H., M. Tsujimoto, S. Kotani, S. Kusumoto, M. Inage, T. Shiba, S. Nagao, I. Yano, S. Kawata, and K. Yokogawa. 1979. Mitogenic effects of bacterial cell walls, their fragments, and related synthetic compounds on thymocytes and splenocytes of guinea pigs. Infect. Immun. 25: 645-652.

161. Takada, H., S. Nagao, S. Kotani, S. Kawata, K. Yokogawa, S. Kusumoto, T. Shiba, and I. Yano. 1980. Mitogenic effects of bacterial cell walls and their components on murine splenocytes. Biken J. 23: 61-68.

162. Wood, D. D., and M. J. Straruch. 1981. Control of the mitogenicity of muramyl dipeptide. Int. J. Immunopharmacol. 3: 31-44.

163. Specter, S., H. Friedman, and L. Chedid. 1977. Dissociation between the adjuvant vs mitogenic activity of a synthetic muramyl dipeptide for murine splenocytes. Proc. Soc. Exp. Biol Med. 155: 349-352.

164. Specter, S., R. Cimprich, F. Friedman, and L. Chedid. 1978. Stimulation of an enhanced in vitro immune response by a synthetic adjuvant, muramyl dipeptide. J. Immunol. 120: 487-491.

165. Leclerc, C., I. Lowy, and L. Chedid. 1978. Influence of MDP and of some analogous synthetic glycopeptides on the in vitro mouse spleen cell viability and immune response to sheep erythrocytes. Cell. Immunol. 38: 286-293.

166. Leclerc, C., E. Bourgeois, and L. Chedid. 1979. Enhancement by muramyl dipeptide of in vitro nude mice responses to a T-dependent antigen. Immunol. Commun. 8: 55-64.

167. Löwy, I., and L. Chedid. 1979. Effect of cell division inhibitors on polyclonal activation can vary according to the target cell used. Immunol. Commun. 8: 479-494.

168. Löwy, I., C. Leclerc, and L. Chedid. 1980. Induction of antibodies directed against self and altered-self determinants by synthetic adjuvant, muramyl dipeptide and some of its derivatives. Immunology 39: 441-450.

169. Saito-Taki, T., M. J. Tanabe, H. Mochizuki, T. Matsumoto, M. Nakano, H. Takada, M. Tsujimoto, S. Kotani, S. Kusumoto, T. Shiba, K. Yokogawa, and S. Kawata. 1980. Polyclonal B cell activation by cell wall preparations of gram-positive bacteria. In vitro responses of spleen cells obtained from Balb/c, nu/nu. Nu/+, CH/He, C3H/HeJ and hybrid (CBA/NxBalb/c)F1 mice. Microbiol. Immunol. 24: 209-218.

170. Löwy, I., C. Leclerc, B. Bourgeois, and L. Chedid. 1980. Inhibition of mitogen-induced polyclonal activation by a synthetic adjuvant, muramyl dipeptide (MDP). J. Immunol. 124: 320-325.

171. Sugimura, K., M. Uemiya, I. Saiki, I. Azuma, and Y. Yamamura. 1979. The adjuvant activity of synthetic N-acetylmuramyl-dipeptide: evidence of initial target cells for the adjuvant activity. Cell. Immunol. 43: 137-149.

172. Leclerc, C., D. Juy, and L. Chedid. 1979. Inhibitory and stimulatory effects of a synthetic glycopeptide (MDP) on the in vitro PFC response: factors affecting the response. Cell. Immunol. 42: 336-343.

173. Watson, J., and C. Whitlock. 1978. Effect of a synthetic adjuvant on the induction of primary immune responses in T cell-depleted spleen cultures. J. Immunol. 121: 383-389.

174. Azuma, I., T. Taniyama, K. Sugimura, A. A. Aladin, and Y. Yamamura. 1976. Mitogenic activity of the cell walls of mycobacteria, nocardia, corynebacteria and anaerobic coryneforms. Jpn. J. Microbiol. 20: 263-271.

175. Azuma, I., K. Sugimura, M. Yamawaki, M. Uemiya, and Y. Yamamura. 1977. Mitogenic activity of cell-wall components in mouse spleen cells. Microbiol. Immunol. 21: 111-115.

176. Sugimura, K., M. Uemiya, I. Azuma, M. Yamawaki, and Y. Yamamura. 1977. Macrophage dependency of T-lymphocyte mitogenesis by Nocardia rubra cell-wall skeleton. Microbiol. Immunol. 21: 525-530.

177. Räsänen, L., and H. Arvilommi. 1981. Cell walls, peptidoglycans, and teichoic acids of gram-positive bacteria as polyclonal inducers and immunomodulators of proliferative and lymphokine responses of human B and T lymphocytes. Infect. Immun. 34: 712-717.

178. Prunet, J., J. L. Birrien, J. Panijel, and P. Liacopoulos. 1978. On the mechanism of early recovery of specifically depleted lymphoid cell populations by nonspecific activation of T cells. Cell. Immunol. 37: 151-161.

179. Ishihara, Y., H. Takada, S. Kotani, S. Kusumoto, T. Shiba, S. Kawata, and K. Yokogawa. 1982. Stimulation of polymorphonuclear leukocytes by bacterial cell wall components and related synthetic compounds, p. 217-220. In Y. Yamamura, S. Kotani, I. Azuma, A. Koda and T. Shiba (eds.), Immunomodulation by microbial products and related synthetic compounds. Excerpta Medica, Amsterdam.

180. Jones, J. M., and J. H. Schwab. 1970. Effects of streptococcal cell wall fragments on lymphocytsosis and tissue culture cells. Infect. Immun. 1: 232-242.

181. Musher, D. M., H. A. Verbrugh, and J. Verhoef. 1981. Suppression of phagocytosis and chemotaxis by cell wall components of Staphylococcus aureus. J. Immunol. 127: 84-88.

182. Narita, T. 1974. Comparative studies on biological and immunological properties of bacterial and fungal cell walls, and solubilization and modification of active principle(s) by cell wall lytic enzymes. J. Osaka Univ. Dent. Soc. 19: 81-99. (In Japanese with English summary).

183. Staber, F. G., R. H. Gisler, G. Schumann, L. Tarcsay, E. Schläfli, and P. Dukor. 1978. Modulation of myelopoiesis by different bacterial cell-wall components: induction of colony-stimulating activity (by pure preparations, low-molecular-weight degradation products, and a synthetic low-molecular analog of bacterial cell-wall components) in vitro. Cell. Immunol. 37: 174-187.

184. Ogawa, T., H. Takada, S. Kotani, S. Kusumoto, T. Shiba, S. Kawata, and K. Yokogawa. 1982. Basophile leukocyte stimulation by bacterial cell walls and related compounds, p. 221-224. In Y. Yamamura, S. Kotani, I. Azuma, A. Koda and T. Shiba (eds.), Immunomodulation by microbial products and related synthetic compounds. Excerpta Medica, Amsterdam.

185. Kimura, Y., Y. Norose, T. Kato, M. Furuya, M. Hida, Y. Banno, S. Kotani, S. Kusumoto, and T. Shiba. 1982. Histamine releasing activity from rat mast cells and platelets by peptidoglycan extracted from streptococcal cell walls and the related synthetic compounds, p. 225-228. In Y. Yamamura, S. Kotani, I. Azuma, A. Koda and T. Shiba (eds.), Immunomodulation by microbial products and related synthetic compounds. Excerpta Medica, Amsterdam.

186. Raskova, H., M. Ryc, J. Rotta, and K. Masek. 1971. Release of 5-hydroxy-tryptamine and morphological changes in blood platelets induced by mucopeptide of staphylococcal cell walls. J. Infect. Dis. 123: 587-594.

187. Ryc, M., and J. Rotta. 1975. The thrombocytolytic activity of bacterial peptidoglycans. Z. Immunitaetsforsch. 149(Suppl.): 265-272.

188. Rotta, J., M. Ryc, K. Masek, and M. Zaoral. 1979. Biological activity of synthetic subunits of staphylococcus peptidoglycan. I. Pyrogenic and thrombocytolitic activity. Exp. Cell Biol. 47: 258-268.

189. Harada, K., S. Kotani, H. Takada, M. Tsujimoto, Y. Hirachi, S. Kusumoto, T. Shiba, S. Kawata, K. Yokogawa, H. Nishimura, T. Kitaura, and T. Nakajima. 1982. Liberation of serotonin from rabbit blood platelets by bacterial cell walls and some related compounds, enzymatically prepared or synthesized. Infect. Immun. (in press).

190. Dewhirst, F. E. 1982. N-acetyl muramyl dipeptide stimulation of bone resorption in tissue culture. Infect. Immun. 35: 133-137.

191. Bokisch, V. A. 1975. Interaction of peptidoglycans with anti-IgGs and with completment. Z. Immunitaetsforsch. 149(Suppl.): 320-330.

192. Tauber, J. W., M. J. Polley, and J. B. Zabriskie. 1976. Nonspecific complement activation by streptococcal structures. II. Properdin-independent inhibition by alternative pathway. J. Exp. Med. 143: 1352-1366.

193. Greenblatt, J., R. J. Boackle, and J. H. Schwab. 1978. Activation of the alternative complement pathway by peptidoglycan from streptococcal cell well. Infect. Immun. 19: 296-303.

194. Peperson, P. K., B. J. Wilkinson, Y. Kim, D. Schmeling, S. D. Douglas, P. G. Quie, and J. Verhoef. 1978. The key role of peptidoglycan in the opsonization of Staphylococcus aureus. J. Clin. Invest. 61: 597-609.

195. Wilkinson, B. J., Y. Kim, and P. K. Peterson. 1981. Factors affecting complement activation by Staphylococcus aureus cell walls, their components, and mutants altered in teichoic acid. Infect. Immun. 32: 216-224.

196. Kawasaki, A. 1982. Activation of human complement system by bacterial cell walls, their water-soluble enzymatic digests and related synthetic compounds. J. Osaka Univ. Dent. Soc. 27: 46-61. (In Japanese with English summary).

197. Kotani, S., H. Takada, M. Tsujimoto, T. Ogawa, K. Kato, T. Okunaga, Y. Ishihara, A. Kawasaki, I. Morisaki, N. Kono, T. Shimono, T. Shiba, S. Kusumoto, M. Inage, K. Harada, T. Kitaura, S. Kano, S. Inai, K. Nagai, M. Matsumoto, T. Kubo, M. Kato, Z. Tada, K. Yokogawa, and S. Kawata. 1981 Immunomodulating and related biological activities of bacterial cell walls and their components, enzymatically prepared or synthesized, p. 231-273. In H. Friedman, T. W. Klein and A. Szentivanyi (eds.), Immunomodulation by bacterial and their products. Plenum Press, New York.

198. Ogawa, T., S. Kotani, M. Tsujimoto, S. Kusumoto, T. Shiba, S. Kawata, and K. Yokogawa. 1982. Contractile effects of bacterial cell walls, their enzymatic digests, and muramyl dipeptides on ileal strips from guinea pigs. Infect. Immun. 35: 612-619.

199. Stewart-Tull, D. E. S., M. Davies, and D. M. Jackson. 1978. The binding of adjuvant-active mycobacterial peptidoglycans and glycopeptieds to mammalian membranes and their effect on artificial lipid bilayers. Immunology 34: 57-66.

200. Shiba, T., S. Okada, S. Kusumoto, I. Azuma, and Y. Yamamura. 1978. Synthesis of 6-O-mycoloyl-N-acetylmuramyl-L-alanyl-D-isoglutamine with antitumor activity. Bull. Chem. Soc. Jpn. 51: 3307-3311.

201. Kusumoto, S., M. Inage, T. Shiba, I. Azuma, and Y. Yamamura. 1978. Synthesis of long chain fatty acid esters of N-acetylmuramyl-L-alanyl-D-isoglutamine in relation to antitumor activity. Tetrahedron Lett. 49: 4899-4902.

202. Imada, I., I. Azuma, S. Kishimoto, Y. Yamamura, and H. Morimoto. 1972. The effect of ubiquinone-7 and its metabolites on the immune response. Int. Arch. Allerg. Appl. Immunol. 43: 898-907.

203. Sugimura, K., I. Azuma, Y. Yamamura, I. Imada, M. Watanabe, and H. Morimoto. 1977. Effect of ubiquinone and related compounds on immune response, p. 151-163. In K. Folkers and Y. Yamamura (eds.), Biomedical and clinical aspects of coenzyme Q. Elseviers/North Holland Publishing Co., New York.

204. Imada, I., M. Watanabe, and H. Morimoto. 1978. Metabolism of ubiquinone, and biological activities of its metabolites and related compounds. Vitamins (Kyoto) 52: 493-501.

205. Brunner, K. T., J. Mauel, H. Rudolf, and B. Chapuis. 1970. Studies of allograft immunity in mice. I. Induction, development and *in vitro* assay of cellular immunity. Immunology 18: 501-515.

206. Kotani, S., H. Takada, M. Tsujimoto, T. Kubo, T. Ogawa, I. Azuma, H. Ogawa, K. Matsumoto, W. A. Siddiqui, A. Tanaka, S. Nagao, O. Kohashi, S. Kanoy, T. Shiba, and S. Kusumoto. 1982. Nonspecific and antigen-specific stimulation of host defense mechanisms by lipophilic derivatives of muramyl dipeptides. In International colloquium on "bacteria and cancer" at Cologne, West Germany. Academic Press, London. (in press).

207. Tsujimoto, M. 1982. Fundamental studies to utilize the adjuvant activity of 6-*O*-acyl-muramyldipeptides to potentiate cellular and humoral immune responses for practical purpose. J. Osaka Univ. Dent. Soc. 26: 63-83. (In Japanese with English summary).

208. Morisaki, I. 1980. Species and strain differences in responsiveness of laboratory animals to immunopotentiating activities of bacterial cell walls and their related adjuvants. J. Osaka Univ. Dent. Soc. 25: 229-249. (In Japanese with English summary).

209. Matsumoto, K., H. Ogawa, T. Kusama, and O. Nagase. 1982. Enhancement of nonspecific resistance to bacterial infection in mice induced by muramyl-dipeptide derivatives, p. 237-240. In Y. Yamamura, S. Kotani, I. Azuma, A. Koda and T. Shiba (eds.), Immunomodulation by microbial products and related synthetic compounds. Excerpta Medica, Amsterdam.

210. Matsumoto, K., T. Otani, T. Une, Y. Osada, H. Ogawa, and I. Azuma. Stimulation of nonspecific resistance to infection induced by MDP analogs substituted in the γ-carboxyl group, and evaluation of MDP-Lys(L18). Infect. Immun. (submitted).

CLINICAL PHASE I INVESTIGATION OF INTRAVENOUS OIL ATTACHED MYCOBACTERIAL COMPONENTS AS IMMUNOTHERAPEUTIC AGENTS

Gerald Vosika[1], Tim Trenbeath[1], Cathy Giddings[1], Gary R. Gray[2]

The Department of Medicine[1], University of North Dakota Medical School, and the Veterans Administration Hospital[1], Fargo, North Dakota (USA). The Department of Chemistry[2], University of Minnesota, Minneapolis Minnesota (USA)

INTRODUCTION

Nonspecific immunostimulation with mycobacterial agents, especially BCG, have been widely utilized (1) in an effort to increase host resistance to malignancy. Crude viable and/or killed mycobacterial agents are heterogenous preparations (2, 3), which have a significant incidence of morbidity. From an immunotherapeutic viewpoint, BCG has been shown (4, 5), in high doses, to cause splenic suppressor cells in mice, and has been implicated in causing tumor enhancement (6). Because of these problems, major interest has centered on the purification and use of microbial components.

In the guinea pig, oil attached mycobacterial cell wall skeleton and trehalose dimycolate is as effective (7, 8) as viable BCG in causing tumor regression and systemic immunity. We have shown (9, 10) that similar results can be obtained using these materials intralesionally in patients with malignant melanoma.

The potential use of systemic intravenous microbial agent is appealing from the standpoint of ease of administration, lack of local toxicity, and the potential for inducing a systemic augmentation. Among microbial agents, *Corynebacterium parvum* has been extensively studied (11) as a systemic intravenous immunomodulator.

As part of our program in the study of the potential use of mycobacterial components, a Phase I study of the toxicity and immunological effects of intravenous cell wall skeleton and trehalose dimycolate attached to oil droplets was performed.

METHODS

Preparation Of Microbial Components

Mycobacterium smegmatis cell wall skeleton (CWS) was prepared (12) as for BCG CWS. CWS of *M. smegmatis*, which was initially erroneously classified as *M. phlei*, has (13) tumor regression properties in the guinea pig model equivalent to BCG CWS. Trehalose dimycolate was purified by microparticulate chromatography from cord factor of *M. tuberculosis* (Agoma B strain) and has been designated as TDM.

The final vaccine was prepared using sterile techniques as previously described (13). Briefly, CWS and TDM, dissolved or suspended in chloroform-methanol (95:5), were placed in a glass grinder (30 to 55 ml). The chloroform-methanol was dried under nitrogen and the tube placed in a vacuum dessicator overnight. The following day, oil (Drakol 6VR, Penreco) was added and the mixture placed in a 56°C water bath for five minutes. The mixture was then ground with a teflon pestle for 2-3 minutes at 800-1000 rpm. The resulting material was then emulsified in saline containing 0.2% Tween 80 by grinding at 800-1000 rpm using 50 strokes of the pestle. The final vaccine contained 1 mg/ml CWS, 0.5 mg/ml TDM, 2% oil, and 0.2% Tween-saline. The material was aliquoted into stoppered vials and frozen to -70°C. Frozen vials were thawed prior to use. Unused, thawed vaccines were discarded. For administration, the appropriate amount of vaccine was diluted into 50 cc of normal saline and given intravenously over 30 minutes.

Treatment Program

For this Phase I study two or three patients were treated intravenously at dose levels of 100, 250, 500, 1000, and 2000 $\mu g/M^2$. Initially, treatment was planned at intervals of every two weeks for a period of eight weeks. Because the material was generally well tolerated, the program was changed to weekly treatment for eight weeks. Therefore, the latter group of patients were treated twice as intensely.

In selecting patients for the program, we preferentially sought newly diagnosed patients for whom there is no consistently effective or standard therapy. Such patients with non small-cell lung cancer, and metastatic colon cancer were treated with immunotherapy prior to other agents. This was done since it is recognized that the relatively less tumor burden and better immunocompetence of the previously untreated patients would be factors favorable to an immunotherapy response.

Clinical Monitoring

All patients admitted to these studies were off all chemotherapy for at least four weeks. No patients received any concurrent chemotherapy, hormonal therapy, or glucocorticoids. All patients were evaluated initially with a complete physical examination, chest roentgenogram, liver-spleen scan, complete blood counts, liver and renal function test and other tests to determine the extent of disease. Pulmonary function test and diffusion capacity were obtained prior to and following treatment to detect pulmonary fibrosis. All blood tests were repeated at two week intervals. Chest x-rays and liver-spleen scan and other tests as indicated were repeated at the end of the treatment program. During the first treatment, patients receiving intravenous therapy were hospitalized and the vital signs watched for 8 hours to detect acute toxicity. Skin tests were performed on all patients with PPD, Trichophyton and Candida prior to treatment. Skin tests were repeated at four to eight week intervals. Results were reported as the maximum induration in millimeters at 48 hours. Serum electrophoresis and quantitative immunoglobulins were performed prior to study at two week intervals.

RESULTS

Patient Populations

Thirteen patients received from 100 $\mu g/M^2$ every two weeks up to 2000 $\mu g/M^2$ weekly, as shown in Table 1. Nine patients (No. 1-9) received a total of 4 treatments given every two weeks. The last four patients were treated weekly and the number of treatments increased to eight. Eleven patients received their full planned course of therapy. Patient No. 13 received only three of the anticipated eight weeks. In that patient, immunotherapy was discontinued and irradiation given because of bronchial obstruction. Patient No. 5 had rapidly progressing disease and died prior to the fourth treatment. Six of the thirteen patients had a definitive surgical procedure. Only three had prior radiation therapy and four had prior chemotherapy.

Side Effects

The side effects are shown in Table 2 as a function of dose level. Mild nausea occurred in three patients at the 1000 and 2000 $\mu g/M^2$ level. Fever and shaking chills occurred in one patient at the 1000 $\mu g/M^2$ level and was essentially universal at the 2000 $\mu g/M^2$ level. The chills usually occurred between one and 24 hours

Table 1. Diagnosis, prior therapy and treatment schedule of the patient population

Patient	Diagnosis	Prior[1] Therapy	Dose (μg/M^2)	Frequency of Treatment	Number of Treatments	Total Received (μg/M^2)
1	Hypernephroma	S	100	2 weeks	4	400
2	Hypernephroma	S,C	100	2 weeks	4	400
3	Thyroid carcinoma	S,C,R	100	2 weeks	4	400
4	Prostate cancer	B,R	250	2 weeks	4	1000
5	Lung (Large cell)	B,C,R	250	2 weeks	3	750
6	Colon cancer	S,R	500	2 weeks	4	2000
7	Hypernephroma	S	500	2 weeks	4	2000
8	Hypernephroma	S,C	500	2 weeks	4	2000
9	Colon cancer	S	1000	2 weeks	4	4000
10	Lung (Adenocarcinoma)	B	1000	weekly	4	4000
11	Lung (Squamous)	B	2000	weekly	8	8000
12	Colon cancer	B,I	2000	weekly	8	8000
13	Lung (Squamous)	B	2000	weekly	3	3000

[1] S - Surgery; C - Chemotherapy; R - Radiation; I - Immunotherapy; B - Biopsy.

Table 2. Systemic side effects associated with intravenous CWS/TDM/oil

Dose level μg/M^2	Patient	Courses Received	Courses associated with			
			Nausea	Vomiting	Fever	Chills
100	1	4	0	0	0	0
	2	4	0	0	0	0
	3	4	0	0	0	0
250	4	4	0	0	0	0
	5	3	0	0	0	0
500	6	4	0	0	0	0
	7	4	0	0	0	0
	8	4	0	0	0	0
1000	9	4	0	0	0	0
	10	4	1	1	4	4
2000	11	8	1	0	8	8
	12	8	1	1	6	8
	13	3	0	0	3	3

after receiving the material. Intravenous meperidine hydrochloride (25 mg) was effective in alleviating the chills. Fever in patients receiving 1000 or 2000 μg/M^2 was maximum at four to six hours following injection. The maximum temperatures recorded for the 5 patients at those dose levels was 37.1 to 38.6°C.

The change in hematological, renal, and hepatic parameters are given in Table 3, which shows the mean change in each parameter occurring in patients treated at each dose level. The significance of the mean difference prior to and following treatment was determined where there was adequate data. In only one case was the mean change significant and that was for the BUN in patients receiving 100 μg/M^2. This single statistically significant change is felt to be due to chance.

Similar analysis of the protime, partial thromboplastin time, serum proteins, and serum immunoglobulins revealed no consistent or significant changes. Pulmonary function tests prior to and following therapy showed no consistent changes in lung volumes, diffusion capacity or blood gasses.

Efficacy

Of the total 13 patients, one response was seen. This response occurred in one of the two patients receiving a full eight weeks of therapy at 2000 μg/M^2. This patient (No. 11) had a newly diagnosed squamous cell carcinoma of the bronchus diagnosed on bronchoscopy (Figure 1) where it appeared as a cauliflower mass at a minor carina. The patient, due to poor general pulmonary status, was considered unresectable. The patient received 2000 μg/M^2 of therapy intravenously for 6 weeks after which he had a repeat bronchoscopy (Figure 2). At that time there was complete disappearance of the mass with only a nodularity remaining (Figure 2). The patient received a further two weeks of therapy after which no further therapy was given. A third bronchoscopy was performed two months after stopping treatment. A nodularity remained which on biopsy showed inflammation and squamous metaplasia.

In our prior intralesional immunotherapy studies, we observed (9, 10) that response occurred only in skin test positive patients. There is an insufficient response rate in the present study for correlation, however, the patient who did respond showed activity prior to therapy to PPD and Candida.

DISCUSSION

The current study was initiated as part of our investigation of the potential clinical use of surface attached purified and/or synthetic mycobacterial components. The potential applicability of

Table 3. Mean change in clinical parameters with therapy[1]

Dose level	HB	WBC ($x10^{-3}$)	Platelets ($x10^{-6}$)	BUN	CR	SGOT	ALK PTASE	LDH	GGT
100	0.76	-0.06	8.33	-3.30[2]	-0.03	0	-1.00	2.66	2.66
250	0.50	2.10	-3.00	4.00	-	-1.50	168.00	13.00	37.00
500	-0.60	0.90	-23.30	3.3	.50	1.00	8.00	20.30	43.00
1000	1.25	-0.35	29.00	0	-.05	1.00	-4.00	15.00	3.50
2000	-1.06	0.63	21.00	-1.6	-.00	1.00	-2.00	-2.30	-18.00

[1] Numbers indicate the average amount of increase or decrease of each clinical value for each patient group.

[2] Significant at the $p < 0.05$ level.

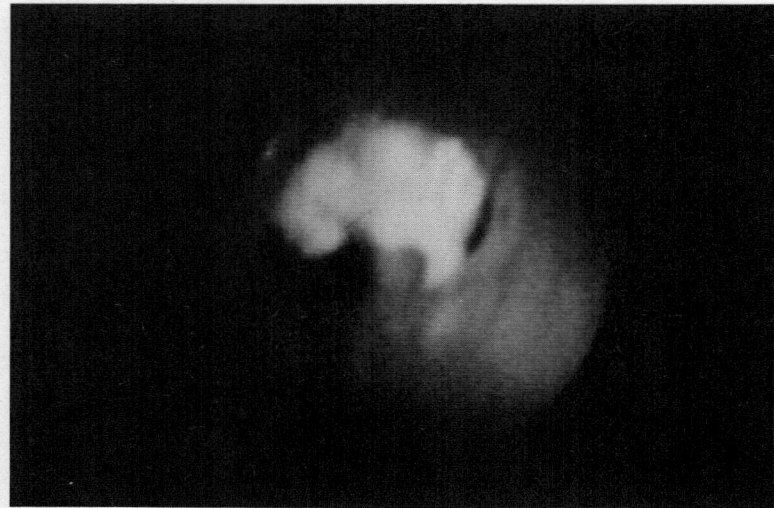

Fig. 1. Photographs obtained via bronchoscopy of an exophytic lesion in the left lower bronchus of patient No. 11. The lesion is at the subcarina of the left lower lobes.

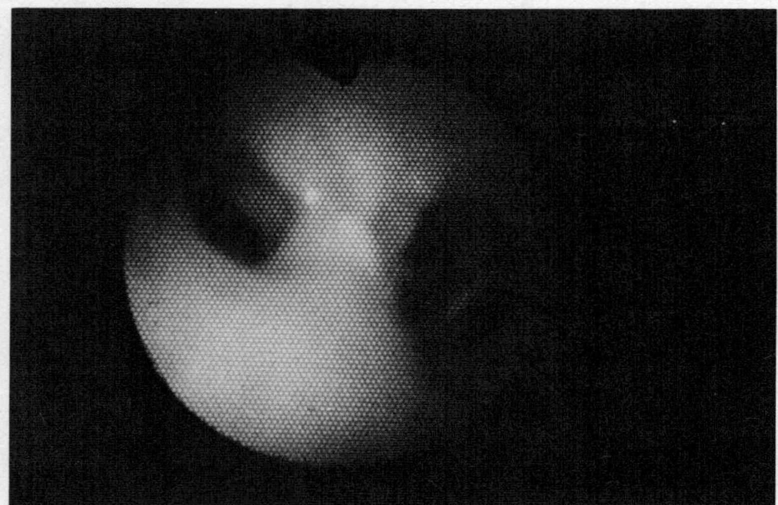

Fig. 2. Photographs obtained at same area as shown in Figure 1 following six weeks of intravenous CWS/TDM/Oil therapy. Repeat bronchoscopy and biopsy eight weeks later showed only inflammation cells and squamous metaplasia.

of intravenous therapy appeared especially suited to patients with hypernephroma, malignant melanoma, soft tissue sarcoma, and colon carcinoma as well as other malignancies which develop predominantly pulmonary and/or hepatic metastasis.

The rationale for intravenous mycobacterial therapy is several fold. First, oil attached CWS and TDM given intralesionally causes (14) tumor regression and tumor specific systemic immunity. One route by which to reach noncutaneous lesions and the regional lymphatics would be via the vascular system. Second, the intravenous use of another microbial adjuvant, Corynebacterium parvum, has demonstrated (15) activity against experimental pulmonary metastasis in mice and visceral metastasis in man. Finally, considerable interest exists in the development and systemic use of agents which can activate macrophages to become tumoricidal.

In the current study the CWS/TDM/Oil was well tolerated. The major side effects were chills and fever. There was no renal injury. There was no evidence of hepatic change. The finding of no apparent hepatic toxicity is in contrast (16) to our previous findings of changes in hepatic enzyme in patients receiving aqueous suspensions of intravenous CWS and TDM not attached to oil. The attachment of the components to a surface may lead to preferential lymphatic uptake, thus preventing hepatic toxicity and facilitating their immunological activity.

The current study demonstrated in a single patient that these materials are active given intravenously. In the guinea pig model, it is necessary (14) for the adjuvant to be given in the area of the tumor. Whether the important factor is proximity to a regional lymph node or association with tumor antigen, is unknown. The efficacy of the vaccine in the present patient may be due to its "embolization" in the tumor or to its uptake by regional lymph nodes.

The demonstration of a total response following a limited course of therapy in a patient with squamous cell carcinoma of the lung, among three lung cancer patients treated at that dose level is enticing. The early results warrant continued development and investigation of totally synthetic and/or highly purified active surface associated mycobacterial components as promising immunotherapeutic agents.

SUMMARY

The toxicity and immunological effects of suspensions of mycobacterial cell wall skeleton (CWS) and trehalose dimycolate (TDM) attached to oil droplets and given intravenously in doses of 100 to 200 μg/M^2 every one or two weeks was investigated. The major limiting side effect was fever and chills at a dose of 2 mg/M^2. There was no major hematopoietic, renal, hepatic toxicity, or pulmonary toxicity.

Intravenous therapy with CWS/TDM/Oil was associated with complete regression of a bronchial squamous cell arcinoma in one of three patients receiving 2000 μg/M^2 weekly. The continued development and clinical study of surface attached purified and/or synthetic microbial adjuvants is a promising area of investigation.

ACKNOWLEDGEMENT

Supported in part by NIH grant numbers CA25307, CA29597 and the Phi Beta Psi Sorority.

REFERENCES

1. Bast, R. C., B. Zbar, T. Boros, and H. G. Rapp. 1974. BCG and cancer. N. Engl. J. Med. 290: 1413-1419 and 1458-1468.

2. Aungst, C. W., J. E. Sokol, and B. V. Jager. 1975. Complications of BCG vaccination in neoplastic disease. Ann. Int. Med. 82: 666-669.

3. McKhann, C. F., C. G. Hendrickson, L. E. Spitler, A. Gunnarson, D. Bannerjee, and W. R. Nelson. 1975. Immunotherapy of melanoma with BCG - two fatalities following intralesional injection. Cancer 35: 514-520.

4. Florentin, I., R. Huchet, M. Bruley-Rosset, O. Halle-Pannenko and G. Mathe. 1976. Studies on the mechanism of action of BCG. Cancer Immunol. Immunother. 1: 31-39.

5. Gefford, M., and S. Orbach-Arbuoys. 1976. Enhancement of T suppressor activity in mice by high doses of BCG. Cancer Immunol. Immunother. 1: 41-45.

6. Bornstein, R. R., M. J. Mastrangelo, N. Sulit, D. Chee, J. W. Yarboro, L. Prehn, and R. J. Prehn. 1973. Immunotherapy of melanoma with intralesional BCG. Nat. Cancer Inst. Monog. 39: 213-215.

7. McLaughlin, C. A., S. M. Strain, W. D. Bickel, M. B. Goren, K. Azuma, K. Milner, J. L. Cantrell, and E. Ribi. 1978. Regression of line 10 hepatocellular carcinomas following treatment with water-soluble microbial extracts combined with trehalose or arabinose mycolates. Cancer Immunol. Immunother. 4: 61-68.

8. Milas, L., N. Hunter, and H. R. Withers. 1975. Combination of local irradiation with systemic applications of anaerobic corynebacterium in therapy of a murine fibrosarcoma. Cancer Res. 35: 1274-1277.

9. Vosika, G. J., J. Schmidtke, A. Goldman, E. Ribi, R. Parker, and G. R. Gray. 1979. Intralesional immunotherapy of malignant melanoma with mycobacterium smegmatis cell wall skeleton combined with trehalose dimycolate. Cancer 44: 495-503.

10. Vosika, G. J., J. Schmidtke, A. Goldman, E. Ribi, and G. R. Gray. 1979. Phase I-II study of intralesional immunotherapy with oil-attached mycobacterium smegmatis cell wall skeleton and trehalose dimycolate. Cancer Immunol. Immunother. 6: 135-142.

11. Halpern, B. (ed.). 1975. Corynebacterium parvum: Applications in experimental and clinical oncology. Plenum Press, New York.

12. Azuma, I., E. Ribi, T. J. Meyer, and B. Zbar. 1974. Biologically active components of mycobacterial cell walls. I. Isolation and composition of cell wall skeleton and component P3. J. Nat. Cancer Inst. 52: 95-101.

13. Gray, G. R., E. Ribi, D. Granger, R. Parker, I. Azuma, and K. Yamomoto. 1975. Immunotherapy of cancer: Tumor suppression and regression by cell walls of mycobacterium phlei attached to oil droplets. J. Nat. Cancer Inst. 55: 727-730.

14. Ribi, E., M. C. Milner, D. Granger, M. T. Kelly, K. Yamomoto, W. Brehmer, R. Parker, R. F. Smith, and S. M. Strain. 1976. Immunotherapy with non-viable microbial components. Ann. N. Y. Acad. Sci. 277: 228-238.

15. Israel, L., R. Edelstein, A. DePierre, and N. Dimitrov. 1975. Daily intravenous infusion of corynebacterium parvum in twenty patients with disseminated cancer. A preliminary report of clinical and biological findings. J. Nat. Cancer Inst. 55: 29-33.

16. Vosika, G. J., Schmidtke, A. Goldman, E. Ribi, R. Parker, and G. R. Gray. 1978. Local and systemic immunotherapy of human cancer with mycobacterial cell wall skeleton and trehalose dimycolate (P3), p. 33-51. In E. M. Hersh, M. A. Chirigos and M. J. Mastrangelo (eds.), Augmenting agents in cancer therapy. Raven Press, New York, N. Y.

IMMUNOMODULATING EFFECTS OF A SHORT-TERM ORAL TREATMENT WITH C 1821 IN UNTREATED CANCER PATIENTS: A CONTROLLED STUDY

J. M. Lang[2], A. Aleksijevic[2], C. Giron[1], S. Levy[2], A. Falkenrodt[2], S. Mayer[2], J. C. Stoclet[3] and F. Oberling[1]

Service des Maladies du Sang, Hopital de Hautepierre[1] Centre de Transfusion Sanguine[2], and UER des Sciences Pharmaceutiques[3], Strasbourg, France

INTRODUCTION

C 1821 is a purified glycoprotein extract from Klebsiella pneumoniae serotype 2 (Laboratories Cassenne and Centre de Recherche Roussel UCLAF, Paris, France). Both gel filtration chromatography and ultracentrifugation of C 1821 yield a single peak. Its molecular weight is about 350,000. Chemical analysis has been performed by J. Montreuil and B. Fournet (Laboratory of Biological Chemistry, University of Lille I, France) and the compound is now chemically fairly well defined (manuscript in preparation). It is thought to be a component of the bacterial outer membrane. C 1821 has been found to enhance immune responses in animals when given orally and to modulate assays of human lymphocyte functions when added in vitro (1). The oral route of administration may be safely used in humans, as shown by toxicity studies. To study the immunomodulating properties of C 1821 further we entered upon a controlled trial on changes of in vivo and in vitro immune parameters after short-term oral administration of C 1821 in untreated cancer patients. In this small series of patients, no significant modifications of peripheral blood natural killer (NK) activity and lymphocyte subpopulation distribution were observed both at the start of the trial when compared to normal controls, and at the end of the trial which could be attributed to C 1821. Therefore, we will limit this presentation to the effects of C 1821 on delayed cutaneous hypersensitivity (DCH) to recall antigens and lymphocyte cyclic nucleotide levels.

METHODS

Patients

Cancer patients were chosen for the present study because of frequent association with defective parameters of cell-mediated immunity and possible prognostic significance of their immune status. Only patients unlikely to show spontaneous recovery or increase of immune reactivity during the trial were selected. They were either untreated patients tested during evaluation of their cancer, or patients developing metastases following previous therapy, or patients with Hodgkin's disease in complete remission. Consecutive patients were alternately allocated to receive either C 1821 or placebo. Tablets were given at a single, uniform, daily dose of 4 mg each morning for 14 days without any associated treatment and in the absence of overt morbid association which could interfere with the results.

Skin Testing

DCH was assayed using a plastic disposable multipuncture device which simultaneously administers a battery of seven standardized glycerinated recall antigens (tuberculin, tetanus toxoid, diphtheria toxoid, streptococcus, candida, trichophyton and proteus antigens) and a glycerin solution as a negative control (Multitest system, Institut Mérieux, Lyon, France). Reported advantages of this system are standardization of test materials, uniformity between batches, easy quantitative evaluation of the reactions, and reproducibility on repeated applications (2). Skin testing was performed 48 h before and immediately after C 1821 or placebo treatment. Reactions were evaluated after 48 h by measuring two diameters of the induration. A mean diameter of 2 mm or more is considered positive with this system. For each individual a score was calculated, which was the sum of the mean diameters of all positive reactions (total score). Anergy is defined by the absence of any positive reactions (score 0). A score of 5 or less defines hypoergy. The Mann-Whitney test was performed to compare variations between study groups.

Peripheral Blood Lymphocyte Separation

Mononuclear cells were prepared by density sedimentation of defibrinated heparinized blood on Ficoll-Triosil, according to the method of Böyum (3) and washed three times in HBSS. Mononuclear cells were resuspended in RPMI 1640 supplemented with 10% heat-inactivated fetal calf serum (HIFCS) and incubated for 10 minutes at 37°C on a glass wool column. Nonadherent cells were eluted from the column with RPMI 1640 supplemented with 10% HIFCS which had been warmed to 37°C. The nonadherent population contained 98 ± 2% lymphocytes and 2 ± 2% monocytes. There was no significant loss of B lymphocytes as shown by membrane markers analysis. Lymphocyte suspensions were washed twice with RPMI 1640 and resuspended in 0.2 ml cold perchloric acid (PCA), rapidly frozen in liquid nitrogen and stored at $-20^{o}C$ until cyclic nucleotide assay.

Cyclic Nucleotide Assay

Cyclic AMP and cGMP were assayed according to the radioimmunoassay described by Cailla et al. (4, 5). This radioimmunoassay was performed by equilibrium dialysis between succinylated cellular cyclic nucleotides and ^{125}I-succinylated cyclic nucleotides against the corresponding specific anticyclic nucleotide antibody kindly provided by M. A. Delaage (Marseille-Luminy). Each dosage was done at least in duplicate.

C 1821 Dependent Lymphocyte cAMP Production In Vitro

Aliquots of cell suspensions containing 10^6 viable monocyte-depleted lymphocytes in 0.1 ml Krebs-Ringer-bicarbonate buffer with 10^{-5} M of the specific phosphodiesterase inhibitor isobutylmethylxanthine (IBMX) were introduced in round bottomed polypropylene tubes. The tubes were centrifuged 5 min. at 250 g and 4° C. Assays were started by addition of C 1821 in a volume of 0.1 ml Krebs-Ringer-bicarbonate buffer to give final concentrations ranging from 10^{-3} to 10^3 µg/10^6 lymphocytes. The tubes were incubated for 7 min. at $37^{o}C$ in humidified 5% CO_2 atmosphere. Supernatants were discarded and reactions stopped by addition of 0.2 ml ice cold PCA to cell pellets. Cells were immediately frozen in liquid nitrogen and stored at $-80^{o}C$ until cyclic nucleotide assay. Each measurement was done at least in duplicate.

RESULTS

Delayed Cutaneous Hypersensitivity (DCH)

Evolution of the multitest total score is given in Table 1 for the control group and in Table 2 for the C 1821 group. Nine patients were given placebo and eight received C 1821. The two groups were comparable in terms of diagnostic make-up, mean age, sex distribution, and multitest total score at the start (mean - 8.9 + 9.4 in the control group; 11.2 $\pm$ 8 in the C 1821 group). In the majority of the patients given placebo either the score did not change significantly, or there was marked diminution of the skin reactions probably related to underlying disease. A mean decrease of 2.7 was observed in this placebo group which was statistically not significant (Wilcoxon's test). In the C 1821 group DCH was clearly enhanced in five patients and in the whole group a mean enhancement of 8.5 in the total score was noted ($p < 0.05$, Wilcoxon's test). In spite of the small number of patients the difference between the two

Table 1. Evolution of delayed cutaneous hypersensitivity (Multitest total score in millimeters) in patients given placebo for 14 days

Age	Sex	Diagnosis	Status	Multitest total score Before	After
37	F	Hodgkin	Remission	4	8
25	F	Hodgkin II_B	Untreated	9	0
25	M	Hodgkin III_A	Untreated	30	16
33	M	Hodgkin I_A	Untreated	0	0
56	F	Lymphoma	Untreated	7	6
65	F	Lymphoma	Untreated	0	0
75	M	Lymphoma	Untreated	6	0
54	F	Lymphoma	Untreated	17.5	16
53	M	Solid tumor	Untreated	7	10

groups was statistically significant ($p < 0.02$) as shown by the Mann-Whitney test.

Lymphocyte Cyclic Nucleotides

Thirteen patients have been evaluated, five in the placebo group and eight in the C 1821 group. There was a statistically significant decrease of lymphocyte cAMP and cGMP basal levels in the patients compared to normal controls (data not shown). Basal levels of both cyclic nucleotides were relatively stable under placebo administration (Figures 1 and 2), whereas patients given C 1821 showed an increase of both cAMP and cGMP that seems more pronounced for cGMP (Figures 1 and 2). No statistical analysis was performed in view of the small number of patients in the placebo group.

C 1821 Dependent Lymphocyte cAMP Production In Vitro

Kinetic studies (data not presented) showed that cAMP levels in lymphocytes stimulated with C 1821 at the single dose of 0.1 $\mu g/10^6$ cells reached a maximum after 7 minutes of incubation at 37^oC. The concentration-effect relationships illustrated in Figures 3 and 4 were therefore studied 7 minutes after addition of C 1821.

Table 2. Evolution of delayed cutaneous hypersensitivity (Multitest total score in millimeters) in patients given C 1821 for 14 days

Age	Sex	Diagnosis	Status	Multitest total score	
				Before	After
37	F	Hodgkin	Remission	8	4
31	M	Hodgkin III_A	Untreated	6.5	8.5
55	M	Hodgkin II_B	Untreated	20	38
24	M	Hodgkin II_B	Untreated	7	14
60	M	Lymphoma	Untreated	26.5	42.5
69	F	Lymphoma	Untreated	4	27.5
70	F	Lymphoma	Untreated	5	10
61	F	Solid tumor	Metastasis	13	14

In normal human lymphocytes (Figure 3) the maximal effect of C 1821 was obtained with 500 $\mu g/10^6$ cells and represented about 2 to 3 times the control levels; the ED_{50} values were close to 100 $\mu g/10^6$

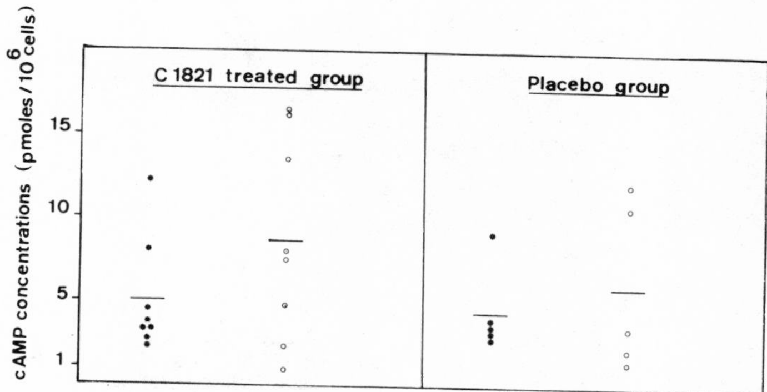

Fig. 1. Evolution of cAMP basal levels in lymphocytes from untreated cancer patients receiving either C 1821 or placebo for 14 days. The mean ± S.D. level of cAMP in lymphocytes from normal subjects is 6.6 ± 3.2 p moles/10^6 cells. (*), before treatment; (0) after treatment.

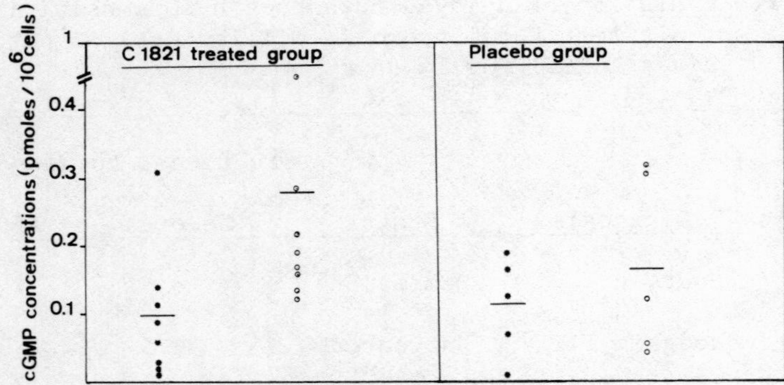

Fig. 2. Evolution of cGMP basal levels in lymphocytes from untreated cancer patients receiving either C 1821 or placebo for 14 days. The mean $\pm$ S.D. level of cGMP in lymphocytes from normal subjects is 0.18 $\pm$ 0.11 pmoles/10^6 cells. (*), before treatment; (0) after treatment.

cells indicating that lymphocytes from healthy donors present a poor sensitivity to C 1821 stimulation. Cancer patient lymphocytes (Figure 4) showed two types of responses. The left panel of Figure 4 demonstrates that lymphocytes from two patients showed classical S-shaped concentration-effect curves, the maximal effect of C 1821 was obtained with 100 µg/10^6 cells and represented about 2 to 3 times the control levels with an ED_{50} value close to 10µg/10^6 cells. The

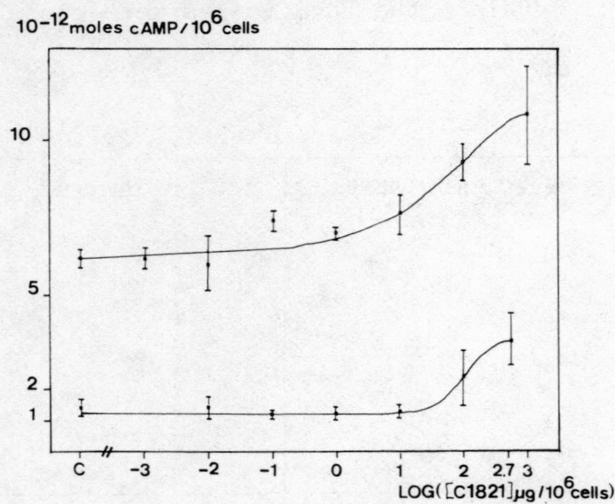

Fig. 3. The in vitro effect of varying doses of C 1821 on cAMP levels of cultured lymphocytes from two normal subjects. "C" refers to control (without C1821) levels. Each data point is the mean of three determinations.

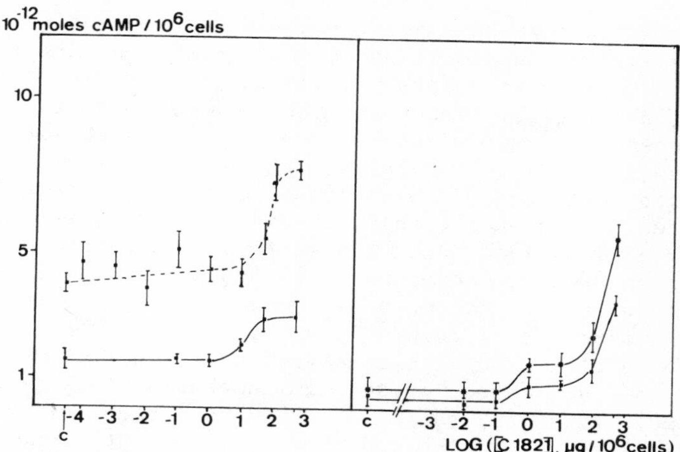

Fig. 4. Experiment similar to that reported in Figure 3 utilizing lymphocytes from four cancer patients. The left panel shows S-shaped concentration curves obtained with lymphocytes from two cancer patients. The right panel shows a variation in the shape of the concentration curves from two other cancer patients.

right panel shows nonclassical concentration-effect curves obtained with lymphocytes from two other cancer patients. After a first increase of cAMP concentrations obtained with 1 μg/10^6 cells and representing about 2-3 times the initial levels with an ED_{50} value close to 0.5 μg/10^6 cells, a second stimulation of cAMP production occurred at C 1821 concentrations ranging between 10 and 10^3 μg/10^6 cells and representing 10 times the control values. Higher concentrations could not be tested due to problems of C 1821 solubility.

DISCUSSION

Cancer may be associated with impaired cell-mediated immunity, the degree and frequency varying widely depending upon site of tumor, histologic types, clinical stage, and other factors (6 - 12). Since some defective general parameters of cell-mediated immunity have been shown to be of prognostic significance in cancer (7, 8, 10, 11), immunorestoration may soon become a significant part of therapeutic strategies, even at an early phase of the treatment.

The present trial clearly indicates that C 1821 given for 14 days significantly increases DCH in cancer patients before any anticancer treatment in spite of active disease and even in patients with untreated Hodgkin's disease. Controlled trial of DCH enhancement with an immunomodulatory drug given orally for a short period of time has been rather limited. A randomized study in a cancer population unresponsive to dinitrocholobenzene (DNCB) failed to show any significant increase of the conversion rate from DNCB-negative to DNCB-positive with levamisole given during DNCB challenge (13). At the present symposium G. Renoux et al. reported the dose-dependent positive results we have obtained with diethyldithiocarbamate (DTC) given orally, once a week for four weeks, in children with unmaintained remission of different types of malignant diseases (see Renoux et al, this volume). Clearly, serial testing of DCH to recall antigens and studies involving sensitization to the neoantigen DNCB in cancer patients provide clinical immunopharmacology with an apparently simple and easy assay to screen for alleged immunomodulating agents in vivo, with the reservation of an appropriate control group. Lymphocyte cyclic nucleotide determinations were included in the present immunopharmacology trial for two main reasons. First, there is increasing evidence for an important regulatory influence of cAMP and cGMP on lymphocyte functions. The differences between changes in cAMP and cGMP during lymphocyte activation and the modulating effects of added exogenous cyclic nucleotides or agents which selectively increase intracellular levels of cAMP or cGMP have suggested an inhibitory role for cAMP whereas cGMP would be involved in positive regulation (14-17). Second, it has been recently shown in our laboratory that lymphocytes from patients with untreated Hodgkin's disease (18) and to a lesser degree those with other lymphomas (manuscript in preparation) exhibited a profound defect of lymphocyte cAMP and cGMP. From the small number of patients in this trial it would appear that in patients given C 1821 resting levels of lymphocyte cAMP and particularly cGMP increased to normal and even supra normal concentrations. Unfortunately we did not look yet for functional correlations. To study further the effects of C 1821 on lymphocyte cyclic nucleotides we incubated control and patient lymphocytes with increasing doses of C 1821 in vitro. In contrast with the data obtained in vivo, cGMP was not affected whereas a dose-dependent increase of cAMP was observed in both control and patient lymphocytes. The difference in ED_{50} concentrations of C 1821 indicates that lymphocytes from the patients are more sensitive to the compound than normal lymphocytes. The mechanism of action of C 1821 on the metabolism of cAMP is only speculative. A decreased activity of the catabolizing enzyme phosphodiesterase is unlikely since the study was performed in presence of the phosphodiesterase inhibitor IBMX. Increased synthesis of cAMP by adenylate cyclase is more likely. As to the secondary marked increase of cAMP observed in some patients with the highest concentrations of C 1821 it is also unexplained. These in vitro data have to be considered preliminary.

SUMMARY

C 1821 is a purified glycoprotein extract from _Klebsiella pneumoniae_ serotype 2 with a molecular weight of about 350,000. It enhances immune responses in animals when given orally and the oral route of administration is devoided of any toxicity even in humans. The present controlled trial showed that C 1821 given per os at the single daily dose of 4 mg for 14 days in untreated cancer patients (mostly lymphomas) significantly enhanced delayed cutaneous hypersensitivity to recall antigens using the Multitest system (7 antigens). It also increased basal levels of lymphocyte cAMP and particularly of cGMP which were decreased in these patients. When incubated in vitro with lymphocytes from either normal controls or patients, C 1821 showed a dose-dependent stimulation of cAMP synthesis which was more pronounced in patients than in controls.

REFERENCES

1. Griscelli, C., B. Grospierre, J. Montreuil, B. Fournet, G. Bruvier, J. M. Lang, C. Marchiani, R. Zalisz, and R. Edelstein. 1982. Immunomodulation by glycoprotein fractions isolated from klebsiella pneumoniae. In Y. Yamamura and S. Kotani (eds). Immunomodulation by microbial products and related synthetic compounds. Excerpta Medica, Amsterdam.

2. Kniker, W. T., M. D. Anderson, and M. Roumiantzeff. 1979. The Multitest system: A standardized approach to evaluation of delayed hypersensitivity and cell-mediated immunity. Ann. Allergy 43: 73.

3. Böyum, A. 1968. Isolation of leucocytes from human blood. Scand. J. Clin. Lab. Invest. 21 (supple. 97): 1.

4. Cailla, H. L., M. S. Racine-Weisbuch, and M. A. Delaage. 1973. Adenosine 3', 5' - cyclic monophosphate assay at 10^{-15} mole level. Anal. Biochem. 56: 394.

5. Cailla, H. L., C. T. Vannier, and M. A. Delaage. 1976. Guanosine 3', 5' - cyclic monophosphate assay at 10^{-15} mole level. Anal. Biochem. 70: 195.

6. Catalona, W. J., W. F. Sample, and P. B. Chretien. 1973. Lymphocyte reactivity in cancer patients: Correlation with tumor histology and clinical stage. Cancer 31: 65.

7. Eilber, F. R., J. A. Nizze, and D. L. Morton. 1975. Sequential evaluation of general immune competence in cancer patients: Correlation with clinical course. Cancer 35: 660.

8. Lee, Y. T. N., F. C. Sparks, F. R. Eilber, and D. L. Morton. 1975. Delayed cutaneous hypersensitivity and peripheral lymphocyte counts in patients with advanced cancer. Cancer 35: 748.

9. Lichtenstein, A., J. Zighelboim, F. Dorey, S. Brossman, J. L. Fahey. 1980. Comparison of immune derangements in patients with different malignancies. Cancer 45: 2090.

10. Mujacic, H., M. Deskovic, B. Malenica, M. Bistrovic, P. Nola, and J. Krusic. 1980. The significance of tuberculin immunity testing in cancer patients. Cell. Mol. Biol. 26: 111.

11. Pinsky, C. M., H. Wanebo, V. Mike, and H. Oettgen. 1976. Delayed cutaneous hypersensitivity reactions and prognosis in patients with cancer. Ann. N. Y. Acad. Sci. 276: 407.

12. Teasdale, C., L. E. Hughes, R. H. Whitehead, and R. G. Newcomb. 1979. Factors affecting pretreatment immune competence in cancer patients. I. The effects of age, sex, and ill health. II. The corrected effects of malignant disease. Cancer Immunol. Immunother. 6: 89.

13. Hirshaut, Y., C. M. Pinsky, I. Frydecka, H. J. Wanebo, S. Passe, V. Mike, and H. F. Oettgen. 1980. Effect of short-term levamisole therapy on delayed hypersensitivity. Cancer 45: 362.

14. Diamantstein, T., and A. Ulma. 1975. The antagonistic action of cyclic GMP and cyclic AMP on proliferation of B and T lymphocytes. Immunology 28: 113.

15. Hadden, J. W. 1977. Cyclic nucleotides in lymphocyte proliferation and differentiation. In R. A. Good and S. B. Day, (eds.), Comprehensive immunology 3. Plenum Medical Book Company, New York.

16. Watson, J. 1977. Involvement of cyclic nucleotides as intracellular mediators in the induction of antibody synthesis. In R. A. Good and S. B. Day, (eds.), Comprehensive immunology 3. Plenum Medical Book Company, New York

17. Strom, T. B., Lundin, A. P. and C. B. Carpenter. 1977. The role of cyclic nucleotides in lymphocyte activation and function. Prog. Clin. Immunol. 3: 115.

18. Aleksijevic, A., J. M. Lang, C. Giron, J. C. Stoclet, S. Mayer and F. Oberling. Alterations of peripheral blood lymphocyte cyclic AMP and cyclic GMP in untreated patients with Hodgkin's disease. Clin. Immunol. Immunopathol. (in press).

CLINICAL EFFICACY OF LENTINAN ON NEOPLASTIC DISEASES

Tetsuo Taguchi[1], Hisashi Furue[2], Tadashi Kimura[3], Tatsuhei Kondo[4], Takao Hattori[5] and Nobuya Ogawa[6]

Research Institute for Microbial Diseases, Osaka University, Osaka[1]; Department of Internal Medicine, Teikyo University, Tokyo[2]; Department of Surgery, National Medical Center Tokyo Hospital, Tokyo[3]; IInd Deparment of Surgery, Nagoya University, Nagoya[4]; Department of Surgery, Research Institute for Nuclear Medicine and Biology, Hiroshima University, Hiroshima[5]; and Department of Pharmacology, Ehime University, Matsuyama[6], Japan

INTRODUCTION

Lentinan, a β-(1-3)-glucan with some β-(1-6)-gluco-pyranoside branchings, has been extracted and purified from <u>Lentinus edodes</u> a most popular edible mushroom in Japan. This substance has been shown to act as an immunostimulating agent through host defense mechanisms as reported by Chihara et al (1, 2). Lentinan exerts it's antitumor activity on both syngeneic and spontaneous tumors. The cellular mechanisms of antitumor activity have been clarified by Hamuro et al (3), in that lentinan appears to stimulate host defense mechanisms to induce cytotoxic T cells, natural cytotoxicity and/or augmented macrophages against tumor cells. This suggests that lentinan may be effective for patients with malignant diseases. Based on the results of Phase I and II clinical trials conducted by Taguchi et al (4), the administration conditions for lentinan have been determined to be intravenous administration at doses of 0.5 to 1.0 mg/person/day once or twice a week in combination with chemotherapeutic agents for patients with advanced or recurrent cancer. In order to clarify the clinical efficacy of lentinan administration a Phase III randomized control trial has been conducted on patients with advanced or recurrent gastric or colorectal cancer.

METHODS

As control therapy, the following two kinds of chemotherapies were employed. One was combined administration of mitomycin C plus 5-fluorouracil (MF) and the other was a single administration of tegafur (FT). Mitomycin C (i.v.) and 5FU (i.v. or p.o.) were administered at doses of 4 and 500 mg/person/day, respectively. The schedule for this was twice a week for the first 2 weeks and once a week thereafter. Tegafur (p.o., i.v., or suppository), as a rule, was administered at doses of 600 mg/person/day everyday, however, the dosage of FT was varied at times according to the clinical conditions of the patient. Lentinan was administered at doses of either 1 mg/person/day twice a week or 2 mg/person/day once a week intravenously in combination with either MF or FT. The lentinan formulation is lyophilized lentinan (1 mg) containing 100 mg of mannitol and 2 mg of dextran-40. The eligibility conditions of patients entered into the trial were the following: those with advanced or recurrent gastric or colorectal cancer proven with a histopathological diagnosis; those without intense disturbances in renal, hepatic and/or bone marrow functions, and having no serious complications; those having more than 4 weeks therapy-free interval after prior treatment and presenting no residual influences; and those younger than 81 years old. Evaluations of clinical efficacy of lentinan administration were prolongation effect, antitumor effect, improvement of host immune response and side effects. Life span prolongation was assessed by Kaplan-Meier's survival curve with statistical examination of generalized Wilcoxon's test. Effective antitumor effect was defined as more than 50% regression of tumor size over four weeks.

RESULTS AND DISCUSSIONS

Eligible Patients

Table 1 shows that for patients with gastric cancer, sixty cases were considered eligible in the MF group, 76 cases in the combined treatment group of MF with lentinan, 72 cases in FT group and 77 cases in the combined treatment group of FT with lentinan. In colorectal cancer patients, 17 cases were eligible in the FT group while 23 cases were eligible in the combined treatment of FT with lentinan.

Table 2 shows that there was no significant bias observed between the FT group and combined treatment group (FT with lentinan) in terms of stratification of sex, age and Zubrod's performance status. However, a slight bias was observed between the MF group and the combination treatment group (MF with lentinan) in terms of stratification of performance status.

Table 1. Number of eligible cases entered into the trial

Types of Cancer \ Therapies	MF	MF+LNT	FT	FT+LNT
Gastric Cancer	Cases 60	Cases 76	Cases 72	Cases 77
Colo-rectal Cancer	——	——	17	23

Life Span Prolongation Effect

Significant ($p < 0.05$ and $p < 0.01$) life span prolongation was observed in patients with advanced or recurrent gastric cancer when treatment combinations of lentinan with MF or FT were employed (Figure 1). In patients with advanced or recurrent colorectal cancer, significant life span prolongation was indicated by combination treatment of lentinan with FT (Figure 2). Life span prolongation effects corresponding to the stratification of performance status are shown in Figure 3 and Figure 4. The combined treatment of lentinan with FT (Figure 4) significantly ($p < 0.05$) prolonged the life span of patients with advanced or recurrent gastric cancer in terms of stratification of every performance status (p.s. 1, 2, 3). In treatment combinations of lentinan with MF, however, a significant ($p < 0.05$) life prolongation effect was observed only in the stratification of performance status 3 (Figure 3).

Table 2. Characteristics of patients.

	Gastric Cancer				Colo-rectal Cancer	
	MF	MF+LNT	FT	FT+LNT	FT	FT+LNT
Male/Female	44/16	47/29	52/20	49/28	10/7	10/13
	(P=0.22)		(P=0.34)		(P=0.52)	
Age						
<30	2	3	1	1	1	0
30~50	12	13	13	16	1	5
50~70	38	46	35	40	12	14
70~80	8	14	23	20	3	4
	(P=0.34)		(P=0.31)		(P=0.23)	
Zubrod's Performance Status						
0	3	1	6	5	1	2
1	9	16	12	15	7	6
2	22	38	21	27	6	9
3	25	20	31	30	3	6
4	1	1	2	0	0	0
	(P=0.17)		(P=0.34)		(P=0.49)	

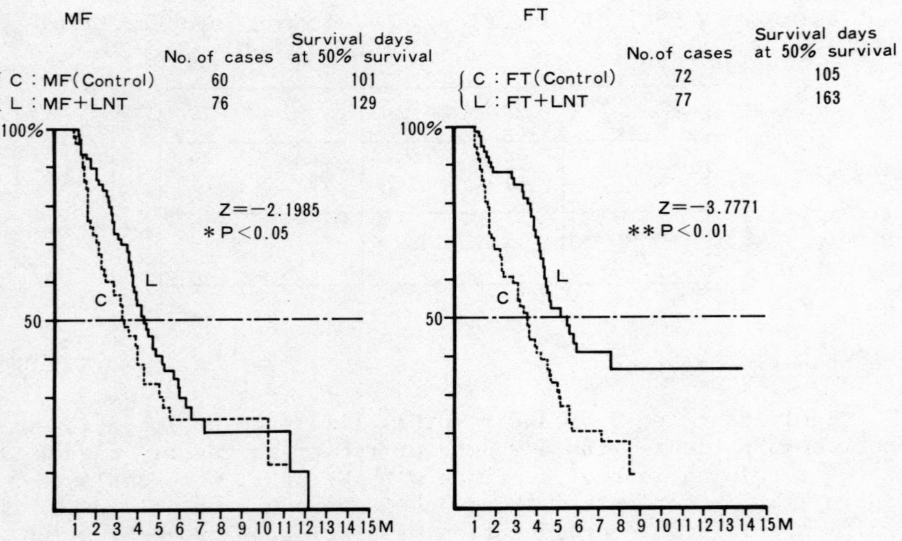

Fig. 1. Effect of lentinan (LNT) on survival curve

Antitumor Effect

The combined administration of lentinan with MF or FT resulted in effective antitumor activity (Table 3). The combined administration of lentinan with FT in gastric cancer patients, in particular, resulted in remarkable antitumor effects with statistical significance of ($p < 0.05$).

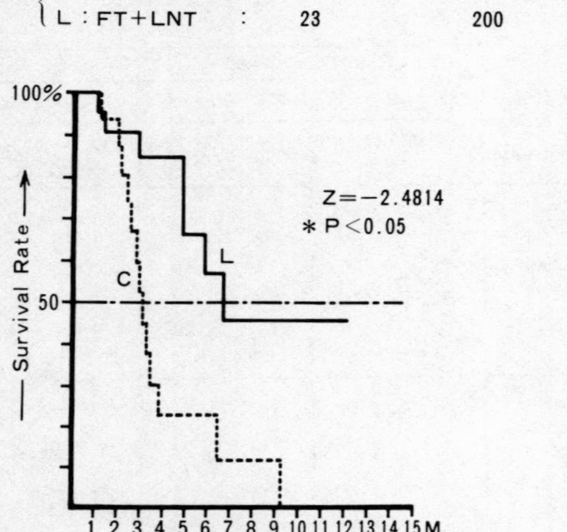

Fig. 2. Effect of lentinan (LNT) on survival curve in patients with advanced or recurrent colorectal cancer.

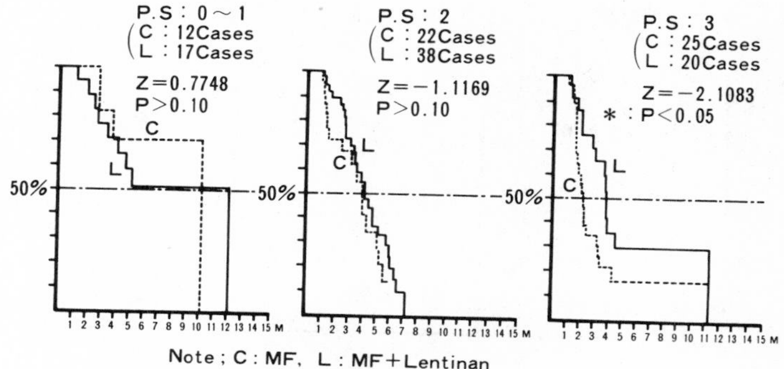

Fig. 3. Life span prolongation effect of lentinan in combination treatment with MF corresponding to the stratification of Zubrod's performance status (p.s.) on patients with gastric cancer

Improvement Of Host Immune Response

The evaluation of host immune responsiveness was examined employing PPD skin tests (Figure 5) and peripheral blood lymphocyte counts (Figure 6) as immunoparameters. These studies indicated

Table 3. Effect of lentinan (LNT) on regression of solid tumor in patients with measurable or evaluable lesions.

	Therapies	A No. of cases	B No. of PR or CR cases	Rate of positive response $\frac{B}{A} \times 100(\%)$	Statistical Examination (Fisher's test)
Gastric Cancer	MF	39	2	5.1	P=0.4585
	MF+LNT	52	6	11.7	
	FT	55	1	1.8	*P=0.0114
	FT+LNT	48	8	16.3	
Colo-rectal Cancer	FT	11	0	0	P=0.4923
	FT+LNT	15	2	13.3	

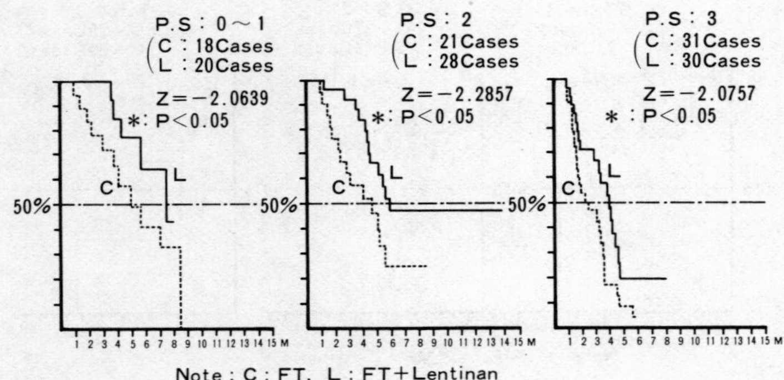

Fig. 4. Life span prolongation effect of lentinan in combination treatment with FT corresponding to the stratification of Zubrod's performance status (p.s.) on patients with gastric cancer.

that the combined treatment of lentinan with FT improved host immunoparameters compared to FT only.

Side Effects

A total of 18 cases (13 patients) displayed side effects associated with lentinan administration. These included, a feeling of heaviness in the chest (4 cases), nausea and vomiting (3 cases), and so on. These side effects were similar to those experienced in Phase I and Phase II studies and every side effect was transitory and not serious.

CONCLUSION

These results have indicated that lentinan should be effective for patients with advanced or recurrent gastric or colorectal

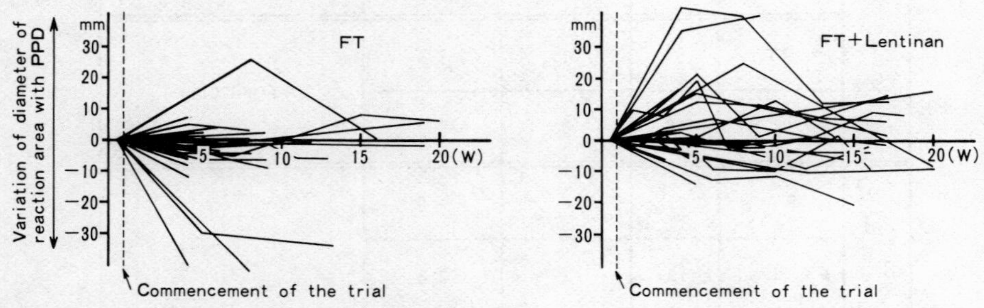

Fig. 5. Variation of diameter of reaction area with PPD skin test (PPD).

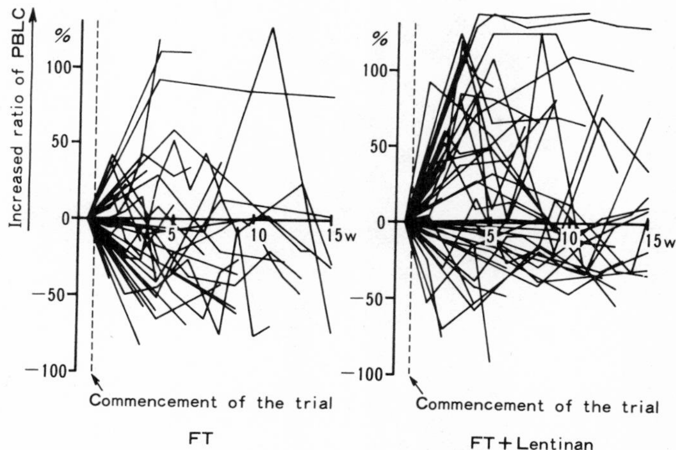

Fig. 6. Variation of peripheral blood lymphocyte counts (PBLC)

cancer as an immunostimulating agent in combination with MF or FT.

REFERENCES

1. Chihara, G., Y. Y. Maeda, J. Hamuro, T. Sasaki, and F. Fukuoka. 1969. Inhibition of mouse sarcoma 180 by the polysaccharides from Lentinus edodes (Berk). Sing. Nature 222: 687-688.

2. Maeda, Y. Y., J. Hamuro, Y. Yamada, K. Ishimura and G. Chihara. The nature of immunopotentiation by the antitumor polysaccharide Lentinan and the significance of biogenic amines in its action, p. 259. In G. E. W. Solstenholme and J. Knight (eds.), Immunopotentiation. Chiba Foundation Symposium, 18, Excerpta Medica, Amsterdam.

3. Hamuro, J., and G. Chihara. 1982. Chapter 29. In A. Szentivanyi and J. R. Battisto (eds.), A comprehensive treatise. Plenum Press, New York.

4. Taguchi, T., T. Aoki, H. Furue, and H. Mazima. Phase I and Phase II studies of lentinan. In T. Aoki, I. Urushizaki and E. Tsubura (eds.), Manipulation of host defense mechanisms. Excerpta Medica, Amsterdam.

PRECLINICAL EVALUATION OF LENTINAN IN ANIMAL MODELS

Goro Chihara

National Cancer Center Research Institute, Tokyo, 104-Japan

INTRODUCTION

Lentinan obtained from the fruit-body of *Lentinus edodes*, the most popular edible mushroom in Japan, is a fully purified β-1,6;β-1,3-D-glucan, and its physicochemical properties are strictly characterized (1-3). This polysaccharide has prominent antitumor activity in syngeneic and even autologous hosts, and its immunopharmacological characteristics are well defined as T-cell oriented immunopotentiators different from the well-known immunostimulants such as BCG, *C. parvum*, LPS or levamisole. Lentinan appears to represent an unique class of immunological adjuvant and has only little toxic side effects. Therefore, lentinan is worth considering as one of the most useful immunopotentiators for cancer patients, and this article concerns preclinical evaluation of lentinan in experimental and animal models for cancer immunotherapy in humans.

ANTITUMOR ACTIVITY OF LENTINAN

Lentinan has marked antitumor activity against various kinds of tumors in syngeneic and even autochthonous hosts as well as allogeneic hosts, and prevents chemical and viral carcinogenesis, as shown in Table 1. Several interesting characteristics have been observed in the antitumor action of lentinan. First, lentinan does not show any direct cytotoxicity against tumor cells and its antitumor action is host-mediated. Second, there exists an interesting phenomenon of optimal dose in administration of lentinan. A higher dose of lentinan administration does not show any antitumor effect and tumor grows as in that of control mice. This phenomenon of optimal dose is also observed in various immune responses to lentinan. Finally, the antitumor effect of lentinan differs among

Table 1. Antitumor effect of lentinan in syngeneic hosts and its prevention of chemical and viral carcinogenesis

Tumors*	Host	Dose**	Timing***	Inhibition**** Ratio(%)	References
Syngeneic tumors:					
A/Ph,MC,S1 sarcoma	A/PH(A/J)	1 x 10 (i.p.)	1 to 11	100	(14)
P-815 mastocytoma	DBA/2	5 x 4 (i.v.)	8,10,15,17	82	(46)
L-5178Y lymphoma	DBA/2	10 x 3 (i.v.)	7,14,21	89	(46)
MM-46 carcinoma	C3H/He	5 x 1 (i.v.)	13,15	100	(46)
MM-102 carcinoma	C3H/He	10 x 1 (i.v.)	7	60	(46)
Lewis lung cancer	C57BL/6	1 x 6 (i.p.)	1 to 7	59	(13)
Prevention of carcinogenesis:					
MC-induced	SWM/Ms	1 x 10 (i.p.)	21 to 31	83 → 33%+	(13)
Adenovirus-induced	C3H/He	10 x 3 (i.p.)	14,16,18	79 → 40%++	(19)

* All tumors are solid form implanted subcutaneously.

** mg/kg x days.

*** Days of lentinan administration after tumor (or MC, Ad) inoculation.

**** Tumor inhibition ratio = $\frac{C - T}{T} \times 100$; (C = average tumor weight of control mice, T = that of lentinan treated mice).

\+ Determination at 30 weeks after MC-inoculation.

++ Determination at 90 days after Adenovirus type-12 inoculation.

various strains of mice. A/J, DBA/2, SWM/Ms or CD-1/ICR mice are high responders and BALB/c or CBA mice are low responders to lentinan action, and C3H/HeN or C57BL/6 mice are medium. Using suitable mice with a suitable dose and strictly planned timing of lentinan administration, lentinan is very effective to many kinds of cancer, even autologous, in experimental animal models. For example, lentinan regresses completely 3-methylcholanthrene-induced A/Ph.MC. S1-fibrosarcoma in high responder A/Ph(A/J) syngeneic host at a dose of 1 mg/kg administered intraperitoneally for ten days (4). Lentinan, however, has no effect against syngeneic Meth-A fibrosarcoma transplanted in low responder BALB/c mice.

As shown in Table 1, lentinan inhibits the growth of MM-46 and MM-102 carcinoma, L-5178Y and EL-4 lymphoma, P-815 mastocytoma and Lewis lung cancer in syngeneic hosts without any combination therapy when it is administered to mice with suitable timing (3). Lentinan is also effective against 3-methylcholanthrene (MC)-induced primary tumor in combination therapy with cyclophosphamide (CY) (5). When the tumor induced by MC has attained a diameter of about 8 mm, 100 mg/kg of CY is administered, and 1 mg/kg of lentinan is injected i.p. once a day for twenty days from three weeks after CY injection. This results in a prolongation of survival time of greater than 200% ($p < 0.01$) compared with control C3H/HeN mice. Such a prolongation of survival time is not observed when lentinan is given either before cyclophosphamide or at the same time.

Lentinan is able to prevent carcinogenesis. When 1 mg/kg of lentinan is administered i.p. once a day for ten days beginning three weeks after MC inoculation in SWM/Ms mice, the incidence of tumor is about 30% compared with 83% in the control mice. Lentinan also prevents viral oncogenesis by adenovirus Type-12(Ad-12) in C3H/He mice. When infected with 1×10^7 $TCID_{50}$ of Ad-12 at birth, the incidence of tumor in this strain of mice is about 80% compared to only 40% in the mice treated with 10 mg/kg of lentinan on 14, 16 and 18 days after Ad-12 infection (6).

Lentinan does not appear to merely stimulate a foreign graft rejection, because lentinan has prominent antitumor effects in syngeneic and autochthonous host-tumor relationships.

INCREASE OF HOST RESISTANCE BY LENTINAN TO VARIOUS INFECTIONS

Lentinan enhances resistance of the host to various bacterial, viral and parasitic infections. These results suggest that lentinan may be effective against various infections frequently observed among immunosuppressed cancer patients, and against obstinate chronic infections. Kanai and Kondo (7) reported a relapse-preventing activity of lentinan administered after termination of chemotherapy with streptomycin, isoniazid and rifampin in experimental tuberculosis in mice. The later multiplication of latent bacilli in lung has been strongly reduced by lentinan treatment during the post-chemotherapy period. Lentinan also potentiates host resistance to infection with _Listeria monocytogenes_, _Streptococcus pneumoniae_, and _Klebsiella pneumoniae_, and prolongs survival time of the infected mice.

Lentinan is effective against various viral infections (8). Of mice infected with VSV-encephalitis virus, about 100% of mice live after lentinan treatment, while 80% of control mice inoculated with this virus die after 2 weeks. Lentinan is also effective in infection with Abelson virus in that it prolonged the survival of infected animals.

Lentinan potentiates lung granuloma formation against the eggs of _Shistosoma mansoni_ and _Shistosoma japonicum_, or antigen-coated polyacrylamide beads (9). Liver granulomas in cercariae-induced _S. mansoni_ infection are augmented up to 8-fold in volume by lentinan treatment. Lentinan-potentiated granulomas have shown a distinct histopathologic picture characterized by frequent, extensive central necrosis. These phenomena are not observed in nude mice.

IMMUNOLOGICAL CHARACTERISTICS OF LENTINAN

Potentiation of host defense mechanisms by lentinan consists of three kinds of pathways in the mode of action. That is: 1) helper T cell oriented immunopotentiation, 2) complement-macrophage mediated nonspecific immunopotentiation, and 3) nonimmunological potentiation of host defense mechanisms.

T cell Oriented Specific Immunopotentiation

One of the distinct characteristics of lentinan is to act as a T cell immune adjuvant (3). Antitumor activity of lentinan does not appear in neonatal thymectomized mice or in nude mice, and is markedly decreased by the administration of antilymphocyte serum. These results clearly support the concept that the antitumor effect of lentinan requires an intact immunocompetent T cell compartment and that the activity is mediated through thymus dependent immune mechanisms. In particular, lentinan appears to augment or restore helper T cell functions to produce humoral and cell-mediated immune responses in normal and tumor bearing mice. We have found transitory increases of several kinds of serum protein components after in vivo application of lentinan. One of the increased serum factors is functionally assigned as colony stimulating factor (CSF). Upon in vitro incubation of nylon column purified splenic T cells with lentinan CSF is released into supernatants in amounts five times larger than control. This produced CSF possibly acts on immune regulatory macrophages, resulting in augmented production of Interleukin-1, which can activate helper T cell function. This may be the first step of immunopotentiation by lentinan. On the other hand, augmented IL-1 production was also observed when peritoneal macrophages were incubated in vitro with lentinan.

Lentinan augments the reactivity of precursor effector lymphoid cells responding to several kinds of lymphokines, such as Interleukin-2, NK cell activating factor, or macrophage activating factor produced by activated helper T cells after specific immune recognition of target cells. This results in the augmented generation of cytotoxic T lymphocytes, natural killer cells, activated macrophages, or humoral antibody production.

Kitagawa et al. (10) revealed that mice pretreated with cell-free cancerous ascitic fluid were selectively depressed in terms of helper T cell activity for a hapten-carrier antigen. Lentinan was an excellent restorer of helper T cell function, having the ability to restore such suppressed immune response to normal state.

Lentinan markedly increases the generation of cytotoxic T lymphocytes (CTL) to alloantigen or haptenated syngeneic tumor cells both in vitro and in vivo. Hamuro et al. (3) reported that responder CBA spleen cells(H-2^k) and irradiated stimulator spleen cells(H-2^d) from BALB/c when mixed and cultured for 5 days resulted in the destruction of mastocytoma P-815 target cells(H-2^d) labelled with ^{51}Cr. This activity was increased 25 times when lentinan was added to the culture medium. In a syngeneic tumor bearing system such as P-815 mastocytoma-DBA/2, alloreactive killer cells generated from thymocytes is markedly suppressed even in the presence of IL-2. This generation, however, was restored to the level of normal mice by the administration of lentinan, and the generation of killer cells from splenocytes was also restored from null to around 40%. Furthermore, spleen cells harvested from syngeneic tumor-bearing mice (P-815-DBA/2) receiving triple i.p. injections of 10 mg/kg of lentinan at two weeks after P-815 transplantation were able to generate significant levels of anti-syngeneic P-815 tumor killer cells in the presence of IL-2. Lentinan is the first adjuvant that has been proven to increase cytotoxic T lymphocyte responses in vivo.

Concerning NK cells, lentinan does not activate these cells in vitro, in contrast to Poly I:C, polyanions, _C. parvum_ and other immunostimulants. In vivo, however, lentinan can augment NK cell activity in spleen when administered into high-responder C3H/HeN mice, but can not when administered in BALB/c mice. Augmented NK cell generation is also observed when lentinan-treated spleen cells are cultured with interferon inducer Poly I:C or with IL-2. Lentinan might stimulate NK cells via T cell dependent pathway, but not via macrophages or interferons (3).

Complement-Macrophage Mediated Nonspecific Immunopotentiation

On the other hand, the antitumor effect of lentinan is blocked by the antimacrophage agents such as carrageenan or silica. Therefore, the antitumor effect of lentinan requires intact immunocompetent macrophage compartment. Lentinan, nevertheless, does not enhance phagocytic activity of macrophage in vitro or in vivo. *C. parvum*, BCG or zymosan all accelerate phagocytic activity and they are said to be stimulants of reticuloendothelial system. Lentinan should not be called an RES stimulant in this sense (11).

Besides phagocytic function, macrophages have complicated functions such as antigen presenting function, various secretive functions or cytotoxic function in host defense mechanisms. Lentinan enhances markedly the cytotoxic activity of peritoneal exudate cells against tumor cell in vivo, but not in vitro (12). The peritoneal macrophages from CBA mice 10 days after triple injections of 10 mg/kg of lentinan display 76% lysis against mastocytoma P-815, while the lysis in the control mice is only 2.5%. This activation of cytotoxicity of macrophages is considered to be a result of C3 splitting activity of lentinan. Lentinan has the ability to split C3 into C3a and C3b, which can be expressed as 96% reduction of hemolytic activity in vitro. Lentinan activated considerably the alternative pathway of the complement system. This is one of the first reactions of lentinan in the host, which undergoes nonspecific activation of macrophages.

Nonimmunological Potentiation Of Host Defense Mechanisms

Various kinds of serum protein components such as acute phase proteins, complement components and bioactive factors such as colony stimulating factor increase after administration of lentinan (13). One of the most interesting properties of lentinan is the augmented induction of colony stimulating factor in the serum from lentinan treated mice. Lentinan seems to activate a fundamental host defense mechanism according to proliferation of leukocytes, bone marrow cells or various kinds of immunocompetent cells. Lentinan increases haptoglobin, ceruloplasmin and hemopexin values. Ceruloplasmin possesses a protecting effect against the lowering of liver catalase activity triggered by toxohormone and it may be used as a therapeutic agent for human aplastic anemia, cachexia and others. These effects represent a general potentiation of host resistance against cancer and infectious diseases.

MODE OF ACTION MECHANISM OF LENTINAN

Considering the various immunological characteristics of lentinan as revealed here, we can tentatively propose the scheme depicted in Figure 1. as the possible mode of action of lentinan, although there are still many obscure points at the moment. Lentinan is not only a unique T cell oriented adjuvant but is a bioactive substance with a variety of immunological characteristics such as macrophage activation, alternative pathway induction, acceleration of acute phase proteins and others.

TOXICOLOGY OF LENTINAN

The acute and subacute toxicities of lentinan were mainly examined by i.v. injection into mice, rats, dogs and monkeys. In any species tested, the LD_{50} of lentinan was more than 100 mg/kg. In anaphylaxis tests, all guinea pigs previously injected with lentinan were not hypersensitized by i.v. or i.c. injection with lentinan. Chronic toxicity of lentinan was examined by daily i.v. injection for 26 weeks into rhesus monkeys, and the control and lentinan-treated groups did not show any side effects or any histological changes. Accordingly, the regular dose of lentinan in clinical trial, 1 mg i.v., is quite safe.

DISCUSSION

Lentinan is now universally recognized as being the most potent presently known immunopotentiator, and its biological and immunopharmacological characteristics are distinguished from those of other

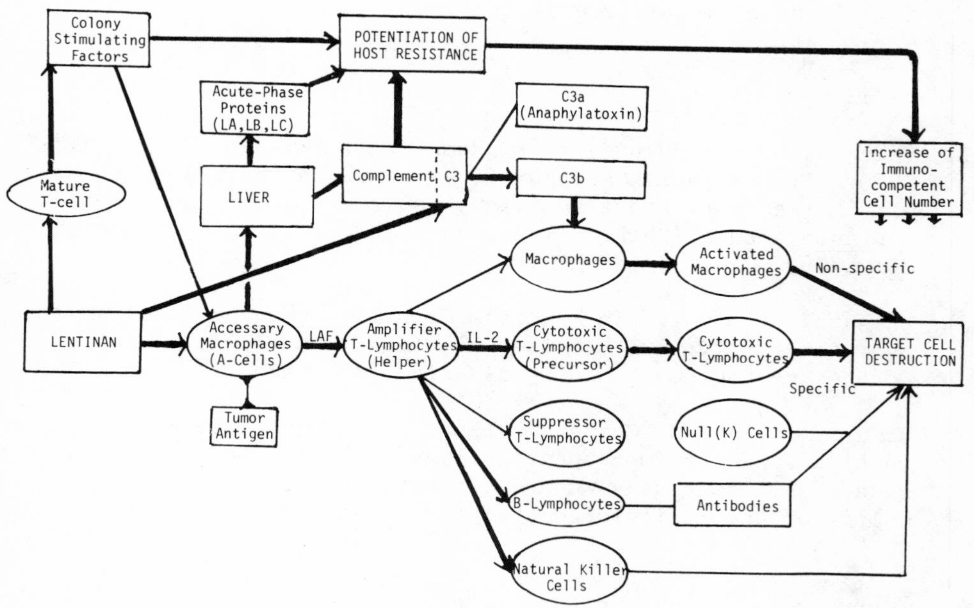

Fig. 1. Possible mode of action of lentinan.

immunostimulants such as BCG and the related substances, *C. parvum*, levamisole, LPS, Poly I:C or interferon. Low toxicity is also an important characteristic of lentinan when compared with other chemotherapeutic agents possessing deterimental toxic side effects. The characteristics of lentinan described in this review are very hopeful for cancer patients.

Nevertheless, cancer immunotherapy is extremely difficult. Lentinan will become effective against human cancer when used in conjunction with other therapy under strictly planned timing and schedules, and only when the host-tumor relationship is in good agreement with such treatment. The basic clinical research in this direction might be the most important and urgent task in this field.

SUMMARY

Lentinan exerts prominent antitumor effects in allogeneic, syngeneic and autochthonous hosts and prevents chemical and viral carcinogenesis, and increases host-resistance to bacterial, viral and parasitic infections. Lentinan augments helper T cell mediated cytotoxic T cell activity, NK cell activity and humoral immune responses, and activates nonspecific cytotoxicity of macrophages in vivo. Lentinan is a representative of a unique class of T cell adjuvants, and has no toxicity. Therefore, lentinan is suitable for clinical application for cancer patients from the results in its preclinical animal model experiments.

REFERENCES

1. Chihara, G., J. Hamuro, Y. Y. Hamuro, Y. Arai and F. Fukuoka. 1970. Fractionation and purification of the polysaccharides with marked antitumour activity, especially lentinan, from *Lentinus edodes* (Berk.) Sing., an edible mushroom. Cancer Res. *30*: 2776.

2. Chihara, G. 1981. The antitumour polysaccharide lentinan: An overview, p. 1. *In* T. Aoki et al. (eds.), Manipulation of host defense mechanisms. Excerpta Medica, Amsterdam.

3. Hamuro, J., and G. Chihara. 1982. Immunopotentiation by lentinan and its immunopharmacology. Chapter 14. *In* J. W. Hadden, A. Szentivanyi and J. R. Battisto (eds.), The pharmacology of the reticuloendothelial system. Plenum Press, New York, N.Y.

4. Zákány, J., G. Chihara and J. Fachet. 1980. Effect of lentinan on tumour growth in murine allogeneic and syngeneic hosts. Int. J. Cancer *25*: 371.

5. Shiio, T., and Y. Yugari. 1981. The antitumour effect of lentinan and tumour recognition in mice p. 29. In T. Aoki et al. (eds.), Manipulation of host defense mechanisms. Excerpta Medica, Amsterdam.

6. Hamada, C. 1981. Inhibitory effect of lentinan on the tumourigenesis of adenovirus type-12 in mice p. 76, In T. Aoki et al. (eds.), Manipulation of host defense mechanisms. Excerpta Medica, Amsterdam.

7. Kanai, K., E. Kondo, P. J. Jacques and G. Chihara. 1980. Immunopotentiating effect of fungal glucans as related by frequency limitation of post chemotherapy relapse in experimental mouse tuberculosis. Jap. J. Med. Sci. & Biol. 33: 283.

8. Chang, K. S. S. 1981. Lentinan-mediated resistance against VSV-encephalitis, Abelson virus-induced tumour, and trophoblastic tumour in mice, p. 88. In T. Aoki et al. (eds.), Manipulation of host defense mechanisms. Excerpta Medica, Amsterdam.

9. Byrum, J. E., A. Sher, J. DiPietro and F. von Lichitenberg. 1979. Potentiation of Shistosoma granuloma by lentinan, A T-cell adjuvant. Am. J. Pathol. 94: 201.

10. Haba, S., T. Hamaoka, K. Takatsu and M. Kitagawa. 1976. Selective suppression of T-cell activity in tumour bearing mice and its improvement by lentinan. Int. J. Cancer 18: 93.

11. Maeda, Y. Y., and G. Chihara. 1973. The effect of neonatal thymectomy on the antitumour activity of lentinan and their effects on various immune responses. Int. J. Cancer 11: 153.

12. Hamuro, J., M. Röllinghof and H. Wagner. 1980. Induction of cytotoxic PE-cells by T-cell immune adjuvant of the β-1,3-glucan type lentinan and its analogues. Immunology 39: 551.

13. Maeda, Y. Y., G. Chihara and K. Ishimura. 1974. Unique increase of serum protein components and action of antitumour polysaccharides. Nature (London) New Biol. 252: 250.

IMMUNOMODULATION BY SMALL MOLECULAR WEIGHT BACTERIAL PRODUCTS

Herman Friedman

University of South Florida College of Medicine
Department of Medical Microbiology and Immunology
Tampa, Florida (USA)

INTRODUCTION

Bacteria are widely recognized for their ability to modulate the immune response as well as stimulate natural defense mechanisms in a nonspecific manner (1, 2). There are many bacterial products which have been investigated in detail concerning their effects on host immunity. In this regard endotoxins derived from gram negative bacteria have been studied in much detail. There are a vast number of biological properties attributed to endotoxin, but their unique capacity to stimulate both immunologically specific and nonspecific host defense mechanisms is unquestionably an important property. In recent years many investigations have been concerned with the mechanisms whereby bacterial products, including the endotoxins, influence the immune response (1, 2). It is now apparent that many microbial cell wall components, including endotoxins, are potent stimulators of interleukin formation by macrophages and/or other lymphoid cells (3, 4). These interleukins undoubtedly serve an important role in modulating the immune response of other lymphoid cells.

Studies performed in this laboratory have shown that not only the lipopolysaccharide (LPS) rich components from cell walls of gram negative bacteria are potent immunomodulators but also the non-lipid-A containing smaller molecular weight polysaccharide (PS) derivative (1, 6, 7). Similarly, lipoteichoic acids (LTA) derived from gram positive organisms have been found to be equally effective in stimulating enhanced antibody responses, both in vivo and in vitro (4). Both lipopolysaccharides and lipoteichoic acids have relatively similar effects on cells of the immune response mechanism since both groups of substances may stimulate interleukin formation which, in turn, affects the responsiveness of other lymphoid cells. There is also evidence that the smaller molecular weight polysaccharide derivative of LPS has the ability to stimulate antibody formation in vitro as well as in vivo, and that this enhancement is also associated with interleukin activities.

In the present report both the intact LPS from Serratia marcescens as well as the nontoxic small weight molecular PS derivatives were found to enhance antibody formation by murine spleen cells, both in vivo and in vitro. Lipoteichoic acids derived from streptococci had almost identical activity. Both bacterial components, i.e., LPS and its PS, as well as LTA, similarly stimulated mice to develop post-treatment serum factors which had immunostimulating activity for cultures of normal spleen cells. Similarly, cultures of splenocytes exposed to LPS or LTA in vitro developed immunoenhancing activity in their supernatants as demonstrated by co-culture procedures. The immunoenhancing factors appear to be derived from macrophages and had as its major target antibody responding B lymphocytes and their precursor.

METHODS

For these experiments inbred Balb/c mice obtained from Jackson Laboratories, Bar Harbour, Maine, were utilized. They were injected either intraperitoneally with sheep red blood cells (SRBC), with or without treatment with endotoxin, or used as a source of nonimmune spleen cells for in vitro immunization. For the latter purpose, the spleen was obtained from normal mice and dispersed cell suspensions prepared for in vitro cultivation. Cultures of 5-8 x 10^6 viable nucleated cells were cultured in microwell plates. The cultures were immunized with 2 x 10^6 SRBC and the numbers of individual hemolytic plaque forming cells (PFC) to the SRBC determined at various times thereafter by the microplaque assay on microscope slides (8). The indirect effects of the bacterial stimulators were assessed by using culture supernatants to treat a second set of spleen cell cultures immunized with 2 x 10^6 SRBC. To obtain post-treatment serum, mice were first injected with BCG (1 x 10^6 organisms per animal) 4 weeks earlier and then challenged by i.p. injection with the bacterial stimulator 2 hours prior to obtaining blood (1, 4). Serum from such animals was considered to be post-treatment sera and were added in graded concentrations to cultures of normal mouse spleen cells being immunized with SRBC. In addition, supernatants obtained from cultures exposed to the bacterial products for 3-5 days were used similarly to treat normal splenocyte cultures. For all experiments the endotoxin was derived from S. marcescens by standard extraction procedures while the PS was prepared by acid hydrolysis with 1 M HCl at 100°C for 30 minutes. The PS consisted of approximately 65% carbohydrate, 10% protein, 0.1% nucleic acid, and less than 0.5% lipid with a molecular weight of approximately 10,000 daltons. The PS preparation contained no measurable endotoxicity when tested by the Limulus lysate assay, chick embryo lethality assay and rabbit pyrogenicity tests. Lipoteichoic acid was prepared from Streptococcus fecalis.

RESULTS

Enhancement of the immune response to sheep RBC occurred after injection of mice with either LPS, PS or LTA (Table 1). A dose of 10 to 100 μg of each of these bacterial components, when injected into mice simultaneously with sheep RBCs, resulted in a 2-3 fold

Table 1. Effect of bacterial cell wall component on antibody response of mice to sheep erythrocytes.

In vivo stimulation[a] (μg)		Antibody response[b]	
		PFC/spleen	Percent of control
None (Control)		795 ± 95	-
LPS	1.0	1280 ± 65	161
	10.0	1850 ± 240	233
	100.0	2130 ± 340	270
PS	1.0	980 ± 110	132
	10.0	1430 ± 460	180
	100.0	1750 ± 165	220
LTA	1.0	820 ± 70	103
	10.0	1200 ± 310	151
	100.0	2100 ± 280	264
MDP	100.0	1970 ± 210	248

[a] Indicated stimulator injected i.p. into groups of mice at same time as i.p. immunization with 4×10^8 SRBC.

[b] Average number of PFC ± SE for spleens from 3-5 mice per group 4 days after an immunization.

enhancement of the antibody response. The highest dose resulted in the highest increase. It should be noted that the LD_{50} for the LPS was approximately 300 μg per mouse whereas for PS it was greater than 2000 μg per mouse. The LTA was toxic at an intermediate dose. As a control, the smaller molecular weight synthetic MDP, at a similar concentration, also resulted in a similar enhancement of the antibody response. As shown previously, modulation of immunity occurred when MDP was given prior to or following SRBC. Similar results were obtained with either LPS, PS or LTA (data not shown). The most consistent enhancement of antibody response was noted when these agents were given simultaneously with sheep red cells.

Although administration of the bacterial products to mice along with SRBC evinced a markedly enhanced antibody response, such experiments, however, did not provide much information concerning the mechanisms involved. In this regard, in vitro studies have been widely utilized to examine not only the adjuvanticity of various substances, including bacterial products, but also to dissect the mechanisms involved. As is evident in Table 2, the bacterial products utilized in this study, i.e., LPS, PS and LTA, had similar immunoenhancing activity for normal mouse spleen cells in vitro. Peak enhancement occurred on day 5 of the in vitro response. However, significant enhancement was evident in treated cultures at an earlier time period, i.e., day 3, and persisted throughout the culture period. The greatest enhancement occurred with 10-50 μg of intact endotoxin, polysaccharide or LTA. Lower doses had less effect, whereas higher doses, i.e., over 100-200 μg per culture, were generally toxic. It is noteworthy that although the peak day of the response was unaffected, its magnitude was markedly influenced by the simultaneous treatment of the cultures with the bacterial product and SRBC.

The concentration of SRBC influenced the magnitude of the immunoenhancement noted (Table 3). Each of the three bacterial products had a polyclonal enhancing effect on spleen cell cultures incubated in the absence of antigen. When SRBC was added to the cultures, there was a markedly lower peak response in untreated spleen cell preparations as compared to those treated with the three bacterial products. In most cases greater enhancement of the response occurred in cultures containing the lower dose of SRBC as compared to those containing the optimal 2×10^8 RBC dose. However, it was noted that the PFC response was not much higher with the highest dose of antigen, either with or without bacterial products. A higher concentration of SRBC did not appreciably increase the antibody response and there was a lower enhancement by the bacterial products (Table 3).

The time of addition of the bacterial modulator to the cultures markedly affected immune responsiveness. As is evident in Table 4, enhancement occurred when the bacterial product, regardless of type, was added to cultures either on the day of culture initiation or one day later. Much less stimulation occurred when the product was

Table 2. Cytokinetics of antibody response to SRBC by spleen cell cultures treated in vitro with bacterial products.

In vitro[a] addition (μg)	Antibody response on day[b]			
	+3	+5	+7	+10
None (control)	185 ± 36	630 ± 45	150 ± 30	120 ± 25
LPS 0.1	296 ± 40	650 ± 80	600 ± 45	250 ± 60
1.0	650 ± 150	960 ± 110	830 ± 110	195 ± 80
10.0	630 ± 210	1980 ± 240	1560 ± 250	2180 ± 55
50.0	500 ± 110	1850 ± 190	1410 ± 110	850 ± 120
PS 0.1	200 ± 38	580 ± 60	480 ± 60	200 ± 45
1.0	350 ± 65	910 ± 150	530 ± 180	325 ± 60
10.0	510 ± 90	2130 ± 340	930 ± 48	610 ± 35
50.0	610 ± 150	1930 ± 35	1290 ± 65	970 ± 140
LTA 1.0	190 ± 30	810 ± 120	800 ± 95	650 ± 67
10.0	430 ± 65	820 ± 250	1160 ± 240	830 ± 95
50.0	550 ± 60	1730 ± 180	1250 ± 180	1010 ± 210

[a] Indicated bacterial product added to cultures of 8 x 10^6 spleen cells from normal mice at time of culture initiation.

[b] Average number of PFC ± SE for 3 - 4 cultures per group on indicated day after in vitro immunization with 2 x 10^6 SRBC.

added on the second day of culture initiation and almost no enhancement occurred when added on day 3 or 4. It is of interest that addition of all three bacterial products simultaneously to spleen cell cultures at an optimal concentration (20-40 μg) failed to induce a higher anti-SRBC response, suggesting that once an optimal dose of the bacterial immunoenhancing product was added to the cultures being stimulated with an optimal dose of SRBC, no further enhancement of the response occurred (data not shown).

Immunoenhancement was observed for both primary IgM PFCs as well as secondary IgM and IgG PFCs (Table 5). It is noteworthy that

Table 3. Effect of antigen concentration on antibody response of mouse spleen cells treated with LPS, PS or LTA.

In vitro[a] stimulator	SRBC Concentration 0	2 x 10^4	2 x 10^6	2 x 10^8	2 x 10^9
None (Control)	58 ± 16	190 ± 30	780 ± 130	930 ± 250	140 ± 110
LPS	240 ± 40	930 ± 130	2250 ± 36	1600 ± 320	835 ± 95
PS	290 ± 45	770 ± 130	2700 ± 370	1900 ± 640	1990 ± 65
LTA	310 ± 50	840 ± 210	1560 ± 510	1630 ± 480	960 ± 90

[a] Indicated bacterial product (50 μg) added to cultures of 8 x 10^6 spleen cells immunized in vitro with indicated concentration of SRBC.

[b] Average number of PFC ± SE for 3-5 cultures per group 5 days after in vitro immunization.

Table 4. Effect of time of addition of bacterial product to mouse spleen cell cultures on antibody response to sheep RBCs.

Time of addition[a] to cultures (day)	Antibody response[b] LPS	PS	LTA
0	2380 ± 280	2960 ± 320	3500 ± 410
+1	1970 ± 170	2365 ± 250	2710 ± 330
+2	1660 ± 210	1130 ± 150	1860 ± 310
+3	1130 ± 320	1100 ± 210	950 ± 185
+4	775 ± 160	860 ± 130	890 ± 210

[a] Indicated bacterial product (50 μg) added to cultures of 8 x 10^6 mouse spleen cells on day indicated after culture initiation and immunization with 2 x 10^6 SRBC.

[b] Average number of PFC ± SE for 3 - 6 cultures per group 5 days after in vitro immunization; cultures without bacterial stimulator gave an average PFC response of 796 ± 58 in the same experiments.

Table 5. Effect of bacterial cell wall components on primary and secondary in vitro antibody response of mouse spleen cells immunized with SRBC.

	Antibody PFC response[b]		
	Primary	Secondary	
Stimulator[a]	IgM	IgM	IgG
None (control)	740 ± 100	530 ± 180	1860 ± 210
LPS	1970 ± 400	1040 ± 260	4870 ± 500
PS	2100 ± 370	1130 ± 270	4150 ± 370
LTA	1760 ± 230	428 ± 310	3870 ± 240

[a] Indicated bacterial product added to cultures of 8 x 10^6 mouse spleen cells immunized in vitro with 2 x 10^6 SRBC.

[b] Average number of PFC ± SE for 3 - 5 cultures per group 4 days after primary or secondary immunization.

[c] Mice primed 4 weeks earlier by i.p. injection with 4 x 10^8 SRBC; IgG PFC detected by anti-globulin facilitation assay.

the bacterial products appeared to stimulate an even greater enhancement of the secondary IgG PFC responses compared to the IgM response. Thus these materials appear to influence a known T cell dependent secondary response to a greater extent than the IgM response.

LPS is considered to be a T-independent bacterial product and it is often assumed that this material does not affect thymus cell responses. Thus it was of interest to determine whether LPS vs. LTA had similar effects on T cell deficient mice. As shown in Table 6, equal enhancement of the antibody response occurred in both conventional Balb/c and athymic Balb/c nu/nu mice when their spleen cells were exposed to either LPS or LTA in vitro (Table 6). It is also of interest that the PS derived from the LPS was equally effective in stimulating an enhanced PFC response for both conventional and nu/nu mice, similar to the effects of the LPS. Although the ability of the nu/nu mice to respond to SRBC was markedly diminished, these bacterial products enhanced the antibody response several fold, although not to the level observed in cultures from normal conventional mice exposed to antigen plus the bacterial product.

It was of equal interest to determine whether the polysaccharide could stimulate an immune response in endotoxin nonresponder mice.

Table 6. Stimulation of spleen cell cultures from conventional and athymic Balb/c mice by bacterial products.

	Mouse strain tested[b]	
Culture treatment[a]	Conventional	Athymic
None (control)	1150 $\pm$ 120	240 $\pm$ 60
LPS	2370 $\pm$ 280	1650 $\pm$ 310
PS	2050 $\pm$ 310	1510 $\pm$ 250
LTA	2860 $\pm$ 300	1890 $\pm$ 400

[a] Indicated preparation of bacterial product (50 μg) added to cultures of 8 x 10^6 spleen cells from conventional or athymic nu/nu Balb/c mice immunized in vitro with 2 x 10^6 SRBC.

[b] Average number of PFC $\pm$ SE for 3 - 5 cultures per group 5 days after in vitro immunization.

It was also of interest to determine whether the LTA, a nonendotoxic cell wall product, could influence endotoxin low responder mice. As is evident in Table 7, addition of LPS or PS to cultures of spleen cells from low responder C3H/HeJ mice failed to enhance their antibody responsiveness to sheep erythrocytes, as occurred when these products were added to cultures of spleen cells from LPS sensitive C3HeB/FeJ mice. In contrast, LTA resulted in an enhanced antibody response by spleen cell cultures derived from both the LPS low and high responder mice (Table 7).

Previous studies have shown that lipopolysaccharides, when injected into mice, stimulates a plethora of immunomodulatory factors, as well as factors which influence tumor destruction, i.e., tumor necrotizing factor, colony forming factors, etc. The major modality to induce these factors is to pretreat responder mice with BCG, followed 3 - 4 weeks later by systemic administration of an endotoxin. Two hours later serum from these animals can be shown to contain a variety of factors, including tumor necrotizing factor. As is evident in Table 8, sera obtained two hours after injection of mice pretreated 4 weeks earlier with BCG and then injected with either LPS or PS had the ability to markedly "help", i.e., enhance, the antibody response of normal mouse spleen cultures in vitro. For example, although relatively small volumes (i.e., 0.01 or 0.1 ml) of sera obtained from normal mice failed to influence the expected antibody response of normal spleen cells immunized in vitro with SRBC, similar volumes of post-LPS or post-PS serum caused an enhanced antibody response by normal spleen cell cultures.

Table 7. Antibody formation of spleen cells from conventional and endotoxin nonresponder mice stimulated in vitro with bacterial products.

	Spleen cells tested[b]	
Culture treatment[a]	C3HeB/FeJ	C3H/HeJ
None (control)	1158 ± 95	946 ± 103
LPS	2486 ± 230	1030 ± 92
PS	2100 ± 350	870 ± 65
LTA	2270 ± 180	1860 ± 210

[a] Spleen cells (8 x 10^6) from either conventional (FeJ) or low responder (HeJ) C3H mice treated in vitro with 50 µg of indicated bacterial product and immunized with 2 x 10^6 SRBC.

[b] Average number of PFC ± SE for 3 - 5 cultures per group 5 days after in vitro stimulation.

As is evident in Table 9, treatment of normal mouse spleen cell cultures for several days in vitro with either LPS, PS, LTA or BCG, induced a helper cell factor for subsequent stimulation of antibody formation by normal mouse spleen cells, but failed to induce migration inhibitory factor capable of inhibiting the migration of normal mouse macrophages in agarose droplets. In contrast, BCG (10^5 organisms per culture) had the ability to moderately stimulate the formation of antibody helper factors in the culture and also had the ability to prime the spleen cell cultures to formation of not only antibody helper factors, but also MIF activity upon simultaneous incubation with LPS, PS or LTA. For example, the culture supernatants from BCG treated spleen cell cultures incubated with any one of these three bacterial modulators had the ability to cause an even greater enhancement of the PFC responses by normal cell cultures and also induced migration inhibition in target cell cultures. It should be noted that if small quantities of these bacterial products, including BCG, were added at time "0" to cultures and then supernatants obtained, no such enhancing activity occurred, indicating that there were not sufficient amounts of the bacterial products in the relatively small volume of culture supernatant being used to affect the immune response of the normal cultures under the conditions prevailing.

The immunostimulatory activity of the post-LPS serum helper factors could be absorbed with mouse bone marrow cells but not with mouse thymus cells (Table 10), indicating that the factor(s) could bind to marrow cells containing precursors of B cells, as well as

Table 8. Effects of LPS or PS post-treatment serum on antibody response of mouse spleen cells in vitro to sheep RBCs.

Treatment[a] (ml)		PFC response[b]	Percent of control
None (control)		670 ± 43	100
Normal serum	0.001	710 ± 40	106
	0.01	705 ± 60	95
	0.1	695 ± 92	104
	0.5	430 ± 110	64
Post LPS serum	0.001	965 ± 130	144
	0.01	1560 ± 230	233
	0.1	1830 ± 195	273
	0.5	990 ± 65	148
Post PS serum	0.001	1010 ± 150	151
	0.01	1310 ± 210	196
	0.1	1250 ± 95	187
	0.5	1130 ± 68	169

[a] Cultures of 8 x 10^6 spleen cells treated in vitro with indicated amount of normal mouse serum or serum collected 2 hrs after i.p. injection with 50 μg LPS or PS.

[b] Average number of PFC ± SE for 3 - 4 cultures 4 days after in vitro vitro immunization with 2 x 10^6 SRBC.

some other cell classes, but not with mature or immature thymus cells. Similar absorption studies with culture supernatants from mouse spleen cells treated with LPS or PS had similar results, i.e., the marrow cells could absorb out activity but not thymus cells. In other experiments (data not shown) it has been found that thymocytes are not involved in production of the bacterial induced factors. The injection of LPS into either conventional or athymic nude mice resulted in formation of a serum helper factor which was equally active in enhancing the antibody response of normal mouse spleen cells and also quite active in stimulating nude mouse spleen cells.

Table 9. Production of MIF and antibody helper activity by spleen cell cultures treated with bacterial product in vitro.

Culture[a] treatment	Percent of control migration[b]	PFC/culture
None (control)	100 ± 12	650 ± 45
LPS (20 μg)	75 ± 16	1840 ± 280
PS (20 μg)	76 ± 10	1680 ± 310
LTA (50 μg)	88 ± 20	2110 ± 265
BCG 10^5	114 ± 5	1230 ± 148
plus LPS	34 ± 12	2730 ± 310
PS	43 ± 12	2150 ± 230
LTA	29 ± 10	2530 ± 188

[a] Indicated bacterial product and/or BCG added to cultures of 2 x 10^7 normal mouse spleen cells. Cell-free supernatants obtained 3 days later.

[b] Average migration inhibition relative to indicator cultures incubated in MIF assay without supernatants.

As is evident in Table 11, 5 day culture supernatants obtained from spleens of normal mice incubated with either LPS, PS or LTA had the greatest immunoenhancing activity for normal mouse spleen cell cultures. Although the 3 day culture supernatant also was immunoenhancing when derived from spleen cells incubated with the bacterial product, they were much less so than the 5 day supernatants. The possible carryover of the bacterial product into supernatants was not a factor since the bacterial product would have been diluted out, or metabolized with time in the cultures. Furthermore, if the presence of the bacterial product was the mediator of the effects noted, then supernatants obtained early after culture initiation would have been more stimulatory, rather than less stimulatory.

Murine splenocytes, as well as macrophages, appeared to be the source of the immunoenhancing factors. As is evident in Table 12, incubation of adherent spleen cells but not nonadherent cells, with LPS resulted in formation of the highest level of immunoenhancing activity. Similarly, peritoneal exudate cells obtained 3 days after stimulation of Balb/c mice by i.p. injection with thioglycollate resulted in a cell population which morphologically consisted of

Table 10. Absorption of post LPS serum helper factor with bone marrow cells.

Culture supernatant absorption[a]	PFC/[b] culture	Percent of control
None (control)	830 ± 65	100
Normal serum - unabsorbed	845 ± 82	102
absorbed with thymus cells	905 ± 72	109
absorbed with marrow cells	810 ± 60	96
Post LPS serum-unabsorbed	1938 ± 158	234
absorbed with thymus cells	1610 ± 210	194
absorbed with marrow cells	878 ± 75	106

[a] Cultures of 8 x 10^6 spleen cells from normal mice treated with 0.01 ml normal or post LPS serum with or without absorption and immunized in vitro with 2 x 10^6 SRBC. Serum (0.1 ml) absorbed with 10^8 bone marrow or thymus cell for 1 hr at 37°C prior to centrifugation.

[b] Average number of PFC ± SE for 5 - 6 cultures per group 5 days after immunization in vitro.

Table 11. Antibody response by normal mouse spleen cells cultured with supernatants from donor mouse spleen cultures treated with bacterial products.

Donor culture treatment[a]	Supernatants for treatment[b]	
	+3 days	+5 days
None (control)	653 ± 90	710 ± 100
LPS	1130 ± 240	2650 ± 270
PS	1210 ± 120	1830 ± 185
LTA	1270 ± 190	2530 ± 280

[a] Cultures of 5 x 10^7 normal mouse spleen cells incubated in vitro with 20 μg of indicated stimulator for 3 or 5 days.

[b] Average number of PFC ± SE for 3 - 5 cultures of normal mouse spleen cells incubated with 0.1 ml of indicated supernatant and immunized with 2 x 10^6 SRBC 4 days earlier.

Table 12. Antibody formation by spleen cell cultures treated with supernatants from cell cultures stimulated in vitro with LPS.

		Antibody response[b]	
Cells cultured[a]	LPS treatment	PFC/culture	Percent of control
Normal spleen	-	768 $\pm$ 128	-
	+	1950 $\pm$ 340	254
Adherent spleen cells	-	930 $\pm$ 65	121
	+	2140 $\pm$ 230	279
Nonadherent cells	-	630 $\pm$ 92	82
	+	840 $\pm$ 110	109
PE cells	-	730 $\pm$ 60	95
	+	1870 $\pm$ 140	242
P388D$_1$ cells	-	935 $\pm$ 112	122
	+	2340 $\pm$ 210	305

[a] Cultures of 5 x 10^7 cells, as indicated, incubated for 4 - 5 days with or without 20 μg LPS.

[b] Average response of 3 - 4 cultures per group 5 days after in vitro treatment with 0.1 ml of indicated cell free supernatant and immunization with 2 x 10^6 SRBC.

about 70-80% phagocytic cells and also responded in a positive manner when incubated with LPS in forming an antibody helper supernatant factor. Similarly, the macrophage-like P388D$_1$ cell line was found to produce a similar immunoenhancing factor when exposed to LPS. In this regard, PS and LTA were also effective (data not shown).

DISCUSSION

Although it is widely recognized that bacteria derived cell surface components are effective stimulators and modulators of immune responses, there is little information available concerning their mechanism of action (7, 10). The results of the studies reported here support the view that immunomodulation induced by microorganisms from which LPS and LTA are derived, is related to their ability to induce soluble mediators, both in vivo and in vitro. It is widely accepted that endotoxins are potent stimulators of interleukin formation by macrophage cultures (1, 2). Similarly, cell wall components from gram positive bacteria, such as LTA, also stimulate interleukin formation (1, 2). It was observed in the present study that both the toxic LPS as well as the nontoxic small molecular weight PS derivative had similar effects on mouse spleen cells in vivo and in vitro and, further, that these bacterial products stimulated lymphoid cell cultures to release factors which could influence in a positive manner the antibody responsiveness of normal mouse spleen cells. Similarly, LTA derived from streptococci had a marked immunostimulatory property in vitro, as evident when relatively small quantities were added to spleen cell cultures. Supernatants from spleen cells exposed to LTA also had immunoenhancing activity. The responsiveness of spleen cells to these bacterial products appear to be T cell independent. In addition LPS nonresponder mice showed immunoenhancement when exposed to LTA, suggesting involvement of a less restrictive genetic control mechanism for recognition to this bacterial product as compared to LPS. Alternately, genes other than those involved in LPS recognition may be important in LTA responsiveness.

Previous studies have suggested that cells most likely to respond to bacterial products are macrophages and that immunoenhancing factors are released by stimulating these cells. Such stimulated cells are similar regardless of whether splenic adherent cells or PE cells are used as a source of soluble factors. Nonadherent lymphoid cells lack the ability to release immunoenhancing factors when exposed to these bacterial products. Bone marrow cells incubated with culture supernatants containing immunoenhancing factors remove most of the activity, whereas thymus cells do not. These and other studies suggest that macrophages are a major if not exclusive source of immunoenhancing soluble factors, and that these factors have many, if not all of the characteristics attributed to interleukins. Thus, it could be concluded that bacterial cell wall components, whether derived from gram negative bacteria such as Serratia or a gram positive one such as streptococci interacted in a similar manner with cells of the immune system, presumably macrophages, resulting in formation of immunoenhancing or at least immunoregulatory factors. Whether the same cell or different cell populations interact with different bacterial products from different sources is not yet known, but further studies of this type should clarify the mechanisms involved.

It is of interest to note that in the past, most activities associated with LPS have been attributed to the lipid-A portion and not the polysaccharide component. However, studies have shown that both the LPS and PS have marked effects on tumors and also in inducing colony stimulating factor. In addition, post LPS as well as PS sera have been shown to contain antitumor factors. The results of the present study extend these observations and show that post endotoxin sera, whether derived from mice injected with LPS or PS, contain similar antibody helper factors. Both bacterial products also enhanced in vitro antibody responses and induced normal spleen cell cultures in vitro to release antibody helper factors. As indicated earlier, this appears due to stimulation of macrophages rather than lymphoid cells. Lack of involvement of T cells in the production of this helper factor also focuses attention on macrophages as the responding cell.

It should be noted that the only difference observed to date with LPS vs PS in stimulating antibody responses is that the latter component apparently required continuous contact with lymphoid cells to induce an enhanced response. Incubation of spleen cell suspension with PS is present throughout the time of culture initiation. In contrast, LPS, when incubated with spleen cell suspensions for only two days, followed by washing the cultures, still resulted in enhanced responses. This suggests that the binding of PS to lymphoid cell surfaces is either a reversible process or that continuous exposure to this stimulator is needed to activate lymphoid cells for enhanced antibody response. It seems likely that further analysis of the interrelationship of smaller molecular weight derivatives of larger complex bacterial cell wall components such as LPS, as well as smaller molecular weight derivatives of LTA such as the peptidoglycans and even possibly MDPs, will be of value in dissecting the pathways whereby these immunomodulators influence the immune response at the cellular level.

SUMMARY

Microbial products are known immunomodulators. Endotoxins derived from gram negative bacteria both enhance and suppress a wide variety of immune responses in vivo and in vitro, depending upon dose, concentration, form, and time of exposure. Studies in this laboratory have shown that a small molecular weight polysaccharide derivative from endotoxin has strong immunomodulatory effects, both in vivo and in vitro, similar to intact LPS. Injection of PS into mice or addition to normal mouse spleen cell cultures results in enhanced responses similar to that observed with LPS as well as with lipoteichoic acid derived from gram positive bacteria. The immunomodulatory activity, both in vivo and in vitro, was related to development of soluble serum factors, most likely interleukins. Similar soluble mediators were observed in vivo since post endotoxin or post LTA serum, when added in small quantities to normal mouse spleen cell cultures, mediated enhanced antibody responses. Normal spleen cell cultures exposed to these materials also released soluble mediators into the supernatants which enhanced the antibody response of normal spleen cell cultures. These observations support the view that similar to larger molecular weight cell wall components, small molecular weight substances such as polysaccharide derivatives, despite lack of toxicity share related mechanisms of enhancing immune responses.

REFERENCES

1. Friedman, H., T. W. Klein, and A. Szentivanyi. 1981. Immunomodulation by bacteria and their products. Plenum Press, New York.

2. Yamamura, Y., S. Kotani, I. Azuma, A. Koda, and T. Shiba. 1982. Immunomodulation by microbial products and related synthetic compounds. Excerpta Medica, Amsterdam.

3. Skidmore, B. J., J. M. Chiller, D. C. Morrison, and W. O. Weigle. 1971. J. Immunol. 114: 770-778.

4. Butler, R. C., and H. Friedman. 1983. Infect. Immun. 39:

5. Butler, R. C., and H. Friedman. 1979. Ann. N. Y. Acad. Sci. 336: 446-455.

6. Frank, S., S. Specter, A. Nowotny, and H. Friedman. 1977. J. Immunol. 119: 855-863.

7. Behling, U. H. and A. Nowotny. 1977. J. Immunol. Method 11: 55-73.

8. Cunningham, A. J. and A. Szenberg. 1968. Immunol. 14: 599-600.

9. Nowotny, A. 1963. J. Bacteriol. 85: 427-435.

10. Nowotny, A. 1969. Bacteriol. Rev. 33: 72-98.

HUMAN MACROPHAGES MAY NORMALLY BE "PRIMED" FOR A STRONG OXYGEN RADICAL RESPONSE

Michael J. Pabst, Nancy P. Cummings, Holly B. Hedegaard and Richard B. Johnston, Jr.

National Jewish Hospital and Research Center/National Asthma Center, Department of Pediatrics and University of Colorado School of Medicine, Departments of Biochemistry and Pediatrics, Denver, Colorado (USA)

INTRODUCTION

In previous work we showed that macrophages must produce oxygen radicals in order to kill pathogenic organisms (1). Oxygen radical production by mouse peritoneal macrophages could be enhanced at least ten-fold if the macrophages were previously "activated". (Throughout this paper we use the term "activated" to mean "primed to release optimal amounts of O_2^- when stimulated"). Macrophages were activated either by infecting the animals with *Mycobacterium bovis*, strain BCG, or by injecting them with bacterial lipopolysaccharide (LPS) or muramyl dipeptide (MDP) (2, 3). Cultured macrophages could also be activated in vitro by addition of LPS or MDP to the cultures (4). Treatment with LPS or MDP enhanced the ability of cultured macrophages to kill bacteria and fungi in vitro (1, 3). Treatment of mice with MDP in vivo enabled them to resist an otherwise lethal challenge infection with *Klebsiella pneumoniae* or *Candida albicans* (3, 5).

To determine whether *human* macrophages could be activated in vitro, we studied superoxide release by macrophages immediately after isolation and following treatment with LPS or MDP for 24 hours. Mouse peritoneal macrophages and blood monocytes were compared with human peritoneal macrophages, milk macrophages and blood monocytes.

METHODS

Activation of Mouse Peritoneal Macrophages by MDP Analogs

Peritoneal macrophages from normal, healthy mice were cultured overnight (18 h) in endotoxin-free Dulbecco's modified Eagle medium in the presence of the indicated concentration of macrophage activator (4). MDP-DD is the inactive analog, N-acetylmuramyl-D-alanyl-D-isoglutamine; B30-MDP is 6-0-(2-tetradecylhexadecanoyl)-MDP; MDP-butyl is N-acetylmuramyl-L-alanyl-D-glutaminyl-α-n-butyl ester; MDP-A-L and MDP-DD-A-L are conjugates of MDP or its inactive isomer with a polyalanine-polylysine carrier. Cultures were then washed, and assayed using 0.08 mM oxidized cytochrome c and 0.5 μg/ml phorbol myristate acetate (PMA) in Earle's balanced salt solution. Cultures were incubated with the assay mixture for exactly 1 h, then the amount of reduced cytochrome c was measured by its absorbance at 550 nm. Adherent cell protein was determined by the Lowry method using bovine serum albumin as standard.

Activation of Human Blood Monocytes by MDP Analogues

Human blood monocytes were isolated by ficoll-hypaque centrifugation and allowed to adhere to tissue culture dishes for 2 h (6). Nonadherent cells were washed away, and the adherent cells were cultured in endotoxin-free medium M199 in the presence of the indicated concentration of the macrophage activators. After 4 days, cultures were assayed for PMA-stimulated O_2^- release.

Superoxide Releasing Capacity of Human and Mouse Macrophages

Human peritoneal macrophages were obtained by saline lavage of trauma victims. (The lavage is routinely performed to diagnose internal bleeding; only lavage fluid that proved to be free from blood was utilized to isolate macrophages). Mouse peritoneal macrophages were obtained by saline lavage from healthy Swiss-Webster mice. Mouse and human blood monocytes were prepared by ficoll-hypaque centrifugation. Human milk macrophages were isolated by centrifuging freshly obtained human milk to pellet the macrophages. All cells were allowed to adhere for 2 h, and then nonadherent cells were washed off. PMA-stimulated O_2^- release was measured after the adherence step, and again after overnight incubation (18 h) in the presence or absence of LPS (10 ng/ml) or MDP (1 μg/ml).

RESULTS

Testing of MDP Analogs for Macrophage Activation

Initially, we studied a variety of MDP analogs to determine

whether any of the new derivatives of MDP might be significantly more effective than MDP or LPS in causing activation of mouse peritoneal macrophages (Table 1) or human blood monocytes (Table 2) in vitro. None of the analogs were superior to LPS in this in vitro system. Therefore, we used only MDP and LPS in our studies with human peritoneal macrophages, which are difficult to obtain in adequate numbers.

Table 1. Activation of Mouse Peritoneal Macrophages by MDP Analogs

Activator	Concentration[a]	O_2^- Released (nmol/hr/mg protein)
Control	-	60 ± 18[b]
LPS	10	431 ± 35
MDP	10	227 ± 10
	1	227 ± 7
	0.1	175 ± 6
MDP-DD	10	54 ± 6
MDP-butyl	100	295 ± 17
	10	217 ± 13
	1	115 ± 11
	0.1	39 ± 6
MDP-A-L	10	248 ± 22
	1	92 ± 7
MDP-DD-A-L	10	604 ± 49
	1	253 ± 78
B30-MDP	100	402 ± 84
	10	162 ± 15
	1	134 ± 3

[a] Concentrations in μg/ml except for LPS which is ng/ml.

[b] Means ± S.E.M., n = 3 to 6.

Table 2. Activation of Human Blood Monocytes by MDP Analogs

Activator	Concentration[a]	O_2^- Released (nmol/hr/mg protein)
Control	-	614 ± 120[b]
LPS	1	1401 ± 148
MDP	1	1651 ± 56
MDP-DD	1	614 ± 48
MDP-butyl	10	1612 ± 7
	1	1324 ± 336
	0.1	1362 ± 14
	0.01	572 ± 108
B30-MDP	1	1657 ± 56
	0.1	1216 ± 89
	0.01	462 ± 194
MDP-A-L	1	1023 ± 96
	0.1	742 ± 112
MDP-DD-A-L	1	1138 ± 248
	0.1	566 ± 192

[a] See Table 1.

[b] Means ± S.E.M, n = 3 to 6.

One interesting feature of these results is the excellent correlation between the ability of the MDP analogs to activate macrophages (measured as enhanced capacity to release O_2^-), as shown here, and the ability of the analogs to enhance non-specific resistance to infection (shown by Prof. Chedid and his colleagues, ref. 5). This is illustrated particularly well by the analog referred to as MDP-DD-A-L, which is a conjugate of the ordinarily inactive D-alanyl isomer of MDP with a polyalanine-polylysine carrier. MDP-DD-A-L is inactive as an adjuvant for both cell-mediated and humoral responses, but is active in enhancing non-specific resistance to infection with *Klebsiella pneumoniae* (5). As shown in Tables 1 and 2, MDP-DD-A-L was capable of producing macrophage activation in vitro, measured as enhanced PMA-stimulated O_2^- release.

Assessment of the State of Activation of Human Macrophages

Unlike peritoneal macrophages in the mouse, human macrophages (blood monocytes, milk macrophages and peritoneal macrophages) appeared to be in an activated state when freshly isolated (Table 3). Mouse blood monocytes also appeared to be initially activated. All the freshly-isolated human macrophage types produced a large amount of O_2^- in response to stimulation by PMA. In contrast with the marked effect of MDP or LPS on mouse cells cultured overnight, LPS or MDP had little or no effect on superoxide release by cultured human cells (Table 3).

DISCUSSION

Freshly isolated human macrophages released large amounts of O_2^- when stimulated with PMA. Subsequent overnight culture of these cells with MDP or LPS failed to enhance their PMA-stimulated O_2^- release. These results suggest that human cells may reside in an "activated" state in vivo. As we have shown (ref 6, 7 and Table 2), human monocytes will eventually become "unactivated" if cultured

Table 3. Superoxide Releasing Capacity of Human and Mouse Macrophages

Macrophage Type	PMA-Stimulated O_2^- Release (nmol O_2^-/hr/mg protein)			
	Freshly isolated	Overnight Culture with Buffer	LPS	MDP
Mouse Peritoneal	148 ± 10[a]	60 ± 18	431 ± 35	246 ± 9
Mouse Blood Monocytes	516 ± 56	24 ± 3	249 ± 7	76 ± 18
Human Peritoneal	1519 ± 50	779 ± 82	721 ± 46	749 ± 13
Human Blood Monocytes	1163 ± 101	1683 ± 119	1523 ± 204	1438 ± 56
Human Milk Macrophages	585 ± 48	362 ± 74	837 ± 38	383 ± 69

[a] Means ± S.E.M, 4 to 10 determinations except for human peritoneal macrophages where n = 6 (duplicate samples from 3 patients).

for 4 days in endotoxin-free medium; such cultured cells will remain activated if MDP or LPS is added to the culture medium. Why human cells appear to be activated in vivo, when mouse peritoneal cells are not, is unclear. Perhaps human cells are more sensitive than mouse peritoneal macrophages to small amounts of endotoxin leaking into the circulation from the gut. Endogenous bacterial products from the gut may play an essential role in maintaining human macrophages in a state of readiness to combat infection. MDP or other macrophage activators may be useful in treating patients whose macrophages are suppressed by drugs or tumors. However, our results raise the possibility that the capacity of MDP and related substances to activate macrophages and to stimulate non-specific resistance to infection in normal people may be limited.

SUMMARY

Human blood monocytes, peritoneal macrophages and milk macrophages, when initially isolated, displayed a vigorous release of superoxide anion (O_2^-), following stimulation with phorbol myristate acetate (PMA). This result contrasts with behavior of mouse peritoneal macrophages, which produce a weak O_2^- response, unless the macrophages are activated by infection or are elicted by injection of inflammatory agents. Treatment of mouse cells in vitro with bacterial products such as lipopolysaccharide (LPS) or muramyl dipeptide (MDP) also "primes" them for a high O_2^- response. Exposure of human macrophages to LPS or MDP for 16 h failed to enhance their O_2^- response. Thus the human cells appeared to be already "primed" for a vigorous oxygen radical response. In this respect, human cells resembled mouse peritoneal macrophages that have been "activated" by infection. These results suggest that MDP or other macrophage "activators" may offer less protection against infection in normal humans than they do in mice.

ACKNOWLEDGEMENTS

This work supported by NIH grants AI 14148 and DE 05494.

REFERENCES

1. Sasada, M., and R. B. Johnston, Jr. 1980. Macrophage microbicidal activity. Correlation between phagocytosis-associated oxidative metabolism and the killing of Candida by macrophages. J. Exp. Med. 152: 85.

2. Johnston, R. B., Jr., C. A. Godzik and Z. A. Cohn. 1978. Increased superoxide anion production by immunologically activated and chemically elicited macrophages. J. Exp. Med. 148: 115.

3. Cummings, N. P., M. J. Pabst and R. B. Johnston, Jr. 1980. Activation of macrophages for enhanced release of superoxide anion and greater killing of Candida albicans by injection of muramyl dipeptide. J. Exp. Med. 152: 1659.

4. Pabst, M. J. and R. B. Johnston, Jr. 1980. Increased production of superoxide anion by macrophages exposed in vitro to muramyl dipeptide or lipopolysaccharide. J. Exp. Med. 151: 101.

5. Chedid, L., M. Parant, F. Parant, F. Audibert, F. LeFrancier, J. Choay, and M. Sela. 1979. Enhancement of certain biological activities of muramyl dipeptide derivatives after conjugation to a multi-poly (DL-alanine)-poly(L-lysine) carrier. Proc. Natl. Acad. Sci. 76: 6557.

6. Pabst, M. J., H. B. Hedesgaard, and R. B. Johnston, Jr. 1982. Cultured human monocytes require exposure to bacterial products to maintain an optimal oxygen radical response. J. Immunol. 128: 123.

7. Hedegaard, H. B., and M. J. Pabst. 1982. Preservation of superoxide anion-generating capacity in cultured human monocytes by treatment with muramyl dipeptide or lipopolysaccharide, p. 205-208. Y. Yamamura et al (eds.), In Immunomodulation by Microbial Products and Related Synthetic Compounds. Excerpta Medica, Amsterdam.

SODIUM DIETHYLDITHIOCARBAMATE (IMUTHIOL) AND CANCER

G. Renoux[1], M. Renoux[1], E. Lemarie[2], M. Lavandier[2], J. Greco[3], P. Bardos[1], J. M. Lang[4], A. Boilletot[4], F. Oberling[4], J. Armand[5], A. Mussett[5], G. Biron[5]

Laboratoire d'Immunologie[1], Service de Pneumologie[2], Service de Chirurgie B[3], CHU Bretonneau-Trousseau, Tours; Service des Maladies[4] du Sang, CHU d'Hautepierre, Strasbourg; Institut Mérieux[5], France

INTRODUCTION

Immune impairment or dysfunction is associated with cancers, and is frequently aggravated by conventional therapies. As a consequence, the development of agents active on the immune system in ways that restore or regulate host defenses, has become a major objective. An overall appreciation of the published data led us to conceptualize the following requirements for suitable immunopharmacologic agents. Absence of carcinogenicity, of tumor promoting influence and of antigenicity or sensitizing effects, is an essential prerequisite since these agents will be administered for long periods of time to patients already at risk. They should have defined influences on populations or subpopulations of immunocompetent cells, as their essential activities. Their toxic levels and pharmacologic effects should be known to delineate the range of doses and predict most side effects. Such requirements will reasonably eliminate most of the inconsistencies which have somewhat dampened confidence in therapies intended to modify the immune system.

The development of sodium diethyldithiocarbamate is based on the aforementioned lines. It was selected from a large series of sulfur-containing drugs (1) in attempts to obviate the ambivalent, time- and dose-dependent effect of levamisole (2), and also to obtain a drug devoid of the sensitizing influence of thiazole or benzol ring structures (3). The term imuthiol will now replace the previous abbreviation "DTC", as the latter could be confused with the chemotherapeutic agent DTIC, dimethyl-triazeno-imidazole-carboxamide. Years of experiments, prior to clinical testing, have evidenced that imuthiol fulfills safety requirements, possesses pharmacologic activities that could be useful to treat cancers or infectious diseases, and exert a unique influence on T cell lineage.

PHARMACOLOGIC ACTIVITIES

Table 1 abstracts from a recent review (4) the main features of imuthiol effects. We would like to stress pharmacologic features that could strengthen the immunopotentiating and immunorestoring activities of imuthiol. Its detoxifying action against drug-induced damages could justify its use in associated chemoimmunotherapies to reduce the toxicity of cytolytic agents, such as *cis*-platinum (5-7), or to increase their activity, such as bleomycin (8). Protection against the lethal effects of ionizing radiations could similarly facilitate their therapeutic use. The antibiotic efficacy of imuthiol, at doses which do not alter normal cells, could help in controlling severe infections that resist antibiotics alone. It might also partially account for immunorestoration in such patients. Anticancer effects (prevention of chemically-induced cancers and reduction in the number of spontaneously arising tumors) could likely be extended to direct effects on some malignant tumors, as it has been shown that imuthiol was cytotoxic for spindle cell carcinoma cells (9), and for melanoma cells (10). An imuthiol-induced reduction of the tumor burden if confirmed in clinical testing, will obviously provide additional chances for cancer cures.

That the administration of imuthiol is safe is clearly shown by a National Cancer Institute study where mice and rats were treated with either 17.5 or 140 mg/kg daily for at least 100 consecutive weeks. In these studies, there were not effects other than a prolonged survival of female mice (11). The data are confirmed by current studies showing the beneficial influence of imuthiol on aged BALB/c mice (Burley-Rosset, personal communication), and on NZB mice where imuthiol prevents lymphomas (M. Renoux).

IMMUNOPHARMACOLOGY

Present findings can be summarized as follows (4, 12, 15, 19). A single administration in a range of 0.5 to 25 mg/kg: elicits a marked increase in IgG plaque-forming cells specific for sheep red blood cells, and abolishes the nonspecific antibody response to horse blood cells; induces the production of IgG specific circulating antibodies as early as 6 days after immunization, and reduces the level of IgM antibodies; creates high and long-standing levels of delayed-type hypersensitivity to sheep red cells (12) or to BGG (16); increases lymphoproliferative responses to T cell mitogens and allogenic antigens at all the days of a 7 day kinetic study; does not modify the number of B cells, nor the response to pokeweed mitogen.

Table 1. Main features of imuthiol effects.

I. Pharmacology

- Virtually nontoxic. No untoward side effects in man.
- Nonantigenic, nonsensitizing and nonpyrogenic.
- No carcinogenicity or tumor-promoting influence.
- No splenomegaly and expansion of the reticuloendothelial system.
- Antibiotic
- Protects against chemically-induced liver damage, cis-platinum toxicity, and against the lethal effects of ionizing radiations.
- Prevents chemically-induced cancerogenesis.
- Kills some neoplastic cells at doses harmless for normal cells.

II. Immunologic Activities.

- Recruits functional T cells from precursors, even in athymic mice.
- Regulates T cell subsets.
- Augments NK activity without production of interferon.
- Restores the responses abrogated by chemotherapies. Prevents immunodepression due to surgical trauma.
- No effect on B cell number, PWM-induced responses, or ADCC to chicken erythrocytes. Decreases circulating IgM antibody levels and immediate hypersensitivity.
- No time- or dose-dependent inhibitory effects.

III. Influence On The T Cell Lineage. - Mechanism of Action

- No *in vitro* activity. Diethylamine or CS alone, are inactive. Acts through the increased production of an inducer of prothymocyte maturation and acquisition of functional activities. Inactive on B cells.
- Replaces a signal missing in athymic mice allowing maturation of functionally active T cells.
- Brain neocortex controls the synthesis of the inducer and the influence of imuthiol.

Current studies show that: oral administration (5 to 500 mg/kg) is as active as s.c. administration, and even if treatment was given 7 days prior to immunization, a dose of 250 mg/kg is as active as 25 mg/kg.

Current studies show also that imuthiol does not modify ADCC to chicken red cells and has no direct influence on macrophages.

Chronic administration of 25 mg/kg, 3 times a week for 4 weeks, stimulates the host to increased T cell associated responses, in contrast with the immunodepression afforded by long-term treatments with other immunomodulating agents (18).

Imuthiol restores to normal values the immune responses abrogated by hydrocortisone or by azathioprine (18). The results affirm the influence of imuthiol on T cells, the activities of which are suppressed by azathioprine.

These effects are not associated with a granulomatous disease or by lymphoproliferative disorders. In brief, imuthiol increases T cell mediated events after either a single administration, a pretreatment or chronic administration. These effects are not associated with direct influences on B cells or macrophages.

Imuthiol activates NK activity depending upon the age of the mice and on the dose, and at time periods differing from those where interferon or interferon inducers are known to be active (Tables 2, 3). As shown by Table 4, the effect on NK activity was not associated with changes in mouse interferon levels (17). The lack of influence on endogenous interferon production was confirmed in a study of 25 patients treated with either 2, 5 or 10 mg/kg imuthiol suspended in 125 ml pyrogen-free isotonic buffer (Table 5). These data show unequivocally that, in man as in animals, imuthiol is not an interferon inducer. It might be of practical as well as basic interest to lay stress on the finding that imuthiol augmented NK activity of 26 week old mice, whose spontaneous response was lowered by age (Table 2). It could be of importance in further clinical studies to verify whether imuthiol will increase NK activity at a different time than that evoked by interferon inducers. Imuthiol was found to act synergistically with interferon against EMC virus infection (Chany, personal communication). Since, even 98% pure interferon is scarcely efficient in cancer patients (20), a combined imuthiol-interferon treatment could be of use against viral infections or cancers.

Imuthiol is inactive in vitro. It promotes or stimulates, even in congenitally athymic mice, the in vivo synthesis of a potent inducer of prothymocyte maturation and acquisition of functional activities. The inducer is active across the species barrier (4, 13, 19, 21-24). The synthesis of the inducer and the influence

Table 2. In vivo modification of NK activity induced in C3H/He mice by 25 mg/kg imuthiol

	8 week old mice		26 week old mice	
Time of[a] treatment	Lytic units per 10^7 cells	%	Lytic units per 10^7 cells	%
0 (saline)	158.3	-	26	-
2 hr	280.8	177[b]	NT	-
6 hr	172.9	109	9.5	38[b]
24 hr	124.6	79	6.8	26[b]
2 d	NT	-	28	107
7 d	NT	-	48.6	187[b]

[a] Four mice per group

[b] p <0.01 in comparison with saline-treated controls.

of imuthiol are controlled by the brain neocortex (13, 25-30). An athymic animal will respond to the agent but not an animal deprived of the right brain neocortex.

Table 3. Influence of age and of dose of imuthiol on NK activity tested four days after treatment in C3H/He mice.

	4 weeks		14 weeks		18 weeks	
Treatment	Lytic units per 10^7 cells	%	Lytic units per 10^7 cells	%	Lytic units per 10^7 cells	%
0	71	-	53	-	14	-
25 mg/kg	58	81	84	158[b]	12	88
2.5 mg/kg	145	254[b]	NT	-	NT	-

[a] Four to 6 mice per group.

[b] Significative at p <0.01 in comparison with saline-treated controls.

Table 4. Serum interferon titers induced by treatment with 25 mg/kg imuthiol

	Time posttreatment					
Strain	0	2	6	24	48	72 hrs
C57Bl/6[a]	< 2	< 2	< 2	< 2	< 2	< 2
C3H/He	< 2	< 2	< 2	< 2	< 2	< 2

[a] Ten mice per group.

SUMMARY OF EXPERIMENTAL FINDINGS

Above data show unique immunological and pharmacological properties of imuthiol. Imuthiol recruits T cells from precommitted precursor cells through an increased, or de novo induced, production of T cell specific inducer. It induces T cells to generate enhanced levels of cytotoxic activities and lymphoproliferative responses. Through its effects on T cells, B cells are induced to secrete antibodies of the IgG class and monocyte/macrophages to participate in delayed-type hypersensitivities. Imuthiol increases NK activity without effects on interferon levels. It has no direct effect on B cells, nor nonspecific polyclonal activities or in vitro enhancing effects. These effects clearly distinguish imuthiol from other thiols, such as 2-mercaptoethanol or levamisole, the activities of which are mediated by a mitogenic, general lymphocyte activator, active both on T and B cells (31).

These actions are evoked in the absence of events initiated by other triggering influences, and contrast with those of promoters which act to increase an already developing immune event, or of adjuvants which augment the response to an antigen. Imuthiol should also be distinguished from most immunomodifiers in that it does not evidence time- or dose-dependent characteristics to augment or inhibit immune responses, and does not give rise to sensitization or to a granulomatous disease.

As a free radical scavanger, also through its regulating influence on lysosomal enzymes, imuthiol evinces detoxifying activities. Likely as an antimetabolite agent against specific tyrosinases, imuthiol shows antibiotic (*M. leprae*, *F. falciparum*) and antitumor (melanocytes) activities. Imuthiol is not a carcinogenic or tumor-promoting agent, and even after prolonged administration, these features, and its low toxicity, favor its safe use in clinical testing.

Table 5. Influence of imuthiol on serum interferon titers in man.

	Time posttreatment						
Dose	0	2 h	6 h	24 h	2 d	7 d	14 d
2 mg/kg							
Ber. M.	<1:2	–	–	<1:2	–	<1:2	–
Ger. M	<1:2	–	–	<1:2	–	1:2	–
Raq. J.	<1:2	–	–	1:6	<1:20	1:6	–
Gicq. R.	1:4	–	–	1:4	1:4	1:4	–
Bour. E.	1:16	–	–	1:16	1:16	1:16	–
Puss. Ch.	1:8	–	–	1:8	1:8	1:8	–
Reig. R.	1:8	–	–	1:2	1:8	1:8	–
5 mg/kg							
Chan. Ed.	15	–	–	15	20	15	–
Lam. M.	40	–	–	40	40	40	–
Sim. R.	40	–	–	40	40	40	40
Len. L.	<25	<25	<25	<25	<25	<25	<25
Rag. J.	<25	<25	<25	<25	<25	<25	<25
Mom. R.	<25	<25	<25	<25	<25	<25	<25
Magn. G.	<25	<25	<25	<25	<25	<25	<25
Mer. J.	<40	–	<40	<40	–	–	–
10 mg/kg							
Piqg. C.	<25	<25	<25	<25	<25	<25	<25
Brou. A.	<25	<25	<25	<25	<25	<25	–
Vill. G.	<25	<25	–	<25	<25	<25	–
Berg. M.	<15	<15	<15	<15	<15	<15	–
Ducl. L.	60	40	30	30	40	40	–
Bla. G.	<15	<15	<15	15	15	15	–
Baus. P.	240	240	–	240	320	240	–
Lanz. J.	15	–	15	15	15	15	–
Gha. B.	15	15	15	20	30	30	–
Chl. M.	20	20	20	20	40	20	1

IMUTHIOL AND CANCER

As we were aware that premature or excessive enthusiasm frequently led to inconsistencies and conflicting data in the general field of therapeutic applications, we deliberately followed a slow pace, waiting for a sufficient body of experimental information prior to clinical testing. Above data indicate that imuthiol could be a useful and safe agent to be employed alone or associated with conventional therapies in the treatment of cancer patients.

Previous phase I-II studies (14, 32), showed that an intravenous injection of 0.5 to 10 mg/kg imuthiol was devoid of side effects, did not modify biochemical parameters, and restored to control values, and even above, the responses to PHA and Con A. They showed also that low doses (0.5 to 2.2 mg/kg) administered prior to surgery for cancer, prevented the immunodepression of surgical trauma and restored to normal levels lymphoproliferative responses to T cell mitogens. Imuthiol was not mitogenic, and did not affect the response to PWM and immunoglobulin levels. The data are currently confirmed by double-blind studies with various time and dose schedules of intravenous or oral administration, the detailed results of which will be published later. No side effects were observed following either administration. In brief, imuthiol is neither a mitogen nor a polyclonal activator in man. It regulates the activities of T cells without apparent direct effects on B cells. Immunostimulant doses are devoid of toxicity, side effects, and synergistic effects with sedative and anaesthetics.

Oral Administration To Cancer-Bearing Children

The effect of imuthiol orally administered was evaluated in a controlled study (Service des Maladies du sang, Centre Hospitalier d'Haute-pierre, Strasbourg). Eleven boys and nine girls between 5 and 19 years of age (mean 10.2), maintained in complete remission (leukemia, nephroblastoma, embryosarcoma or Hodgkin's disease) for more than one year, entered this study. They were randomly assigned to one of the following groups: a) placebo; b) 2.5 mg/kg; c) 5 mg/kg and d) 10 mg/kg imuthiol. Treatment consisted of the oral administration, once a week for four weeks, of gastroprotected pills.

The immune status was evaluated by the delayed-type hypersensitivity (DTH) responses to bacterial or fungal antigens (candida, trichophyton, tuberculin, proteus, streptococcus, tetanus, diphtheria) using Multitest (Institut Mérieux). DTH responses were scored 48 hr after application and total scores evaluated according to the notice of the manufacturer. The first application was made 5 days prior to initiation of treatment, and the second 2 days after the 4th pill ingestion. A five-week clinical surveillance permitted an evaluation of side effects.

Figure 1 summarizes the influence of imuthiol on DTH responses of children affected with cancer, yet in a period of complete remission. A drastic fall in scores, meaning an important inhibition of cell-mediated immunity, was observed in the placebo group. In contrast, a favorable dose effect influence of imuthiol was evidenced (Figure 1). Covariance analysis of the data show significant ($p = 0.07$) differences between the four groups, explained by a linear regression (95% variance at $p = 0.007$) among these groups. This analysis evidences a dose-response relationship. In other words, the oral administration once a week and for 4 weeks of 10 mg/kg imuthiol to cancer children restored better than other dosages tested a cell-mediated immune response (DTH) inhibited in the placebo group. No side effects or clinical changes that could be attributed to imuthiol administration were observed during the study.

This preliminary clinical testing is encouraging, in that it evidences the absence of toxicity or side effects of imuthiol in children and suggests the agent could restore imparied cell-mediated immunity in young cancer patients.

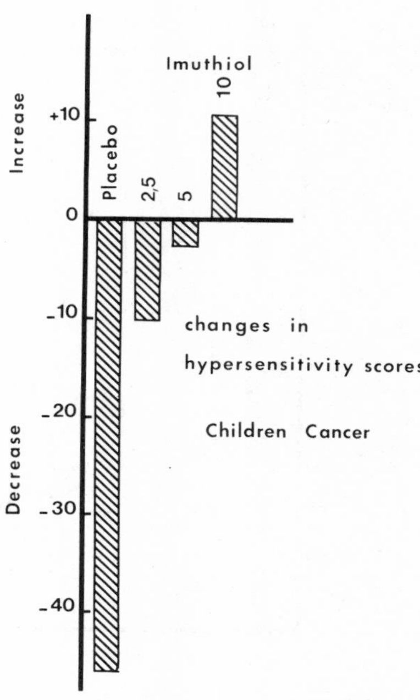

Fig. 1. Influence of imuthiol on cell-mediated immunity of cancer-bearing children. Twenty patients randomly assigned to one of 4 groups of oral treatment (placebo, 2.5 mg/kg, 5 mg/kg or 10 mg/kg imuthiol) once a week for 4 weeks. Skin tests were measured by the Multitest Mérieux, before and two days after treatment.

Influence On Immune Parameters In Lung Cancer Patients

A previous report (15) showed that administering 5 mg/kg imuthiol restored toward normal values the helper/suppressor ratio (% OKT 4^+ cells : % OKT 8^+ cells) within 5 days in 8 patients affected with primary bronchogenic cancers. It has been, however, argued that such changes might be due to a chance day-to-day variation. To test this hypothesis, twelve informed-consent volunteers were randomly assigned to an intravenous injection of 5 mg/kg imuthiol or of isotonic, pyrogen-free buffer as placebo. They were male patients, between 48 and 62 years of age, affected with primary bronchogenic carcinoma. The assay was conducted prior to specific caner therapy. Immunological tests were performed before and 5 days after treatment on blood sampled between 8:30 and 9:00 am to minimize bioperiodicity.

Figure 2 shows that peripheral blood lymphocyte responses to the T cell mitogens, PHA and Con A, were significantly increased ($p < 0.01$, Mann-Whitney U test) above initial values in imuthiol-

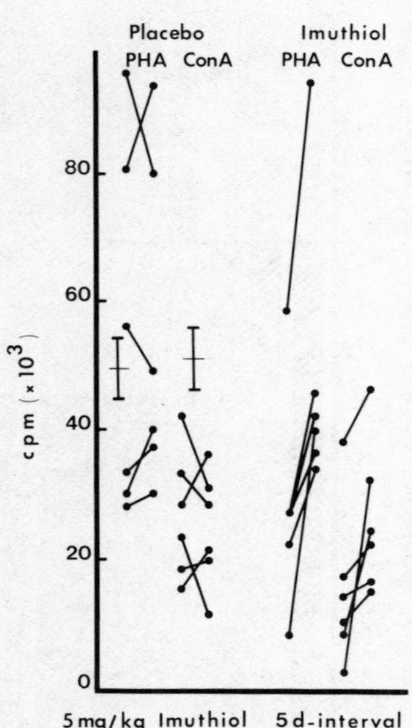

Fig. 2. Lung Cancer. Influence of imuthiol on T cell mitogen reresponses of peripheral blood lymphocytes of lung cancer patients, 5 days after an intravenous injection of 5 mg/kg imuthiol. Vertical bars indicate the values found in 49 healthy controls. No significant changes were observed in the placebo group. Responses to PHA and Con A were significantly increased ($p < 0.01$) in the treated group.

treated cancer patients, whereas these figures remained unchanged in the placebo group. Monoclonal serum analysis of T cell subsets are summaried in Figure 3, where OKT 3^+, OKT 4^+ and OKT 8^+ cells are expressed as percents of the total lymphocyte population. Statistical evaluation shows that counts at day 0 and day + 5 were identical in the placebo group for the three OKT cell populations. In contrast, imuthiol has evoked highly significant increase ($p < 0.01$) in OKT 3^+ and OKT 4^+ cells, accompanied by a significant decrease ($p = 0.06$) in the percentage of the suppressor (OKT 8^+) cell population. Present data therefore confirm in a double-blind study, the feeling previously derived from an open study that imuthiol could regulate in lung cancer patients the relative percents of T cell subsets. They confirm also that an injection of imuthiol increases the responses to T cell mitogens.

Imuthiol And Melanoma

It has been found that imuthiol inhibited melanoma cell development in guinea pigs (10), likely through an antimetabolic effect involving a complex of imuthiol with the copper moiety of the phenolase enzyme abundant in melanoma cells (33). It has been suggested that resistance to the antimetabolic effect of imuthiol by any mutation involving amino acid substitution in the enzyme is not likely to occur as imuthiol would not complex with the enzyme protein itself (33). The data suggest also that imuthiol might be of some interest as an antimetabolic agent against melanoma cells,

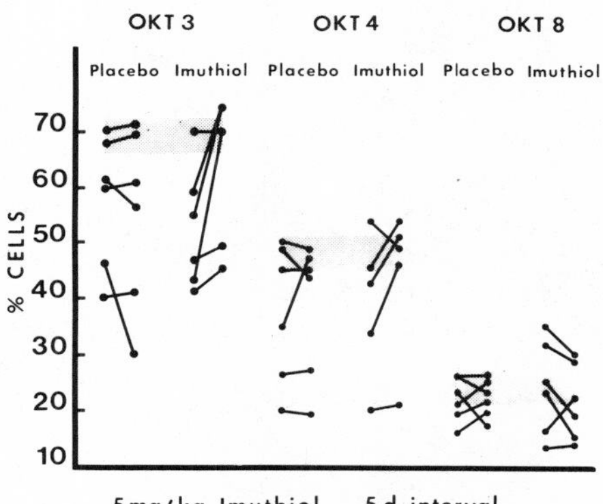

Fig. 3. Lung cancer. Influence of imuthiol on the percentages of T (OKT 3^+ cells, inducer (OKT 4^+) and suppressor-cytotoxic (OKT 8^+) cells of lung cancer patients. Shaded areas indicate normal values. Statistical analysis reveal a significant ($p < 0.01$) increase in OKT 4 percentages and a significant decrease ($p = 0.06$) in OKT 8 percentage in the treated group, and no changes in the placebo group.

in addition to its influence on the T cell lineage. Assays are in progress to test this hypothesis.

We thought it of interest however, to give present data, even if they are largely provisional. As seen in Table 6, one month treatment by 5 mg/kg i.v. once a week increases the responses to PHA and Con A but has little, if any, influence on modifying the relative percentages of T cell subsets (OKT 4^+ and OKT 8^+) in four patients (1 male and 3 female) affected with stage IV melanomas. This response is different from the rapid influence of imuthiol on the T cell subpopulations in lung cancer patients.

The long-term follow-up of a 48-y-old woman, melanoma stage IV, Breslow index >2, is summarized in Figure 4. During the course of combined chemotherapy (DTIC + vincristine), which lowered the responses to mitogens, 10 mg/kg imuthiol were intravenously administered once a week for 1 month and after 2 weeks rest, continuously for 3 months. It permitted chemotherapy to be accepted with minimal side effects. During 1981 and 1982, 250 mg imuthiol was given by the oral route once a week. Two main features emerge from the data. The one is that it takes more than one year of immunotherapy to restore OKT 4^+ counts that were impaired by disease and chemotherapy. The second is that the patient is actually perfectly healthy, weighing 60 kg for 1.64 m, with no apparent symptoms that could be related to melanoma and with biochemical or hematological tests, all at normal values. A two-year survival associated with a normal comfort in life is unusual after a diagnosis of stage IV, Breslow >2, melanoma.

One sparrow does not make a spring, and a more elaborate study, involving various dosages and control groups, is needed before assessing a value for imuthiol in the treatment of melanoma. Nevertheless, the present result is encouraging in that it suggests imuthiol could be associated with chemotherapy. As doses higher than 10 mg/kg are both nontoxic and immunoactive, higher dosages might be tested to evidence or utilize direct effect of the agent on melanoma cells.

DISCUSSION

The present report indicates our trend toward immunotherapy of cancers, i.e., a step-by-step study taking into account the human problems of clinical testing to minimize the danger of a new treatment for volunteer patients. As a biological response modifier, imuthiol demonstrates a unique influence on the T cell lineage and not directly on the other immunocompetent cells. In addition to specific recruiting efficacy, imuthiol has no dose- or time-dependent inhibitory influence and does not induce an expansion

Table 6. Influences of one month (5 mg/kg imuthiol once a week) treatment on immunological tests in stage IV melanoma patients.

	PATIENT							
	No. 1. (male)		No. 2 (female)		No. 3 (female)		No. 4 (female)	
Test	0	1 month	0	1 month	0	1 month	0	1 month
E rosettes	58	56	62	72	62	78	77	70
OKT 3	-	-	50	67	84	76	58	70
4	-	-	35	38	64	46	46	56
8	-	-	40	36	28	31	21	18
PHA (cpm x 10^3)	37	75	40	74	72	105	43	87
Con A (cpm x 10^3)	23	42	23	42	68	71	18	56

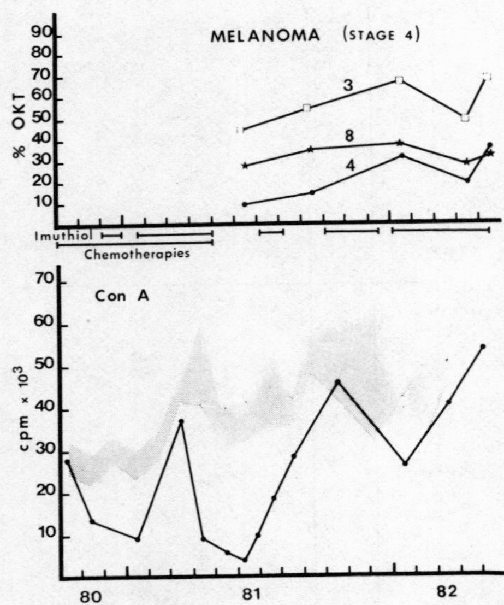

Fig. 4. Influence of a twenty-month treatment with imuthiol on immune parameters of a stage IV, Breslow index >2, melanoma patient. Treatments are summarized in text. Shaded areas correspond to same-day control values for Con A. Responses to PHA are not indicated, as they paralleled those of Con A.

of the reticuloendothelial system that may trigger lymphoid malignancies. These features distinguish imuthiol from other agents (19).

Imuthiol is active after either intravenous or oral administration. Imuthiol is devoid of toxic or deleterious effects in man. It restores to normal values immune parameters altered by cancer, chemotherapy or surgical trauma. In man as in animals, imuthiol might also regulate the ratio among T cell subsets. It seems likely that it could act synergistically with interferon, thus allowing for full efficacy of the two agents employed in combination.

Present findings, although preliminary, suggest that a dose of imuthiol (e.g. 5 mg/kg) might be not equally active on immune responsiveness of patients affected with different cancers. Inasmuch as cancer, in general, is associated with immunodeficiency, one shoul therefore test various doses and schedules of administration to determine the best dose for a given type of cancer, since genetically-induced modulation (34) has little influence on imuthiol activities (35).

We believe that available data are sufficient to suggest the us of imuthiol for the preoperative management of cancer patients to lessen or suppress immune impairment provoked by surgical and anaesthetic trauma, thus reducing the risk of disseminated micrometastases. Its use after radical surgery may prevent recurrences or metastases. Similarly, its administration could protect against the detrimental influence of radiation. Imuthiol could be a rational basis for improved chemoimmunotherapy. Its antibiotic-like effects and influence on the T cell lineage support the clinical testing of imuthiol in bacterial, viral, fungal and parasitic diseases, particularly in immunosuppressed patients. As suggested by studies in athymic mice, imuthiol might be able to correct a genetically determined immunodeficiency. Its regulatory effect on human T cell subsets may well deserve its use in autoimmune diseases.

In conclusion, imuthiol already fulfills the requirements for a biological response modifier of known specific activities, and devoid of untoward side effects, toxicity, carcinogenicity, tumor-promoting influence and antigenicity.

SUMMARY

Sodium diethyldithiocarbamate (imuthiol), a nonantigenic, nontoxic and noncarcinogenic compound, evinces distinctive properties in recruitment and activation of T cells, and no direct influences on B cells or macrophages. The biological attributes of imuthiol (destruction of neoplastic cells, bacteria, fungi and parasites; a detoxifying influence against carcinogens or agents toxic for the liver) could strengthen its activity as a biological response modifier. Preliminary clinic testings show that imuthiol restores T cell activities and regulates the ratio among T cell subsets in cancer patients, without untoward side effects.

ACKNOWLEDGEMENTS

This work was supported by Grants-in-Aids from Institut Mérieux and in parts by INSERM and Ligue Nationale contre le Cancer.

REFERENCES

1. Renoux, G., and M. Renoux. 1974. C. R. Acad. Sci. (Paris) 278 D: 1139.

2. Renoux, G. 1980. Drugs 20: 89.

3. Blacow, N. W. 1972. Martindale the Extra Pharmacopoeia, 26th Edition. The Pharmaceutical Press, London.

4. Renoux, G. 1982. J. Pharmacol. (Paris) 13 (in press).

5. Borch, R. F. and M. E. Pleasant. 1979. Proc. Natl. Acad. Sci. USA 76: 6611.

6. Borch, R. F., J. C. Katz, P. H. Lieder, and M. E. Pleasant. 1980. Proc. Natl. Acad. Sci. USA 77: 5441.

7. Gale, G. R., and L. M. Atkins. 1981. J. Clin. Hematol. Oncol. 11: 41.

8. Lin, P. S., L. Kwock, and N. T. Goodchild. 1980. Cancer 46: 2360.

9. Powell, A. K. 1954. Brit. J. Cancer 8: 529.

10. Blagoeva, P. and I. Stoichev. 1979. Experientia 35: 1389.

11. National Cancer Institute. 1979. Technical Rep. Series 172

12. Renoux, G., and M. Renoux. 1979. J. Immunopharmacol. 1: 247.

13. Renoux, G. 1980. In B. Serrou and C. Rosenfeld (eds.), New trends in human immunology and cancer immunotherapy. Doin, Paris.

14. Renoux, G. and M. Renoux. 1981. In E. M. Hersh, M. A. Chirigos, and M. Mastrangelo (eds.), Augmenting agents in cancer therapy. Raven Press, New York.

15. Renoux, G. and M. Renoux. 1982. In B. Serrou et al. (eds.), Current concepts in human immunology and cancer immunomodulation. Elsevier Biomedical Press, Amsterdam.

16. Neveu, P. J. 1978. Clin. Exp. Immunol. 32: 419.

17. Renoux, G., P. Bardos, D. Degenne, M. Musset. In R. B. Herberman (ed.), Natural cell-mediated immunity. Academic Press, New York (in press).

18. Renoux, G. and M. Renoux. 1980. Clin. Immunol. Immunopathol. 15: 21.

19. Renoux, G. 1982. In M. Rola-Pleszczynski, P. Sirois (eds.). Immunopharmacology. Elsevier/North-Holland.

20. Scherwin, St. 1982. In G. Mathé et al (eds.) Tumor Pharmacology, Paris.

21. Renoux, G. and M. Renoux. 1977. J. Exp. Med. 145: 466.

22. Renoux, G., M. Renoux, J. M. Guiolaumin, and C. Gouzien. 1979. J. IMmunopharmacol. 1: 145.

23. Renoux, G. and M. Renoux. 1980. Thymus 2: 139.

24. Renoux, G., J. L. Touraine, and M. Renoux. 1980. J. Immunopharmacol. 2: 49.

25. Renoux, G., K. Bizière, M. Renoux and J. M. Guillaumin. 1980. C. R. Acad. Sci. (Paris) 290 D: 719.

26. Bardos, P., D. Degenne, Y. Lebranchu, K. Bizière, and G. Renoux. 1981. Scand. J. Immunol. 13: 609.

27. Bizière, K., G. Renoux, and M. Renoux. 1982. Neuroscience 7: 528.

28. Renoux, G., K. Bizière, and M. Renoux. 1982. Bull. Acad. Nat. Med. 166: 88.

29. Renoux, G., K. Bizière, M. Renoux, and J. M. Guillaumin. 1982. Scand. J. Immunol. (in press).

30. Renoux, G., K. Bizière, P. Bardos, D. Degenne, and M. Renoux. 1982. In R. B. Herberman (ed.), Natural cell-mediated immunity. Academic Press, New York (in press).

31. Hewlett, G., H-G. Opitz, and H. D. Schlumberger. 1981. In E. Pick and M. Landy (eds.) Lymphokines, Vol. 4. Academic Press, New York.

32. Renoux, G., M. Renoux, J. Greco, J. Baudouin, M. Lavandier, and E. Lemarié. 1980. In B. Serrou and C. Rosenfeld (eds.), New trends in human immunology and cancer immunotherapy. Doin, Paris.

33. Prabhakaran, K., E. B. Harris, and W. F. Kirchheimer. 1972. Microbios. 5: 273.

34. Renoux, G. 1979. Internatl. J. Immunopharmacol. 1: 43

35. Renoux, G., and M. Renoux. 1982. In R. L. Fenichel (ed.), Immunomodulating agents. Marcel Dekker, New York (in press).

ISOPRINOSINE AND NPT 15392: IMMUNOMODULATION AND CANCER

L. N. Simon[1], F. K. Hoehler[1], D. T. McKenzie[1] and J. W. Hadden[2]

Newport Pharmaceuticals International, Inc., Newport Beach, California[1]; University of South Florida College of Medicine, Tampa, Florida[2] (USA)

INTRODUCTION

In cancer, there appears to be a direct relationship between immunosuppression and the ability of neoplastic cells to flourish. Because the immune system is compromised, tumor growth is unchecked by the normal immune regulatory mechanisms. For this reason it has been suggested that immunomodulators, agents that directly affect immune function, might be used therapeutically in the treatment of cancer. Such compounds could restore the body's capacity to mount an immunologic response leading to the eventual destruction of the neoplasm. Perhaps better supported by clinical evidence, is the possible use of immunomodulators as adjuvants to standard cancer therapies, such as chemotherapy or radiotherapy. The generalized immunosuppression resulting from these procedures often leads to severe problems with opportunistic infections. Used in combination with standard chemotherapy or radiotherapy, immunomodulators might speed the recovery of normal immune function thereby not only reducing the incidence of recurrence but also reducing the likelihood of infection. Immunomodulators, therefore, might be used either as a primary cancer therapy or as an adjuvant to established therapies. In this paper we review recent investigations which support the potential application of two immunomodulators, Isoprinosine and NPT 15392, in cancer therapy.

ISOPRINOSINE

Isoprinosine is a chemical complex of inosine with the p-acetamidobenzoic acid salt of N, N-dimethylamino-2-propanol in a molar ratio of 1:3. Evidence for interaction of the components, including spectral data and measurements of association constants, has been reviewed (11). Based on in vitro results it has been proposed that much of Isoprinosine's biological activity is attributable to the inosine moiety which is liberated upon dissociation of the complex in tissues and biological fluids (37). Despite the drug's eventual dissociation, other studies (17) indicate that, in order to mediate biological activity in vivo, Isoprinosine must be administered as a complex rather than as individual components. The pharmacology and toxicology of Isoprinosine have been reviewed (40), as has its immunopharmacology in animals (11) and, therefore, these topics will not be discussed here.

In Vitro Effects of Isoprinosine on Human Immune Function

Hadden et al. provided the first measure of Isoprinosine's immunomodulatory properties, the augmentation of phytohemagglutinin (PHA)-induced blastogenic responses expressed in vitro by human peripheral blood lymphocytes (13). Since that time the observation that Isoprinosine can influence the blastogenic response of human lymphocytes has been extended to a number of mitogens. Enhancement of the response was seen when Isoprinosine was present at concentrations between 0.1-220 μg/ml. In general, the drug had the greatest impact when added to cultures containing optimal concentrations of mitogen. Hadden et al. (13) and Morin et al. (23) have localized the effect of Isoprinosine in the initiation phase of the response. As shown in Table 1, responses were augmented 1.6-3.4 fold depending

Table 1. In vitro blastogenic responses to Isoprinosine in humans.

Mitogen (antigen)	Increase*	Investigator
Phytohemagglutinin	1.6	Hadden (13)
	1.7	Simon (29)
Concanavalin A	3.4	Morin (23)
Pokeweed Mitogen	1.6	Hadden (16)
	1.6	Morin (23)
Mixed Leukocyte Culture	2.4	Wybran (36)
Tetanus Toxoid	2.7	Morin (23)

* Control = 1.0

on the mitogen. Interestingly, the blastogenic response was augmented regardless of whether the mitogen utilized was specific for T or B lymphocytes. The human mixed leukocyte culture reaction (a measure of histoincompatibility) also expresses enhanced levels of thymidine incorporation in the presence of Isoprinosine (36).

The in vitro effects of Isoprinosine on the differentiation and function of human lymphoid cells have also been documented in a number of systems (Table 2). Confirming results obtained in the mouse, Touraine et al. (32) showed that human T-lymphocyte differentiation antigen (HTLA) was induced in bone marrow cell cultures incubated with Isoprinosine. Differentiation of active T-rosettes and autologous T-rosettes by Isoprinosine has been documented in cultures of human peripheral blood lymphocytes (32). In an assay which suggests an effect of Isoprinosine on B-cell differentiation, pokeweed mitogen (PWM) was found to induce higher percentages of IgG-containing human peripheral blood lymphocytes when mixed with Isoprinosine (1, 23). The Concanavalin A (Con A)-induced suppressor cell levels in unfractionated peripheral blood lymphocytes and in T-lymphocytes purified by E-rosetting technique showed Isoprinosine-induced augmentation (32). Wybran et al. (37) observed that Isoprinosine augmented leukocyte adherence inhibition and increased monocyte phagocytosis of yeast. The production of the monokine Interleukin I was stimulated by Isoprinosine (17).

Overall, concentrations of 1-10 µg/ml Isoprinosine were usually sufficient for generating in vitro augmentation of immune differentiation and function, and the measured effects were greater in magnitude than those produced by levamisole in similar systems.

In Vivo Effects of Isoprinosine of Human Immune Functions

Many of the human and animal immune tests which were influenced by Isoprinosine in vitro were also shown to be affected when the drug was administered to human subjects in vivo (Table 3).

In a study which demonstrated the positive clinical effects of Isoprinosine in herpes simplex virus infections, a parallel increase in PHA-induced lymphoblast transformation was observed (3). Likewise, Corey et al. (4) showed an increase in the PHA response of peripheral blood lymphocytes of herpes genitalis patients. Isoprinosine treatment augmented blast transformation, whereas controls treated with placebo showed depressed responses. There was also an increase in HSV specific blast transformation in Isoprinosine-treated patients as compared to placebo-treated controls.

In an influenza challenge study, Betts et al. (2) reported an increase in influenza virus-induced blast transformation of drug-treated volunteers. Subjects receiving Isoprinosine also expressed

Table 2. In vitro effects of Isoprinosine on human lymphocyte differentiation and functions*

Test	Results	Investigator
Induction of Human T-Lymphocyte (HTLA) Marker in Bone Marrow Cells	Augmentation of T-Cell (HTLA) Marker Acquisition	Touraine (32)
Peripheral Blood Lymphocytes (PBL) Active Rosette Test	Increase in Active Rosettes	Wybran (36)
Autologous Rosette Test (PBL)	Increase in Autologous Rosettes	Wybran (37)
Pokeweed-Mitogen Induction of IgG Containing Peripheral Blood Lymphocytes	Augmentation of Percent IgG Containing Cells	Morin (23) Ballet (1)
Peripheral Blood Lymphocytes Incubated With Con A, Then Assayed in M.L.C.	Augmentation of Con A-Induced Suppressor Cells	Touraine (32)
Rosette-Purified T-Lymphocytes Incubated With Con A, Then Assayed in M.L.C.	Augmentation of Con A-Induced Suppressor Cells	Touraine (32)
Leukocyte Adherence Inhibition (LAI) Test	Increase of LAI	Wybran (37)
Peripheral Blood Monocyte Phagocytosis Assay	Increased Phagocytosis Yeast Cells	Wybran (37)
Macrophage Interleukin I Synthesis	Increased Induction of B-Cell Differentation by Soluble Factor (Interleukin I)	Hadden (17)
Lymphocyte Interleukin Synthesis	Induction of Helper Factor	Wybran (37)

* Adapted from Hadden and Ginsberg (12)

Table 3. In vivo effects of Isoprinosoine on immune functions*

Test	Results	Investigator
Proliferative Response to PHA	Increased LBT in Herpes Simplex Patients	Bradshaw (3)
Proliferative Response to PHA, Herpes Virus	Increased LBT in Initial Herpes Genitalis Patients	Corey (4)
Proliferative Response to Influenza Virus	Increased LBT in Volunteers with Artificial Influenza Infections	Betts (2)
Proliferative Response to Con A, PHA	Increased LBT in Aged Immunodepressed Subjects	Moulias (24)
Lymphotoxin Production	Increased Lymphotoxin Titers in HSV Patients	Bradshaw (3)
Rosettes, Active	Increased in 6/9 Chronic Bronchitis Patients	Wybran (37)
Cutaneous Reactivity	Increased Skin Tests Response in Aged, Immunodepressed Patients	Moulias (24)
Interferon (IF) Levels In Blood	Increased IF Levels in Patients Treated with Isoprinosine. Increased Immune IF Production by Lymphocytes	Kott (20)

* Adapted from Hadden and Ginsberg (12)

higher levels of lymphocyte-mediated cytotoxicity. These immunological reactions were paralleled by symptomatic improvement and reduced virus shedding in nasal secretions. In an experiment using aged, immunodepressed subjects Moulias et al. (24) reported an increased lymphoblast transformation response to Con A and PHA following Isoprinosine administration.

Bradshaw et al. (3) in a study of herpes simplex virus infections, measured lymphotoxin titers present in the supernatant of PHA-stimulated lymphocytes harvested from Isoprinosine-treated patients and compared them to lymphotoxin titers from placebo treated controls. Cells from Isoprinosine-treated patients showed higher titers of lymphotoxin while the levels produced by control cells were depressed. In a study of nine chronic bronchitis patients, Wybran et al. (37) reported an increased level of active rosette formation in two-thirds of the treated patients. In aged and immunodepressed patients anergic skin test responses were reversed following Isoprinosine therapy (24).

In a study of four patients with subacute sclerosing panencephalitis (SSPE), Kott et al. (20) reported that, following treatment with Isoprinosine, previously low or absent circulating interferon levels increased and became measurable. Lymphocytes from these patients also acquired the ability to produce immune interferon in vitro following drug treatment.

Clinical Studies of Isoprinosine in Cancer Patients

The capacity of Isoprinosine to restore immune function in cancer patients has been the subject of several clinical trials. Tsang et al. (35) have recently reported that Isoprinosine added in vitro to cells of 47 patients with melanoma or lung or breast cancer significantly augmented Con A-induced lymphoproliferation, natural killer (NK) activity and monocyte chemotaxis in those patients whose initial values were depressed. Fridman (9) in a study of 106 patients with head, neck, breast or uterine cancer examined the immune function following radiotherapy. The patients were randomized in a double-blind fashion to receive either Isoprinosine or placebo. Overall immune status was assessed through measurement of the following parameters: lymphocyte count, E-rosette and EA-rosette enumeration, PHA and PWM proliferative responses, percent of Ig-positive cells and tuberculin skin-test response. The duration of drug therapy was five months, during which time the above immune parameters were periodically monitored. Recovery of normal immune status occurred faster in patients receiving Isoprinosine than in controls. After three months of treatment, 64% of the Isoprinosine-treated patients and 23% of the control patients had immune responses considered to be normal ($p < 0.05$). At the completion of the study, 89% of the Isoprinosine-treated patients and 66% of the controls were restored to normal immune system function.

Fenton et al. (6) made similar measurements in 29 patients with genital tumors who were undergoing radiotherapy. By the third month of the study, 54% of the patients receiving Isoprinosine were immunorestored compared to 13% in the control group. However, by the fifth month, the percentage of immunorestored patients was the same in both groups (31%). Schaison et al. (27) studied leukemia patients under heavy chemotherapy and at high risk of serious collateral infections. Prophylactic administration of Isoprinosine, gammaglobulin and trimethoprim-sulfamethoxazole prevented the appearance of viral infections.

Talpaz and Mavligit studied the effect of Isoprinosine on the graft versus host (GVH) response in 56 patients with solid tumors (31). Two groups of 20 patients received either 1 g/day or 4 g/day of Isoprinosine for seven days. The remaining patients served as a control group and did not receive immunotherapy. The GVH response was measured in all patients prior to therapy and immediately after its termination. In both groups receiving Isoprinosine, there was a greater than 38% ($p < 0.05$) stimulation of the measured local GVH reaction (Table 4). In contrast there was no significant change in the GVH of the non-treated patient population. In the group receiving 1 g/day of Isoprinosine, 55% showed an elevated GVH reaction following drug therapy while only 5% had a depressed GVH reaction. At the higher dosage level (4 g/day) 35% of the patients had an elevated GVH response while 5% had depressed responses.

NPT 15392

NPT 15392 (erythro-9-(-2-hydroxy-3-nonyl)-6-hydroxy-purine) is a purine immunomodulating compound that was jointly developed by Newport Pharmaceuticals International Inc. and the Sloan-Kettering Institute for Cancer Research. It is a white crystalline powder with good solubility in organic solvents but only slight solubility in water. Once hydrated in aqueous solution it is very stable. A pharmacological and toxicological profile of NPT 15392 has been presented by Simon et al. (30).

In Vitro Effects of NPT 15392 on Immune Function

Table 5 summarizes the in vitro immunopotentiating effects of

Table 4. Effect of Isoprinosine administration in vivo on local graft versus host (GVH) reaction among cancer patients

Dose	# Patients	Local GVH Reaction (mm^3) Before	After	p
4 gr/day x 7 days	20	42.1 ± 20.1	58.9 ± 23.8	< 0.01
1 gr/day x 7 days	20	44.1 ± 19.1	61.0 ± 37.1	< 0.05
No Treatment	16	31.8 ± 17.0	31.1 ± 16.0	> 0.10

*From Talpaz and Mavligit (31).

Table 5. In vitro effects of NPT 15392 on human lymphocyte differentiation and function

Test	Increase*	Investigator
Proliferative response to Con A, PHA and Pokeweed Mitogen	1.1-1.3	Hadden et al. (15)
Generation of Active E-Rosettes	1.5	Wybran et al. (38)
Induction of Suppressor Cells	1.3-1.5	Hadden et al. (15)
Generation of PMN and Monocyte Chemiluminescence	1.2	Maxwell et al.(19)

* Control = 1.0

NPT 15392 on human lymphocyte differentiation and function. An augmented mitogen-induced blastogenic response has been observed in human peripheral blood lymphocytes incubated with NPT 15392 at concentrations ranging from 0.01-0.1 μg/ml (15). The magnitude of augmentation was variable and appeared to be inversely related to the amount of thymidine which the cells were capable of incorporating in the absence of NPT 15392. In support of this contention are observations in mice and hamsters indicating that the most pronounced restorative effect of NPT 15392 is on aged animals who have a diminished mitogen response (18, 34). Increasing the concentration of NPT 15392 to 10 μg/ml or above acted to inhibit the mitogenic response. No effect of NPT 15392 on background thymidine incorporation by peripheral blood lymphocytes has been observed and this compound, like Isoprinosine, acts as a potentiator of the mitogenic response. However, in contrast to Isoprinosine, the magnitude of the maximum stimulatory effect and the active concentration ranges for NPT 15392 are both considerably less.

Simon et al. (28) have reported that NPT 15392, like thymic hormones, increased the percentage of active rosettes in vitro. In support of these findings, both Hadden et al. (15) and Wybran et al. (38) found that NPT 15392 (0.01-20 μg/ml) significantly augmented the number of active T-cell rosettes present in human peripheral blood lymphocytes. In Hadden's study a total of 19 individuals were studied and 16 showed significant increases in T-cell active rosettes with a mean maximal increase of 51%. A comparative measurement of differentiation in mice showed that prothymocytes from eight-week old athymic (nu/nu) animals treated in vitro with concentrations of NPT 15392 between 0.01-10 μg/ml demonstrated the appearance of the T-cell marker Thy-1 (18). A maximum induction of 27-34% was observed at 0.1 μg/ml NPT 15392. This induction is equivalent to the effect of thymic hormones. Touraine et al. (33) have confirmed the thymic hormone-like action of NPT 15392 in human bone marrow cells treated with the drug in vitro.

Hadden et al. (15) reported that in vitro pre-treatment with NPT 15392 (0.01-10 μg/ml) induces suppressor cells in cultures of human peripheral blood lymphocytes. This suppressor activity was manifested in the response of autologous lymphocytes to Con A or to allogeneic stimulation in a one-way mixed lymphocyte culture (MLC). Maximal inhibition (30%) occurred with 1 μg/ml NPT 15392 ($p < 0.01$). NPT 15392 (0.01-1 μg/ml) enhanced the Con A-induced suppression of the MLC by 16% to 27% and the Con A lymphoproliferative response by 8% to 15% ($p < .01$). Optimal interaction with Con A was observed at 0.1 μg/ml NPT 15392. The effect of NPT 15392, either by itself or in combination with Con A was not abolished by indomethacin (10^{-5} M) or cimetidine (3×10^{-5} M) indicating that the suppressor cell effects of NPT 15392 could not be explained by effects on histamine or prostaglandin production. Neither did NPT 15392, with or without Con A, induce detectable levels of interferon which might account for the observed suppression.

In vivo studies (19) with normal human peripheral blood lymphocytes showed that a single oral dose of NPT 15392 (0.01 mg/kg) significantly augmented PHA-induced lymphocyte proliferation (8 normals). A higher dose of NPT 15392 (0.1 mg/kg) augmented active rosettes (7 normals) and decreased PHA-induced lymphocyte proliferation in five out of seven normal subjects.

In Vivo Effects of NPT 15392 in Animals

NPT 15392 has exhibited significant in vivo immunomodulating activity in numerous animal systems which are relevant to cancer immunotherapy. In mice treated with a single dose of NPT 15392 (0.01 mg/kg), a significant augmentation of the Con A-induced lymphoproliferative response was observed in spleen cells from normal animals or animals immunosuppressed with Friend leukemia virus (FLV) (19). In a series of experiments, Jones et al. (19) examined mitogen responses in normal adult Balb/c mice receiving either multiple intraperitoneal (i.p) injections or oral administrations of NPT 15392 (0.1-0.3 mg/kg). When the experimental procedures tended to suppress thymidine incorporation in spleen cells from placebo-treated animals, NPT 15392 enhanced the mitogenic response. Conversely, experiments characterized by enhanced response in the control group showed a slight suppression resulting from treatment with NPT 15392.

Pretreatment of Balb/c mice with a single i.p. dose of NPT 15392 (0.1 mg/kg) significantly augmented their delayed type hypersensitivity (DTH) reaction to a secondary ear lobe challenge with oxazolone (8). The optimal response (a 1.9 fold augmentation) was observed when NPT 15392 was given seven days prior to the initial sensitization.

Plaque formation of spleen cells (PFC), in either the Mishell-Dutton or the Jerne plaque assay, was augmented by NPT 15392 therapy. Merluzzi et al. (21) found that the T-cell dependent PFC responses to sheep red blood cells (SRBC) were elevated 2-3 fold in C57BL/6 mice which had received six daily injections of 0.3-3 μg/kg NPT 15392 prior to in vitro antigen exposure. Jones et al. (19) found that Balb/c mice mounted a 2.5 fold higher PFC response than placebo animals as a consequence of NPT 15392 (0.05 to 0.5 mg/kg i.p.) administration on days 0, 1, 2, 3 relative to SRBC immunization. A similar response was evoked if the drug was given on a single occasion i.p. (0.5 mg/kg) at the time of SRBC immunization or orally (0.05 to 0.5 mg/kg) on days 0, 1, 2 and 3. Florentin et al. (8) measured the PFC response in Balb/c mice given a single i.p. dose of NPT 15392 up to fourteen days prior to SRBC immunization. They observed an enhanced PFC response in spleen cells from NPT 15392-treated animals. On average, the maximum drug-induced increases occurred when NPT 15392 was administered one day prior to antigen. In the Florentin et al. (8) study, effects of NPT 15392 on both T-cell dependent and T-cell independent responses were observed.

NPT 15392 modulates a variety of cytocidal functions in animals which are considered relevant to tumor surveillance. Stimulation of T cell cytotoxicity has been observed (8, 21). NK cell activity was also significantly elevated in spleen or peritoneal cells harvested from Balb/c mice which received a single i.p. or i.v. injection of NPT 15392 (0.1 mg/kg) one to fourteen days prior to testing. In both cell populations the ability to lyse the YAC-1 tumor target cells was increased at least three-fold by NPT 15392. The response was maximal three to seven days after administration of NPT 15392. The degree of augmentation was related to the route of administration. As expected, more NK activity was exhibited by peritoneal cells following an i.p. injection of NPT 15392. Likewise, spleen cells expressed a higher level of NK activity after an i.v. administration of NPT 15392. In an extension of these studies, Florentin has shown that combinations of interferon on NPT 15392 in vivo appear to produce an additive effect in augmenting NK cell activity (Figure 1) (7). In these studies, interferon was always administered i.p. A more significant augmentation was observed when NPT 15392 was given i.p. rather than i.v. Goutner (10) has confirmed these results with human cells in vitro; NPT 15392 potentiated effects of suboptimal doses of exogenous interferon on spontaneous cytotoxicity of human mononuclear cells.

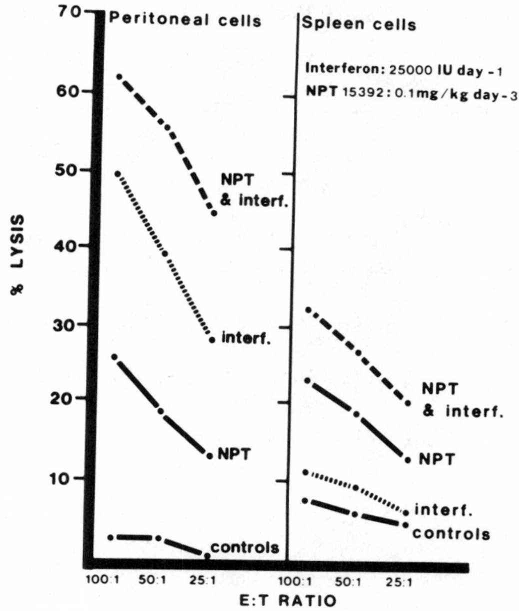

Fig. 1. Effect of combined administration of NPT 15392 and fibroblast interferon on NK cell activity. Balb/c mice received 25,000 I.U. interferon (interf.) intraperitoneally on day minus-one and/or 0.1 mg/kg NPT 15392 (NPT) intraperitoneally on day minus-three. On day zero spleen and peritoneal cells were harvested and their NK cell activity measured in a 4 hour chromium release assay using YAC-1 cells as targets (7).

In Vivo Effects of NPT 15392 in Tumor Models

Table 6 lists the tumor models in which the antineoplastic and immunorestorative properties of NPT 15392 have been evaluated. Florentin, et al. (7) have investigated the effect of NPT 15392 on tumor development and metastatic potential in a Lewis Lung carcinoma model (LLC). Groups of C57BL/6 mice received a single subcutaneous inoculation of 10^5 tumor cells, and were then given 10 i.p. injections of NPT 15392 (0.1 mg/kg) over a 25 day period beginning one day after tumor administration. The mean diameter of the implanted tumor was determined on each day of drug treatment. After 25 days, animals were sacrificed and the mean number of lung metastases were measured in both treated and control animals. NPT 15392 had no demonstrable effect on the rate of tumor growth, but it did produce statistically significant reduction (40-75%) in the

Table 6. Summary of NPT 15392 effects in animal tumor models

Tumor Model	Effect	Investigator
LLC (C57/BL/J6 mouse)	Metastasis (40-75%)	Sato (25), Florentin (7)
SA 180 (ICR mice)	Tumor weight in combination with 5-FU	Sato (25)
AH 41c, 44	Life Span of > 200%	Sato (25)
AH 66, 130	Life Span of 50-150%	Sato (25)
Fibrosarcoma-T241 (C57BL/J6)	Metastasis (30-50%)	Jones (19), Deodhar (5)
L-1210	No effect	Sato (26)
NF (Sarcoma)	No effect	Sato (26)
P-388 (Leukemia)	Life Span (20-30%)	Sato (26)
BC-47	Life Span (21-45%)	Sato (26)

mean number of metastases. These observations have been confirmed by Sato (26).

NPT 15392 has a similar effect on the number of metastases which develop in animals bearing the T-241 fibrosarcoma. Jones et al. (19) and Deodhar (5) implanted the T-241 fibrosarcoma into the dorsal aspect of the foot of C57BL/6 mice. NPT 15392 was given by i.p. injection (0.3 mg/kg) beginning on the day of implantation and continuing until day 28, the day of sacrifice. The number and size of lung metastases were determined on day 28. A control group received saline injections daily. The results indicate that NPT 15392 reduced the frequency of metastasis by 35-64%.

Sato (25) has utilized the AH series of hepatomas as a model system for evaluating NPT 15392 action. Groups of six female Sprague-Dawley rats were inoculated (i.v.) with 10^7 cells from one of ten hepatoma types, followed by a series of i.p. (0.5 mg/kg) or oral (5 mg/kg) administrations of NPT 15392. Survival was observed in control and drug-treated animals for a period of 60 days. The drug was judged of positive efficacy if the increased life span (ILS) was greater than 200% relative to the untreated control and mixed if the improvement was between 50-150%. All untreated animals, regardless of AH tumor type received, died within 20 days.

Orally administered NPT 15392 was found to have a positive effect against AH-44 tumors. The majority of these animals survived for the entire 60-day observation period. Animals with the AH-66 and AH-130 hepatoma types also responded positively to drug treatment. Two animals with AH-66 and one animal with AH-130 remained alive at the end of the study. In animals that received i.p. injections of NPT 15392 the effect on survival was not as dramatic. Animals bearing the AH-44 or AH-66 tumor type were the only ones whose survival curves were improved by NPT 15392.

P-388 is a cultured cell line derived from a methylcholanthracene-induced lymphoid neoplasm of the DBA/2 mouse, which will cause a leukemia when injected into a syngeneic host. In one study by Sato (26), treatment of BDF_1 mice with NPT 15392 (0.01 to 0.1 mg/kg, i.p.) commenced five days prior to an i.p. inoculation of P-388 while, in another, the mouse received eight additional doses of NPT 15392 after tumor cell inoculation. Regardless of the drug administration protocol, all mice treated with NPT 15392 exhibited a greater than 21% increase in the mean survival time relative to the control animals. These effects were statistically significant ($p < 0.01$).

In rats, a chemically induced BC-47 bladder carcinoma was treated with NPT 15392 (26). A significant increase in survival was reliably obtained in animals receiving drug (0.07 mg/kg i.p.) every other day for 15 days after tumor inoculation as compared to saline treated controls. Of the 15 animals receiving NPT 15392, two animals were characterized as long-term survivors (survival > 51 days), whereas none of the controls were so described. Enhancement of the cytotoxic T-cell response against BC-47 carcinoma measured in a spleen cell preparation was significantly elevated in animals receiving NPT 15392.

Sato (25, 26) has also measured drug-induced restoration of immune function in tumor-bearing mice. In all experiments, mice received NPT 15392 i.p. either prior to tumor inoculation or both before and after exposure to the tumor. As a result of drug treatment, the suppressed DTH in the Ehrlich ascitic tumor, Ehrlich lung tumor, sarcoma 180, and L1210 leukemia models was partially reversed. An otherwise depressed mitogenic response in Ehrlich ascitic tumor or L1210 leukemia models was normalized by treatment with NPT 15392. Sato found the PFC response improved in tumor-bearing animals treated with NPT 15392. In mice with Ehrlich lung metastic tumor, the number of plaque forming cells was increased from 27% to 97% (relative to non-treated controls) by NPT 15392. PFC levels, in treated Ehrlich ascitic carcinoma-bearing animals, were elevated 2-3 fold over non-treated tumor-bearing controls. The degree of improvement in PFC depended on the drug dose and administration regimen. In general, the most effective dose of NPT 15392 was 0.1 mg/kg.

Clinical Trials of NPT 15392 in Cancer Patients

The immunomodulating properties of NPT 15392 were evaluted in tumor patients (39). The study was conducted under the auspices of the Tumor Immunology Project Group of the European Organization for the Research and Treatment of Cancer (EORTC) in nine centers throughout Europe. Subjects admitted to the study were high risk patients newly diagnosed as having a solid tumor. They had not received chemotherapy for at least six weeks nor received radiotherapy for at least one year prior to NPT 15392 administration. Sixty patients meeting these criteria received one of two doses of NPT 15392 (0.4 mg or 0.7 mg), on Days 1, 4, 7 and 10 of the study. Immunological parameters were recorded prior to treatment (Days -1 or -2), during treatment (Days 4, 7 or 10) and following treatment (Days 17 or 22).

As shown in Table 7, analyses of the data obtained from the EORTC study identified six immunological parameters that were significantly changed after treatment with NPT 15392. To perform this analysis normal clinical values from published sources were used to classify each initial test value as elevated, normal or depressed. A binomial test was performed to see if there was a statistically significant pattern in the change of the test values that relates to whether the initial value was depressed, normal, or elevated. This is consistent with the hypothesis that NPT 15392 is more effective in

Table 7. Significant effects of NPT 15392 in the EORTC study

Test	Initial value	NPT 15392 causes increase (+) or decrease (-)	Patients responding	Significance (p value)*
IgG	Elevated	-	6/6	.02
B-Lymphocyte #	Normal	+	5/5	.03
Lymphocyte #	Depressed	+	6/7	.06
T-Lymphocyte #	Depressed	+	9/12	.07
E-Rosette	Depressed	+	9/12	.07
NK Activity	Depressed	+	6/6	.02

*One-tailed test

restoring the response of suppressed patients than in modulating normal values.

This hypothesis was further examined by Micksche et al. (22), who determined that patients with low initial NK activity had a significant increase in the levels of NK-mediated cytotoxicity during NPT 15392 therapy. Patients with normal initial NK activity were not affected by the therapy (Table 8). This observation may have important implications for the use of NPT 15392 as an immunomodulating agent in the treatment of cancer.

SUMMARY

These data demonstrate that both Isoprinosine and NPT 15392 are active nontoxic biological response modifiers that qualify for studies in cancer patients. Because of their immunomodulating properties, these agents are expected to be most appropriate in the treatment of immunosuppressed patients who are prone to infection or recurrence following cytoreductive therapy.

Table 8. In vivo Augmentation of NK activity by NPT 15392*

	% Cytotoxicity Against K-562	
	Day 1	Day 4
Control (6)	46.5 ± 5.2	45.2 ± 2.4
Patients with normal NK Activity (4)	45.5 ± 5.2	44.8 ± 5.5
Patients with low NK Activity (8)	13.8 ± 1.4	35.2 ± 6.0**

* From Micksche et al. (22)

** p <0.05

REFERENCES

1. Ballet, J. J., A. M. Morin and M. Agrapart. 1980. Modulation by Isoprinosine of the activation, differentiation and antigen specific responses of human lymphocytes in vitro. 4th Congress of Immunology, Paris, France.

2. Betts, R. F., R. G. Douglas, Jr., S. D. George and C. J. Rinehart. 1978. Isoprinosine in experimental influenza A infection in volunteers. 78th Annual Meeting of the American Society for Microbiology, Las Vegas, Nevada.

3. Bradshaw, L. J. and H. L. Sumner. 1977. In vitro studies on cell-mediated immunity in patients treated with inosiplex for herpes virus infection. Ann. N.Y. Acad. Sci. 284: 190-196.

4. Corey, L., W. Chiang, W. Reeves, W. Stamm, L. Brewer and K. Holmes. 1979. Effect of Isoprinosine on the cellular immune response in initial genital herpes virus infection. Clin. Res. 27: 41A.

5. Deodhar, S. Unpublished observations.

6. Fenton, J., 1981. Etude en double-insu de l'influence de l'isoprinosine sur les tests immunitaire de patients recevant une irradiation pelvienne. Bull. Cancer. 68: 200.

7. Florentin, I., L. Kraus, G. Mathe and J. W. Hadden. 1982. In vivo study in mice of the immunopharmacological properties of NPT 15392. In B. Serrou et al (eds.), Proceedings of the international meeting on human cancer immunology. Elsevier-North Holland (in press).

8. Florentin, I., E. Taylor, M. Davigny, G. Mathe and J. W. Hadden. 1982. Kinetic studies of the immunopharmacologic effects of NPT 15392 in mice. Int. J. Immunopharm. 4: 225-234.

9. Fridman, H., R. Calle and A. Morin. 1980. Double-blind study of Isoprinosine influence on immune parameters in solid tumor-bearing patients treated by radiotherapy. Int. J. Immunopharm. 2: 194.

10. Goutner, A. 1980. In vitro modulation of natural killer cell activity by Isoprinosine, NPT 15392 and interferon. Int. J. Immunopharm. 2: 197.

11. Hadden, J. W. and A. Giner-Sorolla. 1981. Isoprinosine and NPT 15392: modulators of lymphocyte and macrophage development and function. In E. M. Hersh et al (eds.), Augmenting agents in cancer therapy. Raven Press, New York.

12. Hadden, J. W. and T. Ginsberg. 1982. Immunopharmacology of methisoprinol. International symposium on recent advances in immunomodulators. Viarregio, Italy.

13. Hadden, J. W., E. M. Hadden and R. G. Coffey. 1976. Isoprinosine augmentation of phytohemagglutinin-induced lymphocyte proliferation. Infect. Immun. 13: 382-387.

14. Hadden, J. W., E. M. Hadden and R. G. Coffey. 1979. Biological significance of the purine salvage pathway. Transplant. Clin. Immunol. 10: 143-153.

15. Hadden, J. W., E. M. Hadden, T. Spira, R. Settineri, L. Simon and A. Giner-Sorolla. 1982. Effects of NPT 15392 in vitro on human leukocyte functions. Int. J. Immunopharm. 4: 235-242.

16. Hadden, J. W., C. Lopez, R. O'Reilly and E. Hadden. 1977. Levamisole and inosiplex: antiviral agents with immunopotentiating action. Ann. N. Y. Acad. Sci. 284: 139-152.

17. Hadden, J. W. and J. Wybran. 1981. Immunopotentiators II Isoprinosine, NPT 15392 and Azimexone: modulators of lymphocyte and macrophage development and function. In J. Hadden et al (eds.), Advances in immunopharmacology. Pergamon Press, New York.

18. Ikehara, S., J. W. Hadden, R. A. Good, D. G. Lunzer and R. N. Pahawa. 1981. In vitro effects of two immunopotentiators, Isoprinosine and NPT 15392, on murine T-cell differentiation and function. Thymus 3: 87-95.

19. Jones, E. C., B. Binko, R. Settineri and K. Maxwell. 1982. Influence of NPT 15392 on mouse and human lymphocyte responses (in preparation).

20. Kott, E., N. Gadoth, S. Levin, T. Hahn, V. Bergman, R. Avidor and C. Braun. 1981. Stimulation of the interferon system by Isoprinosine (inosiplex) in subacute sclerosing panencephalitis (SSPE). 13th Symposium of Israeli Immunological Society.

21. Merluzzi, V. J., M. M. Walker, N. Williams, B. Susskind, J. W. Hadden and R. B. Faanes. 1982. Immunoenhancing activity of NPT 15392: a potential immune response modifier. Int. J. Immunopharm. 4: 219-224.

22. Micksche, M., E. M. Kokoschka, H. Rainer and A. Uchida. 1982. Augmentation of natural killer (NK) cell activity in cancer patients by NPT 15392. Int. J. Immunopharm. 4: 283.

23. Morin, A., J. L. Touraine, G. Renoux and J. W. Hadden. 1980. Isoprinosine as an immunomodulating agent. Symposium of New Trends in Human Immunology and Cancer Immunotherapy, Montpellier, France.

24. Moulias, R., J. Proust, M. Marescot, M. Piette and A. Devulecharbrolle. 1978. Action of Isoprinosine (inosiplex) on the immunological parameters of aged people. 7th International Congress of Pharmacology. Paris, France.

25. Sato, S. and M. Tsurufuji. 1980. NPT 15392: immunorestorative effects in tumor-suppressed mice. Int. J. Immunopharm. 2: 200.

26. Sato, S. Unpublished observations.

27. Schaison, G., E. Gluckman, J. F. Souilllet and J. M. Turc. 1980. Isoprinosine curative and prophylactic treatment of viral infections in patients with malignant hematologic disorders. 4th International Congress of Immunology. Paris, France.

28. Simon, L. N., A. Giner-Sorolla and J. W. Hadden. 1980. NPT 15392 a novel immunomodulating agent. 4th International Congress of Immunology. Paris, France.

29. Simon, L. N. and A. J. Glasky. 1978. Isoprinosine: an overview. Cancer Treatment Report. 62: 1963-1969.

30. Simon, L. N., R. Settineri, E. P. Pfadenhauer, C. Jones, K. Maxwell and A. J. Glasky. 1980. NPT 15392: a pharmacologic and toxicologic profile. Int. J. Immunopharm. 2: 200.

31. Talpaz, M. and G. Mavligit. 1982. Immune restoration augmentation by Isoprinosine in cancer patients. 2nd International Conference of Immunopharmacology. Washington, D. C.

32. Touraine, J. L., J. W. Hadden and F. Touraine. 1979. Isoprinosine-induced T-cell differentiation and T-cell suppressor activity in humans. 19th International Conference on Antimicrobial Agents and Chemotherapy., Boston, Mass.

33. Touraine, J., G. Gay-Ferret, K. Sanadji, O. Othmane, G. Fournie and F. Touraine. 1982. Syngergistic effect with NPT 15392 in vitro and activity on suppressor T-lymphocytes in autoimmune mice in vivo. Internal Symposium on New Trends in Human Immunology and Cancer Immunotherapy. Montpellier, France.

34. Tsang, K. Y., C. B. Phillips, M. J. Gnagy and H. H. Fudenberg. 1982. In vivo and in vitro effects of NPT 15392 on the immune responses of hamsters. Fed. Proc. 41: 812.

35. Tsang, K. Y., M. J. Gnagy, C. B. Phillips and H. H. Fudenberg. 1981. In vitro effects of Isoprinosine (Iso) on the immune responses of cancer patients. Proceedings 13th International Cancer Congress. Seattle, Washington.

36. Wybran, J. 1978. Inosiplex, a stimulating agent for normal human T-cells and human leukocytes. J. Immunology. 121: 1184-1187.

37. Wybran, J. 1981. Immunomodulatory properties of Isoprinosine in man: in vitro and in vivo data. International Symposium on New Trends in Human Immunology and Cancer Immunotherapy. Montpellier, France.

38. Wybran, J. 1980. NPT 15392, a new synthetic immunomodulatory agent: human, in vitro and in vivo (cancer patients) effects. Int. J. Immunopharm. 2: 193.

39. Wybran, J. 1982. Immunomodulatory properties of NPT 15392 in man: in vitro and in vivo. Int. J. Immunopharm. 4: 292.

40. Wybran, J., J. P. Famaey, R. Gortz, I. Dab, A. Malfroot and T. Appelboom. 1982. Inosiplex (Isoprinosine): a review of its immunological and clinical effects in disease. In Advances in pharmacology and therapeutics II. Pergamon Press, New York.

IMMUNOMODULATION BY NPT 15392 IN CANCER PATIENTS UNDER CHEMO-THERAPY

R. Favre, D. Bagarry-Liegey, B. Jeanroy, T. Pignon, G. Meyer, and Y. Carcassonne

Institut J. Paoli-I. Calmettes, 232, Bd de Ste Marguerite 13273 Marseille - France

INTRODUCTION

Many investigators have tried to define the immunologic properties of Biologic Response Modifiers (BRMS). We studied a BRM, NPT 15392 (Newport Pharmaceuticals International, Inc.) (2, 3) known to have properties of immunomodulation. We explored the potential of this agent in respect to immunorestoration and immunostimulation in ten cancer-bearing patients presenting signs of immunosuppression and treated by repeated chemotherapy courses.

METHODS

NPT 15392 is a new synthetic drug developed in a joint program by the Sloan-Kettering Institute for Cancer Research and Newport Pharmaceutical International, Inc. Its formula is erythro-9-(-2-hydroxy-3-nonyl)-6-hydroxy-purine. It is thus a purine derivative like isoprinosine (4, 5).

Patients

Six advanced head and neck cancer patients comprising five males and one female, ages 45 to 58 years were studied. Chemotherapy was either 5-fluorouracil + adriamycin + cisplatinum or an association of methotrexate and L. disin alternated with bleomycin and cisplatinum.

Three mammary carcinomas with liver and bone metastases comprising two female and one male aged 37, 57 and 58 years and treated subcutaneously with adriamycin + vincristine + cyclophosphamide + 5-fluorouracil. One 69 year old female patient with well differentiated lymphoma was treated with cyclophosphamide + vincristine + prednisolone.

Immune Assessment

A battery of ten immunological tests was used comprising three categories. Firstly, skin tests (IDR) with tuberculin (one and ten units), candidine (1/1000 and 1/10,000) and PHA (1 μg and 10 μg). The latter test was read at 24 and 48 h.

Secondly, the study of the patients' lymphocytes including peripheral lymphocyte count (no/mm^3), E. rosetting, membrane immunofluorescence and L.B.T. (PHA and PWM). Finally, serum levels of the C'3 fraction of complement and IgA were evaluated. The patients for whom 70% of the tests were negative were classified as immunodepressed.

The Clinical Protocol Of The NPT 15392 Trial

The patients received courses of repeated chemotherapy usually every three to four weeks. In order to define more accurately our immunodepressed population we performed an immune assessment between two chemotherapy courses (forty-eight hours after the end of a course and three to four weeks later, just before the following course).

We included in the trial either patients presenting immunodepression (at least 70% of negative tests at one of these two assessments) or those presenting a relatively low immune state at the time of the initial assessment but frankly immunodepressed at the time of the second assessment. Conversely, we excluded patients with a satisfactory, stable immune state at the time of both assessments, as well as those who had become immunodepressed after a course or who underwent immunorestoration before the following course. We also excluded from this trial patients presenting a viral or microbial infection, detectable clinically, before treatment. We did not associate corticoid treatment during the trial. NPT 15392 treatment consisted of a 7 ml ampoule orally (i.e. 0.7 mg) every three days for ten days, i.e. D1, D4, D7 and D10 after a chemotherapy course (Figure 1).

Successive immune assessments were done on days 3, 6 and 9 with respect to NPT 15392 intake then on day 17 and day 30, which was prior to the next chemotherapy course. Most of the time, two additional immune assessments were done on days 37 and 58.

Ten immunosuppressed patients approximately comparable to ten patients who had received NPT 15392 also underwent immunologic assessment (four to six immune assessments total). Although we are

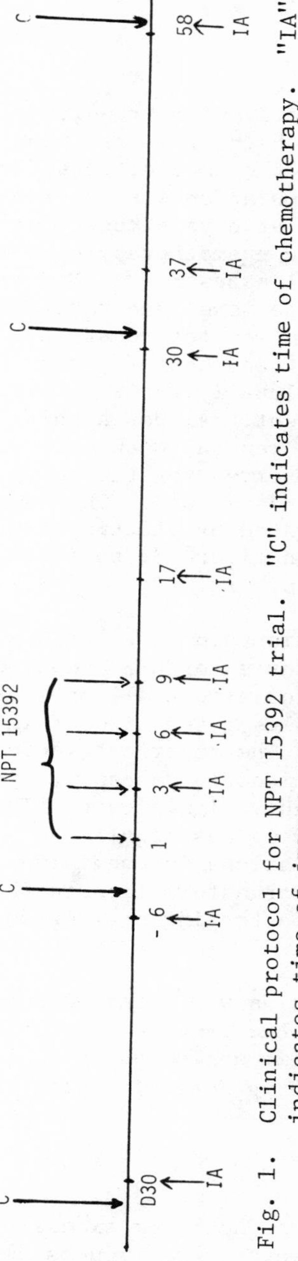

Fig. 1. Clinical protocol for NPT 15392 trial. "C" indicates time of chemotherapy. "IA" indicates time of immune assessment.

aware that these patients cannot be considered true controls, we used their responses as guidelines.

RESULTS

We observed no toxic symptoms resulting from NPT 15392 including no digestive troubles or baldness. As illustreated by Figure 2, representing the mean of the immune tests for ten patients, immunorestoration or immunostimulation was observed during or after NPT 15392 treatment, notably at days 6 and 17 or occasionally day 30. Then, after the following chemotherapy course (D37) the level dropped below that of the initial assessment. Finally, at the time of the last assessment (D58), the level had returned to a relatively good mean but this observation was not constant. This effect of immunorestoration was transient and not effective for all the tests. Thus, each patient individually was stimulated during and/or immediately after treatment. Although this stimulation was fleeting it was comparable to the general mean curve. Such a variation in immune status was not observed for the ten patients who did not receive NPT 15392 (data not shown). The same phenomenon of stimulation could be demonstrated by plotting the curves of individual patients. For example in Figure 3, the response curves for patients No. 1 and No. 4 are given.

In detail, tuberculin skin tests at one and ten units are almost negative. Conversely, tests for C'3 complement fraction were positive and varied little for almost all patients. We did analysis of variance with two variables : the time of immune testing and the different patients (4). The recurrent individual variations in E-rosetting, membrane immunofluorescence, lymphocyte counts and even IgA levels were very highly significant. The variation in PHA skin reactions at doses of 10 μg was significant. Conversely, the recurrent, individual variations in candidine skin testing (1/100 and 1/10,000) lymphoblastic transformation to PHA and PWM, serum levels of C'3 fraction, PHA skin testing at 1 μg doses (with early reading) were not significant.

Clearly, a stimulation was observed during and/or immediately after NPT treatment for the lymphocyte count, percentage of E-rosetting and membrane immunofluorescence, IgA level and diameter of skin test to PHA at a 10 μg dose with late reading.

DISCUSSION

NPT 15392 orally does not seem excessive since no toxic side-effects were noted. However, the immunostimulatory and immunorestorative action, although evident, seemed transient and the administration schedule should be reassessed.

The importance of this point can be appreciated if one considers that when immunosuppressive chemotherapy and NPT 15392 treatment were associated, immunodepression was observed in four cases

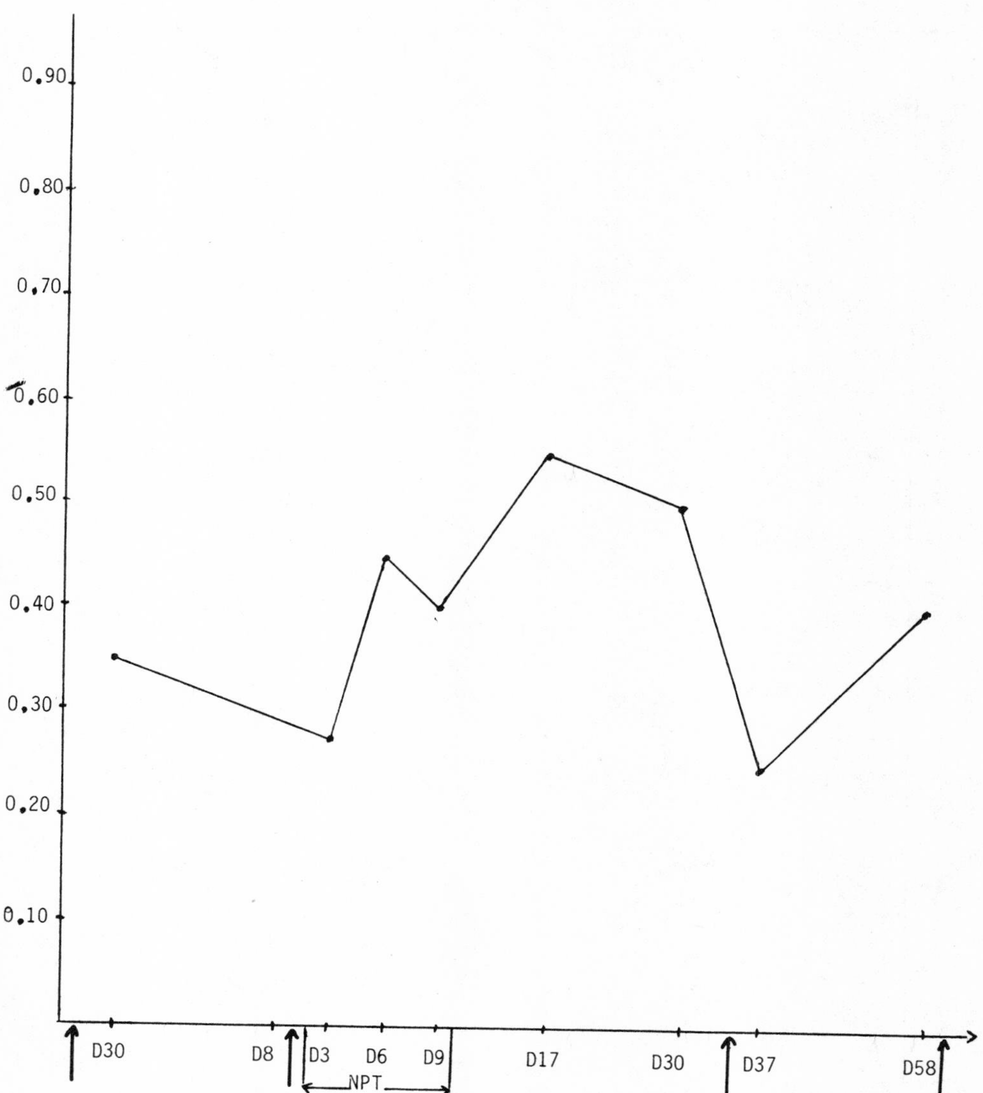

Fig. 2. Immunorestoration by NPT 15392 treatment. Data points represent the mean value of 10 patients. The ordinate refers to the percentage of positive immune tests for each patient (see methods) and the arrows indicate the time of chemotherapy.

after a course of chemotherapy i.e. following the recommendations for prescription of this BRM. Such a late immunosuppression took the form of an infectious syndrome which was concomitant with a drop in lymphocyte count. This finding may be considered as indirect proof for the action of NPT 15392 but draws attention to the precautions that should be used when prescribing an active BRM which

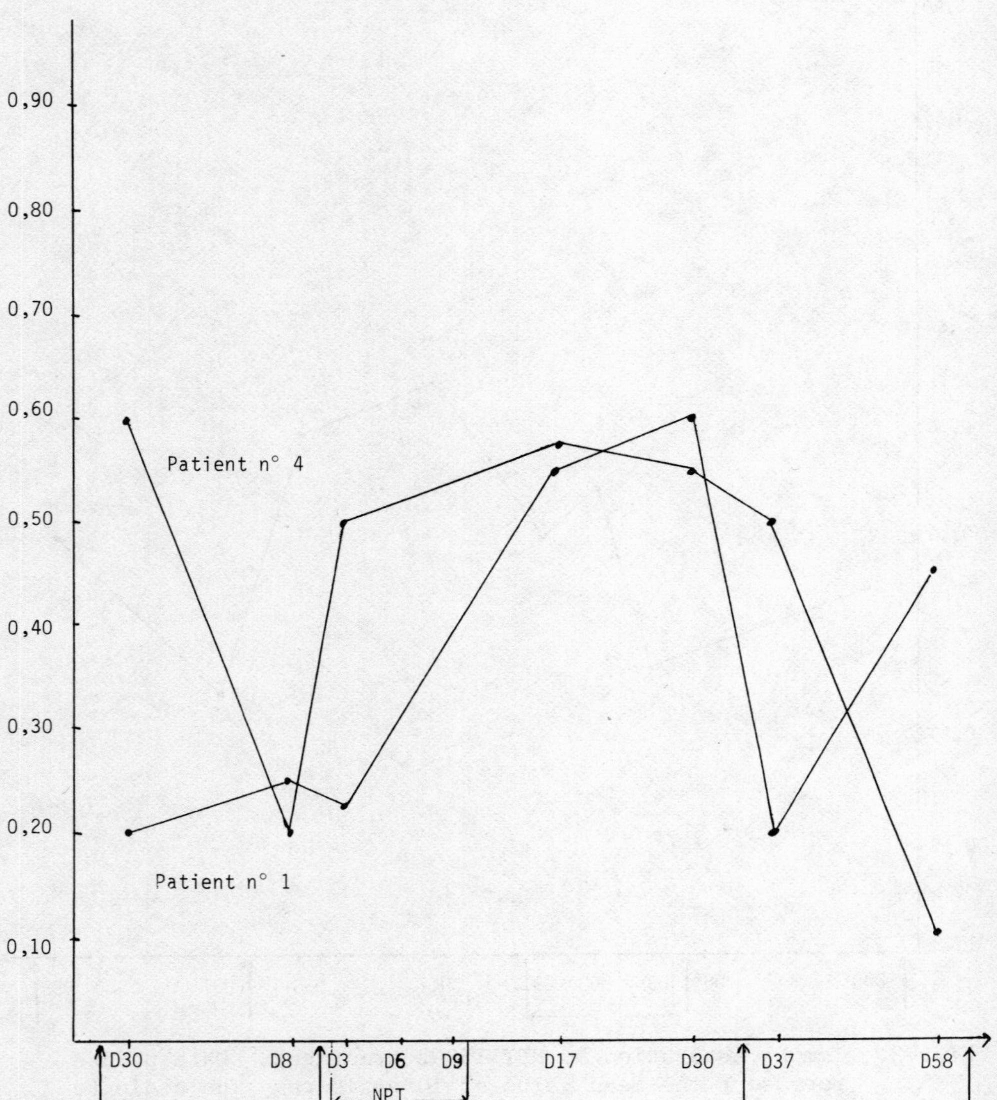

Fig. 3. Immunorestoration by NPT 15392 treatment in two select patients (1 and 4). See legend of Figure 2 for details.

stimulates lymphocytes and subsequently renders them more sensitive to chemotherapeutic action.

To obtain an idea of the type of lymphocyte stimulated by NPT 15392 after initial chemotherapy, the percentage of E-rosetting diminished drastically while the lymphocyte count and percentage of postive cells with membrane immunofluorescence increased in parallel. It therefore would seem that T lymphocytes are more particularly destroyed by chemotherapy. During and immediately after NPT 15392 T lymphocytes increased considerably in comparison to the number of B lymphocytes and the total lymphocyte count. NPT 15392 should therefore mainly act on cell mediated immunity.

SUMMARY

A clinical trial of NPT 15392, a purine derivative, was run in ten head and neck cancer patients presenting signs of immunosuppression and undergoing repeated chemotherapy. A battery of ten tests was used to assess the immune status of the subjects. Those tests included skin tests, lymphocyte investigations (count, E-rosetting, membrane fluorescence and lymphoblastic transformation) and determination of serum levels of C'3 fraction of complement and IgA. The drug induced transitory, immune stimulation during or after treatment without any side effects. NPT 15392 seemed to selectively exert an action on T lymphocytes. Inasmuch as transitory, immune stimulation and secondary immune depression were noted after treatment, the therapeutic protocol for use of this drug should be reexamined.

ACKNOWLEDGEMENT

We thank Mesdames J. Masse and M. Mouren for efficient technical assistance and Drs. L. Simon and S. Ginsberg for efficient help.

REFERENCES

1. Favre, R. and Y. Carcassone. 1980. Les modificateurs de la réponse biologique. Méditerranée medicale 236: 21.

2. Florentin, I., E. Taylor, G. Mathé and J. W. Hadden. 1980 In vitro immunomodulating properties of NPT 15392. Int. J. Immunopharmacol. 3: 240.

3. Ikehava, S., J. W. Hadden, R. A. Good, D. G. Lunzer and R. N. Pahwa. 1981. In vitro effects of two immunopotentiators, isoprinosine and NPT 15392, on murine T cell differentiation and function. Thymus 3: 87.

4. Jeanroy, B. 1982. Contribution à l'étude de l'action du NPT 15392 sur la relation hôte-tumeur. Doctor of Medecine Thesis, Marseille, France.

5. Wybran, J. 1980. NPT 15392, a new synthetic immunomodulatory agent : human in vitro and in vivo (cancer patients) effects. Int. J. Immunopharmacol. 2: 193.

EFFECT OF CHRONIC ADMINISTRATION OF A SYNTHETIC AROMATIC RETINOID (Ro 10-9359) ON THE DEVELOPMENT OF LUNG SQUAMOUS METAPLASIA AND EPIDERMOID CANCER IN RATS

D. Nolibe[1], R. Masse[1], J. Lafuma[1] and I. Florentin[2]

Commissariate a l'Energie Atomique (CEA), IPSN, Department de Protection[1], Laboratoire de Toxicologie Experimentale, BP 561, 92542 Montrouge Cedex, France

Institut de Cancerologie et d'Immunogenetique (ICIG), Department de'Immunopharmacologie Experimentale[2], Hopital Paul Brousse, 94804 Villejuif Cedex, France

INTRODUCTION

Since the first studies of Saffioti et al. (1) suggesting the preventive effect of high doses of vitamin A on squamous metaplasias of trachea and bronchis, several authors have used synthetic analogs of vitamin A, like retinoic acid, in chemoprevention and chemotherapy of tumors. Successful results were reported with skin (2) bladder (3) and mammary carcinogenesis (4). However for cancers of the respiratory tract the findings of Saffioti have not been confirmed in mice (5) hamsters (6) or rats (7). In our laboratory we have developed a model of lung carcinogenesis by using the combined effect of inhalation of radioactive particles and intratracheal instillation of benzopyrene. This model was used to examine the preventive and curative effect of a synthetic aromatic retinoid (Ro 10.9359) on the induction of development of metaplasia and epidermoid lung cancer. For this purpose, the compound was administered chronically at various times after carcinogen exposure.

METHODS

Animals

Pathogen free male Wistar rats, 8 weeks of age and weighing 200 to 220 g were obtained from Iffa Credo (L'arbresle, France).

Lung Carcinogenic Treatment

At day -15, animals were submitted to a nose only inhalation of plutonium dioxide ($^{239}PuO_2$) particles (median aerodynamic diameter, 2.06 μm, σ, 1.28) according to an already described procedure (8).

Initial lung burdens were determined by external chest counting 7 days after inhalation using a proportional counter (9). Lung burdens at death were determined in the same way. Less than 0.5% of the initial lung burden was translocated outside the lungs. Lung clearance was measured based on initial and final burdens (10). The data were fitted by a single exponential equation (half-time was 170 days) and the radiation dose delivered to lungs was calculated according to McClellan (11). At day 0, an intratracheal instillation of benzopyrene hematite (5 mg each) in 0.2 ml of saline solution was performed under halothane anesthesia, according to Saffioti et al. (1).

Retinoid Treatment

The aromatic retinoic acid analog Ro 10.9359, ethyl all-trans-9- (4-methoxy-2,3,6-trimethylphenyl)-3-7-dimethyl-2,4,6,8-nonatetraenoate (Hoffman La Roche), was presented as a hydrosuspendable galenical preparation. At different times after carcinogen exposure, depending upon the aim of experiment, i.e., metaplasia prevention, established metaplasia therapy or lung tumor therapy, rats received a chronic treatment with Ro 10.9359 given by stomach tube once a week. The doses used varied from 25 to 200 mg/kg per gastric administration.

Histopathology

The animals were autopsied after sacrifice at predetermined times in metaplasia prevention or therapy assays or after natural death in the lung cancer therapy assay. Organs presenting tumors or metastasis were studied histologically. In particular, lungs were removed in bloc and fully expanded by Bouin fixative and later embedded in paraffin. Lung tumors and lung metaplasia were diagnosed using large slices of whole organ sectioned along the longitudinal axis. The area of metaplasia was evaluated by a random observation of ten fields in different lobes using a grid ocular divided in 400 squares. For each field, the percentage of squares with metaplasia was checked, and results were expressed as the percent of positive squares for a mean number of 12.000 squares examined per lung. Lung tumors were diagnosed microscopically using also large slices of whole tissue and cancer staging was performed according to our previous studies (8).

RESULTS

Metaplasia prevention assay

Two groups of 20 rats were given 25 mg/kg Ro 10.9359 weekly from day 0 (day of the end of the carcinogenic treatment) to day 30 or 70, at which times lungs were examined for the presence of metaplasia and compared to their respective control groups. As shown in Table 1, the percentage of animals free of metaplasia was not significantly different in groups treated with retinoid as compared to untreated rats. Animals with metaplasia were divided into three classes corresponding to metaplasia area of respectively 0.1, 0.1 to 1 and more than 1 percent of the total checked lung surface. The distribution of animals in these three classes was not significantly different in retinoid-treated or untreated groups. However, a decrease in the percentage of animals presenting the largest metaplasia area was observed.

Metaplasia therapy assay

Groups of 25 rats received a weekly administration of 25, 75 or 200 mg/kg Ro 10.9359 starting from day 50 after carcinogen exposure. Untreated and retinoid-treated rats were sacrificed on day 150 or otherwise examined at natural death and compared for lung metaplasia extent. Results presented in Table 2 shows that the percentage of animals without metaplasia is significantly diminished in the groups of rats treated with 75 mg/kg ($p = 0.02$) and 200 mg/kg

Table 1. Comparison of metaplasia area in rats treated or not by aromatic retinoid (Ro 10.9359)

Treatment	Day of Sacrifice	Percent of animals with: No Metaplasia	Mean % of Metaplasia Area*		
		0	<0.1	0.1-1	>1
PuO_2 Inhalation	30	25	13	37	25
Benzo(a)pyrene (IT)	70	33	8	29	29
PuO_2 Inhalation					
Benzo(a)pyrene (IT)	30	16	16	64	4
Aromatic Retinoid	70	27	0	54	18

* Mean squamous metaplasia area in percent of total checked lung area

Table 2. Effect of aromatic retinoid (Ro 10.9359) treatment on 50 days established squamous lung metaplasia.

Aromatic Retinoid Treatment*	Percent of Animals with			
	No Metaplasia	Mean % of Squamous Metaplasia Area**		
	0	<0.1	0.1-1	>1
None	16	13	71	0
200 mg/kg	56	30	14	0
75 mg/kg	28	34	38	0
25 mg/kg	32	11	77	0

* Treatment was given intragastrally weekly from week 1 to week 22 after carcinogen exposure.

** Mean squamous metaplasia area in percent of total checked lung area.

($0.001 < p < 0.01$) of retinoid. In addition, when the animals develop precancerous lesions an inhibitory effect on the size of metaplasia was also observed in these retinoid-treated groups ($p = 0.05$ and $0.01 < p < 0.02$). The chronic administration of the lowest dose of Ro 10.9359 (25 mg/kg) did not significantly affect metaplasia development. It can be stressed that a toxic effect of retinoid treatment was observed which increased with the dose administered since 20% of the control animals died within the 150 days period of observation versus 24%, 68% and 100% in groups treated respectively with 25, 75 and 200 mg/kg.

Lung cancer therapy assay

One of two groups of carcinogen-exposed rats received 25 mg/kg of Ro 10.9359 weekly from day 0 to their natural death. Two additional control groups consisted of normal rats receiving or not the same retinoid treatment. All animals autopsied at natural death except a few lost through cannibalism were examined for lung tumor incidence, tumor size and intrathoracic metastasis. As shown in Table 3, tumor incidence in carcinogen-exposed rats was not significantly modified by the chronic administration of retinoid. Moreover, this treatment resulted in a higher percentage of early deaths since about 25% of retinoid-treated rats died before the first death occurred in the untreated group. However, the mean age of

Table 3. Comparison of lung tumor incidence in rats treated or not by aromatic retinoid (Ro 10.9359)

Treatment	No. of Animals	Median Survival (Days)	Lung Tumor Incidence (%)	Mean Age of Rats Died with Lung Tumor (Days)
0	48	850 (288-1122)	0	-
Aromatic Retinoid Ro 10.9359	24	801 (160-1087)	0	-
PuO_2 Inhalation + Benzo(a)pyrene (IT)	50	317 (154- 635)	72	357 ($\pm$103)
PuO_2 Inhalation + Benzo(a)pyrene (IT) Aromatic Retinoid	46	270 (86- 631)	63	353 ($\pm$157)

animals dying with lung tumors was closely similar in both groups. Similar toxicity of retinoid treatment was observed in rats not exposed to carcinogens.

The staging and local invasiveness of lung tumors are reported in Table 4. The only difference observed between the retinoid-treated group and the control group related to regional lymph node invasion which was significantly reduced ($p = 0.02$) in treated rats.

DISCUSSION

In the present study, we have used the combined effect of α irradiation and benzopyrene-Fe_2O_3 particles for the induction of respiratory tract tumors. Most of them originated from the epithelium of the bronchi. These tumors showed histopathologic characteristics similar to those observed in human lung cancer, all were squamous cell carcinomas. A sequence of changes from normal bronchial epithelium to squamous metaplasia and to squamous tumors was apparent in the histogenesis of these neoplasms.

The results of this work indicate that, at non toxic doses, Ro 10.9359 did not reverse established squamous changes. However, when higher doses (200 mg/kg) were given, a complete inhibition of metaplasia occurred on a significant percentage of animals. This benefit was strongly counterbalanced by the acute toxic effects

Table 4. Comparison of size and invasiveness of lung tumors in rats treated or not by aromatic retinoid (Ro 10.9359)

Treatment	Size (%)				Pleural Invasion (%)	Lymph Nodes Invasion (%)
	T_1	T_2	T_3	T_4		
PuO_2 Inhalation + Benzo(a)pyrene (IT)	8	24	24	44	64	35
PuO_2 Inhalation + Benzo(a)pyrene (IT) Aromatic Retinoid	12	16	22	50	62	12

which seriously diminished the life span of the treated animals. When nontoxic doses of retinoid were given before the establishment of metaplasias and during the post initiation, the growth of transformed cells seemed to slow down since the areas of metaplasia decreased, but this phenomenon was not statistically significant due to very large individual fluctuation.

The third point is that chronic administration of Ro 10.9359 up to the natural death of animals was without effect on the total incidence of lung tumors as well as their development. However an inhibition of the local invasiveness to the regional lymph nodes was observed.

Like others (5,6,7) the present study failed to demonstrate chemoprevention or chemotherapy of respiratory tract cancer by retinoic acid. Several hypothesis can be considered. It was observed by Nettesheim (12) that reversal of transformation by retinoids is limited by the dosage of the carcinogen. In particular, in our model, the carcinogen exposure is prolonged during all the life of animals. Indeed the plutonium particles are known to stay in the lungs for a long biological half life. The total dose delivered to the lungs was high, between 3000 rads and 8000 rads. We cannot exclude that the persistance and dosage of the carcinogens overwhelmed the protection by the retinoid. It must however be taken into account that benzopyrene Fe_2O_3 acted as a promoter in that model and we can thus conclude that, under these conditions, Ro 10.9359 was not an antipromotor. Currently, experiments are in progress in which anticarcinogenic and antitumor effect of Ro 10.9359 are being tested in a model of lung cancer in which carcinogen exposure is short and the tumor latency very long (13).

The general failure of treatment with retinoids in different lung tumor models (5,6,7) in contrast to successful results obtained with other types of epithelial tumors (2,3) may lead to the hypothesis that lung target cells are not sensitive to retinoids. This is unlikely, since in the present study, inhibition of metaplasia development was observed after administration of high but toxic doses, of Ro 10.9359. In addition, chronic administration of this retinoid to heavy smokers was shown to induce the regression of established bronchial metaplasia (14). Another possibility for explaining the negative results is that the quantity of the drug reaching the target cell was too low. To test this hypothesis, it would be interesting to administer the drug by aerosol in order to deliver locally a higher dose of retinoid to transformed cells without increasing its general toxic effects.

The inhibition of metaplasia growth observed after high doses of retinoid may be explained by a direct effect on cellular differentiation. On the other hand, the decrease of local lymph node invasion in retinoid-treated rats bearing tumors would be more likely related to an effect of the drug on the immune system. Indeed, we have previously shown that Ro 10.9359 is able to activate macrophages rendering them highly cytotoxic for tumor cells (15). Moreover, stimulation of specific T cell cytotoxicity and nonspecific natural killer (NK) cell activity was demonstrated with other types of retinoids (16). A high level of NK activity was demonstrated in the lung of normal rats (17) as well as its inhibition during lung carcinogenesis (18). Its restoration during treatment with Ro 10.9359 may be, at least in part, responsible for the antitumor effect of this retinoid. Experiments are in progress to test this hypothesis.

ACKNOWLEDGEMENTS

We thank Dr. Bollag from Hoffman-La-Roche for its generous gift of the synthetic aromatic retinoid (Ro 10.9395).

REFERENCES

1. Saffiotti, U., R. Montesano, A. R. Sallakumar and S. A. Borg. 1967. Experimental cancer of the lung. Inhibition by vitamin of the induction of tracheobronchial squamous metaplasia and squamous cell tumors. Cancer 20: 857.

2. Bollag, W. 1974. Therapeutic effects of an aromatic retinoid acid analog on chemically induced skin papillomas and carcinomas of mice. Eur. J. Cancer 10: 731.

3. Sporn, M., R. Squire, C. Brown, J. Smith, M. Wenk and S. Springer. 1977. 13-Cis-Retinoic acid, inhibition of bladder carcinogenesis in the rat. Science 195: 487.

4. Moon, R., C. Grubbs and M. Sporn. 1976. Inhibition of 7,12 dimethylbenz(a)anthracene induced mammary carcinogenesis by retinyl acetate. Cancer Res. 36: 2626.

5. Smith, W. E., E. Yazdi and L. Miller. 1972. Carcinogenesis in pulmonary epithelia in mice on different levels of vitamin A. Environ. Res. 5: 152.

6. Smith, D. M., A. E. Rogers, B. J. Herndon and P. M. Newberne. 1975. Vitamin A (retinyl acetate) and Benzo(a)pyrene-induced respiratory tract carcinogenesis in hamsters fed a commercial diet. Cancer Res. 35: 11.

7. Nettesheim, P., and M. L. Williams. 1976. The influence of vitamin A on the susceptibility of the rat lung to 3-methylcholanthrene. Int. J. Cancer 17: 351.

8. Nolibe, D., R. Masse and J. Lafuma. 1981. The effect of neonatal thymectomy on lung cancers induced in rats by plutonium dioxide. Rad. Res. 87: 90.

9. Lansiart, A., and J. P. Morrucci. 1965. Nouveau compteur proportionnel destine a la detection in vivo de traces de plutonium dans les poumons, P. 131-141. In Assessment of radioactivity in man, Vol. 1. Intern. At. Energy Agency, Vienna.

10. Metivier, H., R. Masse, D. Nolibe and J. Lafuma. 1977. $^{239}PuO_2$ aerosol inhalation with emphasis on pulmonary connective tissue modifications, p. 583-595. In W. H. Walton (ed.), Inhaled particles IV. Pergamon Press, Oxford.

11. McClellan, R. O. 1972. Progress in studies with transuranic elements at the Lovelace Foundation. Health Phys. 22: 815.

12. Nettesheim, P., M. C. Cone and C. Snyder. 1976. The influence of retinyl acetate on the post initiation phase of preneoplastic lung nodules in rats. Cancer Res. 36: 996.

13. Chameaud, J., R. Perraud, J. Chretien, R. Masse and J. Lafuma. 1982. Lung carcinogenesis during in vivo cigarete smoking and Radon daughter exposure in rats. Recent Results Cancer Res. 82: 11.

14. Gouveia, J., T. Hercend, G. Lemaigre, G. Mathe, F. Gros and G. Santelli. 1982. Degree of bronchial metaplasia in heavy smokers and its regression after treatment with a retinoid. Lancet 19: 710.

15. Hercend, T., M. Bruley-Rosset, I. Florentin and G. Mathe. 1981. In vivo immunostimulating properties of two retinoids: Ro 10.9359 and Ro 13.6298, P. 21-30. In C. E. Ordanos (ed.), Retinoids. Springer Verlag, Berlin.

16. Goldfarb, R. M. and R. M. Herberman. 1981. Natural cell killer reactivity: regulatory interactions among phorbolester, interferon, cholera toxin and retinoid acid. J. Immunol. 126: 129.

17. Nolibe, D., E. Berel, R. Masse and J. Lafuma. 1981. Characterization of a major natural killer activity in rat lungs. Biomedicine 35: 230.

18. Nolibe, D., E. Berel, R. Masse and J. Lafuma. 1982. An argument for the concept of the dose to the lung. Radiosensitivity of intracapillary natural killer cells. In Eighth Symposium on Microdosimetry, Julich, Germany (in press).

A FEASIBILITY STUDY TO DETERMINE IF MICROBICIDAL ACTIVITY CAN BE MEASURED IN DEXAMETHASONE-TREATED MACROPHAGE CULTURES

Robert J. Grasso and Robert C. Guay, Jr.

Department of Medical Microbiology and Immunology
University of South Florida College of Medicine
Tampa, Florida (USA)

INTRODUCTION

Macrophages play a major role in host resistance by ingesting and killing microorganisms. If these normal phagocytic processes are impaired by chemotherapeutic agents, host resistance decreases and susceptibility to infectious diseases increases accordingly. This may be the case with the glucocorticoid steroids since these agents suppress other macrophage functions (1,6,7). However, whether glucocorticoids act directly on macrophages *in vivo* to reduce host resistance by inhibiting their normal phagocytic functions remains to be established.

Therefore, we have employed an *in vitro* model system to study direct glucocorticoid effects on the ingestion of heat-killed *S. cerevisiae* in cultures of murine peritoneal macrophages (2-4). In 6 day-old control cultures, ~90% of the macrophage population is capable of ingesting >20 yeast particles. In contrast, ~25% of the population in 1 μM dexamethasone-treated cultures is capable of ingesting only a limited number of yeasts (*i.e.*, 1 to 3 particles). The suppression of particle ingestion in steroid-treated cultures is a specific glucocorticoid-directed inhibitory response.

It is not known whether dexamethasone action also impairs the ability of the treated phagocytes to kill the few ingested yeasts. In order to explore this possibility, the following two questions must be considered. First, does intracellular killing of living *S. cerevisiae* occur in control macrophages not exposed to dexamethasone? Secondly, can sufficient numbers of living yeast be recovered shortly after their limited ingestion by the few phagocytic steroid-treated macrophages in order to generate survival curves? Thus, the purpose of this preliminary study was to answer these two questions.

METHODS

The preparation of tissue culture medium and stock dexamethasone solutions, the removal of resident peritoneal leukocytes by lavage from male C57BL/6 mice, the establishment of control and 1 μM dexamethasone-treated coverslip cultures of adhered macrophages, yeast phagocytosis assays with heat-killed S. cerevisiae, and statistical analysis of the data collected by light microscopy were described previously (2). Day 0 refers to the day that the macrophage cultures were established. Phagocytes are defined as those macrophages that ingested at least 1 heat-killed yeast particle after 15 min phagocytosis assays.

For experiments with living yeasts, stock cultures of S. cerevisiae were maintained at 30°C on Sabouraud's dextrose agar slants. Three day old slants were washed with Sabouraud's dextrose broth and the released organisms were incubated at 30°C for an additional 3 days. Yeast cells were pelleted by centrifugation and were resuspended at 4×10^7 particles per ml in tissue culture medium containing 20% heat-inactivated (56°C, 30 min) fetal bovine serum. Phagocytosis assays with living yeasts were carried out for 15 min in macrophage cultures at 37°C under the same conditions employed for heat-killed particles. Extracellular yeast cells were removed by extensive washing in PBS. The macrophages containing intracellular yeasts were lysed 20 min after the coverslips were placed in distilled H_2O at ambient temperatures. Liberated yeasts were diluted in PBS and plated on Sabouraud's dextrose agar plates which were incubated at 30°C for 48 hrs. The colonies were counted and the total numbers of viable organisms per macrophage culture were calculated.

RESULTS

In order to establish in this study that dexamethasone action suppresses yeast ingestion, phagocytosis assays with heat-killed particles were performed in control and 1 μM dexamethasone-treated cultures. Relative to controls, ~35% of the macrophage population in the treated cultures was phagocytic on Day 4 (Table 1). Most control phagocytes ingested >20 yeast particles whereas most steroid-treated phagocytes ingested 1 to 2 particles (data not shown). These results confirm our earlier findings that limited numbers of particles are ingested by a minor subpopulation in dexamethasone-treated macrophage cultures (2-4).

Table 1. Limited ingestion of heat-killed *Saccharomyces cerevisiae* in dexamethasone-treated cultures of peritoneal macrophages[a]

Day	Percentages of Phagocytes in		% of Control Cultures
	Control Cultures	1 μM Dexamethasone-Treated Cultures	
0	59.3 ±7.4[b]		
4	80.0 ± 3.7	28.3 ± 2.4	35.4[c]

[a] N = 4

[b] Mean ± S.E.M. percentage of macrophages ingesting at least one yeast particle.

[c] $p < 0.050$.

In order to determine whether intracellular killing of ingested yeasts occurs within macrophages not exposed to dexamethasone, 15 min phagocytosis assays were performed with living organisms in 2 sets of 4 day-old control cultures. After removing extracellular yeast, the macrophages in one set were lysed immediately and the liberated yeasts were plated. The macrophages in the other set were allowed to incubate for an additional 105 min in 4 day-old conditioned medium obtained from other control cultures. After this time, the macrophages in this set were lysed and the liberated yeasts were plated. Table 2 indicates that untreated control macrophages are capable of killing ingested *S. cerevisiae*. These results confirm an earlier report that living *S. cerevisiae* organisms are killed within murine resident peritoneal macrophages (5).

We next examined whether numbers of viable yeasts sufficient for microbicidal studies can be recovered from the minor phagocytic subpopulation in glucocorticoid-treated cultures. Hence, 15 min phagocytosis assays with living yeasts were performed in 4 day-old control and 1 μM dexamethasone-treated cultures. After removing extracellular organisms, the macrophages were lysed and the liberated yeasts were plated. Table 3 clearly demonstrates that ~10^4 viable yeasts per dexamethasone-treated culture were recovered. Assuming that little if any intracellular killing of *S. cervisiae* occurred during the brief 15 min phagocytosis assays, Table 3 also shows that dexamethasone action in the treated cultures produced an 87% phagocytic inhibitory effect with living organisms relative to controls.

Table 2. Intracellular killing of Saccharomyces cerevisiae within cultured peritoneal macrophages[a]

Minutes[b]	10^3 x Total Number of Viable Yeasts Per Culture	% of 15 Min Value
15	15.9 ± 0.3[c]	
120	9.3 ± 0.2	58[d]

[a] N = 6

[b] Total time that macrophages containing intracellular yeast were incubated at 37°C.

[c] Mean values ± S.E.M.

[d] $p < 0.050$

DISCUSSION

Taken together, these results provide answers to the two questions posed above. Intracellular killing of S. cerevisiae occurs in untreated control cultures and numbers of viable yeasts sufficient for microbicidal studies can be recovered from the steroid-treated cultures. Thus, it is feasible to explore whether dexamethasone action impairs the ability of the treated phagocytes to kill the few intracellular viable yeasts that are ingested.

Table 3. Recovery of viable Saccharomyces cerevisiae shortly after their ingestion by control and steroid-treated macrophages

Steroid Treatment	N[a]	10^3 x Total Number of Viable Yeasts Per Culture	% of Control
None (Control)	4	71.3 ± 0.2[b]	
1 μM Dexamethasone	9	9.5 ± 0.1	13[c]

[a] N = Number of macrophage cultures

[b] Mean values ± S.E.M.

[c] $p < 0.050$

SUMMARY

Dexamethasone action severely limits the ingestion of Saccharomyces cerevisiae in cultures of murine peritoneal macrophages. In spite of this inhibitory response, numbers of viable yeasts sufficient for microbicidal studies can be recovered shortly after their limited ingestion from lysed steroid-treated phagocytes.

REFERENCES

1. Fauci, A. 1978-79. Mechanisms of the immunosuppressive and and anti-inflammatory effects of glucocorticosteroids. J. Immunopharmacol. 1: 1-25.

2. Grasso, R. J., T. W. Klein, and W. R. Benjamin. 1981. Inhibition of yeast phagocytosis and cell spreading by glucocorticoids in cultures of resident murine peritoneal macrophages. J. Immunopharmacol. 3: 171-192.

3. Grasso, R. J., L. A. West, R. C. Guay, Jr., and T. W. Klein. 1972. Inhibition of yeast phagocytosis by dexamethasone in macrophage cultures: Reversibility of the effect and enhanced suppression in cultures of stimulated macrophages. J. Immunopharmacol. (in press).

4. Grasso, R. J., L. A. West, R. C. Guay, Jr., and T. W. Klein. 1983. Modulatory effects of heat-labile serum components on the inhibition of phagocytosis by dexamethasone in peritoneal macrophage cultures. Internatl. J. Immunopharmacol. (in press).

5. Hart, P.D'A. 1981. Macrophage antimicrobial activity: Evidence for participation by lysosomes in the killing of Saccharomyces cerevisiae by normal resident macrophages. Infect. Immun. 31: 828-830.

6. Parrillo, J. E., and A. Fauci. 1979. Mechanisms of glucocorticoid action on immune processes. Ann. Rev. Pharmacol. Toxicol. 19:179-201.

7. Spreafico, F., and A. Anaclerio. 1977. Immunosuppressive agents, p. 245-278. In J. W. Hadden, R. G. Coffey, and F. Spreafico (eds.), Immunopharmacology. Plenum Publishing Corp., New York.

IMMUNOLOGICAL STUDIES OF MALE HOMOSEXUALS WITH THE PRODROME OF THE ACQUIRED IMMUNODEFICIENCY SYNDROME (AIDS)

Evan M. Hersh[1], James M. Reuben[1], Peter W. A. Mansell[2] Adan Rios[1], Guy R. Newell[2], Jess Frank[3], and Allan L. Goldstein[4]

Department of Clinical Immunology and Biological Therapy[1], Department of Cancer Prevention[2], Department of Biomathematics[3], M. D. Anderson Hospital and Tumor Institute, 6723 Bertner Avenue, Houston, Texas (USA) and Department of Biochemistry[4], The George Washington University School of Medicine and Health Sciences, Washington, DC (USA)

INTRODUCTION

During the last three years, a syndrome of opportunisitic infection and Kaposi's sarcoma has been described in young male homosexuals in the United States (1-3). More recently this syndrome has also been described in other countries (4) and in a limited number of heterosexuals from both the United States and other countries. It has also been described in a small number of subjects in other patient groups, such as individuals with hemophilia (5). In addition to opportunistic infection and Kaposi's sarcoma, small numbers of cases of other malignancies are beginning to appear in this group, such as oral squamous cell carcinoma (6) and malignant lymphoma (7).

Immunological studies of patients with frank opportunisitic infection or Kaposi's sarcoma have indicated that the patients are lymphopenic, have impaired delayed hypersensitivity and impaired in vitro lymphocyte blastogenic responses to mitogens and antigens (1-3). Almost all have low helper T cells with an inverted helper:suppressor T cell ratio (1-3).

The etiology of this new syndrome, or set of syndromes, is obscure but there are possible relationships to recurrent viral infections, multiple sexual partners, multiple sexually transmitted diseases, gastrointestinal introduction of germ cells and intensive use of steroid creams and recreational drugs, particularly nitrites.

In the current study we have evaluated a group of individuals with the homosexual life style and with some indications that they were at a high risk of developing this syndrome. These indications included a history of one or more of the following: fever, weight loss, lymphadenopathy, or recurrent diarrhea. These patients were referred by their private physicians for immune evaluation at M. D. Anderson Hospital. Observations made in this latter group of patients have indicated that a significant degree of immunodeficiency can be detected in the majority of them, indicating an underlying and preceeding status of immune deficiency, prior to the development of opportunistic infection, Kaposi's sarcoma or other unusual malignancies. The findings are important because they indicate a basis for the development of preventive immunorestorative therapy.

METHODS

Thirty-three homosexual male subjects, with a normal performance status, aged 25-36 and a similar number of heterosexual controls were evaluated in these studies. Five of the thirty-three had or developed limited Kaposi's sarcoma. Delayed type hypersensitivity to recall antigens was done as previously described (8). Recall skin test antigens included dermatophytin, candida, varidase, mumps, and PPD. Peripheral blood leukocytes were studied to determine the lymphocyte blastogenic responses to the mitogens phytohemagglutinin (PHA), concanavalin-A (CON-A), and pokeweed mitogen (PWM) (9). In addition, peripheral blood leukocytes were evaluted for their natural killer cell activity (10), for their ability to mediate antibody dependent cellular cytotoxicity (ADCC) (11), and to determine the numbers of strongly adherent macrophage precursors (12). The following T lymphocyte cell surface markers were measured: E-rosettes, OKT 3, OKT 4, and OKT8 (13). B cells were measured by determining the number of surface immunoglobulin of the IgM/IgD types (14). Serum lysozyme was measured using the Worthington Biologicals Kit. Serum thymosin α_1 levels were measured by a radioimmunoassay (15). Suppressor cell activity was measured by co-culturing nonirradiated or irradiated patient lymphocytes with normal lymphocytes stimulated with PHA, CON-A, and PWM (16). For the delayed hypersensitivity responses, the control group represents a large number of normal subjects (397) seen for evaluation of delayed hypersensitivity concurrent with a visit of a family member to M. D. Anderson over the last several years (8). Controls for the surface markers and cellular immune parameters were concurrent age-matched heterosexuals seen at M. D. Anderson at the same time that the homosexual patients were evaluated.

RESULTS

Table 1 summarizes the results observed in this patient group. Delayed hypersensitivity was markedly impaired in the patients compared to the controls. Only 7% of the patients, compared to 49% of the controls, reacted to dermatophytin, only 26% of the patients compared to 71% of the controls reacted to varidase, only 30% of the patients compared to 60% of the controls reacted to mumps, and only 7% of the patients compared to 29% of the controls reacted to PPD. There was a modest reduction in the candida reactivity of the patients compared to the controls, but 52% of the patients did develop positive delayed hypersensitivity reactions to this antigen.

In regard to cell surface markers, there was a modest deficiency in the percentage of T cells measured by the E-rosette method, a marked deficiency in the helper cells measured with the monoclonal antiserum to the OKT 4 antigen and a modest but significant elevation in the proportion of suppressor cells measured with monoclonal antibody to the OKT 8 antigen. This resulted in an inverted helper:suppressor ratio. The ratio was .85 in the patients compared to 1.92 in the controls.

There was also significant but selective abnormalities in parameters associated with cell-mediated immunity and/or cell associated host defense mechanisms. Thus, while the lymphocyte blastogenic responses to phytohemaglutinin were slightly reduced on average compared to controls, the difference between patients and controls was not statistically significant. However, the blastogenic responses of the patients to CON-A and and PWM were markedly and significantly reduced compared to the controls. Cell-mediated cytotoxicity, measured by the natural killer cell reactivity to the K562 cell line and antibody dependent cell-mediated cytotoxicity to isoantibody coated human erythrocytes, was normal in essentially all of the patients. Monocyte adherence, which measures the numbers of strongly adherent monocytes, which can stick to plastic and transform to macrophages in 7 days, was depressed in the patients compared to the controls. There were 2 striking serological findings related to cell mediated immunity. First, the serum thymosin $\alpha 1$ levels were markedly and significantly elevated compared to the controls. Second, serum lysozyme levels were also markedly and significantly elevated compared to the controls.

Table 1. Immunological findings in homosexual males with the prodrome of the acquired immune deficiency syndrome (AIDS)[a].

Delayed Type Hypersensitivity			Cell Surface Markers			Cellular Immune Parameters		
Parameter	Patient	Control	Parameter	Patient	Control	Parameter	Patient	Control
Dermatophytin	7*	49	E-rosettes	59.8*	68.8	PHA	75.1	90.7
Candida	52	82	OKT 3	43.7	52.9	CON-A	32.2*	56.3
Varidase	26*	71	OKT 4	18.0*	34.6	PWM	30.7*	60.1
Mumps	30*	60	OKT 8	29.6*	21.3	NK	13.6	16.5
PPD	7*	29	OKT 4/8	0.85*	1.92	ADCC	9.6	9.8
			SIg	7.5	6.6	Monocyte Adherence	8.2	16.2
						Thymosin α_1	147.3*	52.4
						Lysozyme	11.6*	4.9

[a] For delayed hypersensitivity, the percent positive patients and controls are shown. For cell surface markers, the percent positive cells are shown. E-rosettes are the total T cells, OKT 3 is the monoclonal antibody to the pan-T antigen, OKT 4 to helper cells, OKT 8 to suppressor cells and SIg is the cell reactivity to anti IgM/D. PHA, CON-A, and PWM responses are reported in cpm/culture x 10^3. NK targets were K562 cells. ADCC targets were isoantibody coated human RBC; both NK and ADCC are reported in % target cell lysis. Monocyte adherence was the number of adherent cells per ml of blood x 10^4, Serum thymosin α_1 by radioimmunoassay was reported as picograms per ml and lysozyme in μg/ml. An * indicates that the patients were statistically significantly different than the controls.

Of the parameters described above, four were abnormal compared to the controls in essentially all of the patients. These included the percentage of OKT 4 positive cells, the OKT 4/8 ratio, the serum thymosin α_1 level and the serum lysozyme level. In the remainder of the assays, a proportion of the subjects were normal while only a proportion were abnormal.

Table 2 shows data generated relating to suppressor cell activity in these patients. Twenty-one individuals were studied using our previously reported co-culture system and twelve showed suppressor cell activity. The median values of normal and patient cells cultured alone, normal plus patient cells in co-culture and normal plus patient cells in co-culture where the patient cells were irradiated prior to co-culture are shown. The cultures were then stimulated with PHA, CON-A or PWM as previously described. The data shown are on the twelve of the twenty-one patients who showed suppressor cell activity. It is clear that these patients' cells showed low blastogenic responses compared to the controls, that the addition of patient lymphocytes to normal lymphocytes suppressed the proliferative responses of the latter and that after irradiation of the patient cells, the proliferative response of the normals recovered or were restored.

Table 2. Evidence for suppressor cell activity in homosexual males with the prodrome of the acquired immune deficiency syndrome (AIDS)[a]

Responder Cells in Cultures	Mitogen Responses (mean cpm/culture x 10^3)		
	PHA	CON-A	PWM
Normal	82.9	38.7	46.5
Patient	3.8	2.7	3.8
Normal + Patient	0.9	20.6	21.5
Normal + [Patient irrad.]	63.3	39.5	44.0

[a] Data shown is for 12 pairs of controls and patients. Normal and patient cells were each cultured at concentrations of 1.5×10^5 cells per well. Cultures were harvested for ^{3}H-thymidine incorporation. In some experiments, patient cells were irradiated with 4000 rads. In each instance the co-culture of normal plus patient was significantly suppressed compared to normal alone.

DISCUSSION

The data reported in this paper confirm and extend observations made by others on the acquired immunodeficiency syndrome predominantly seen in homosexuals. The unique aspect of the current study is that most of the patients did not have severe opportunistic infection or malignancy, were not hospitalized and had a normal performance status. The majority had been selected because they manifested one or more components of a prodrome of the syndrome, such as weight loss, fever of unknown origin, lymphadenopathy or chronic diarrhea. It is interesting in this regard, that these patients had a definable syndrome of immune deficiency characterized by delayed hypersensitivity, skin test hyporeactivity, diminished helper cells with an inverted helper:suppressor ratio, impaired lymphocyte blastogenic responses, a suppressor cell for lymphocyte blastogenesis, impaired monocyte adherence, and elevated levels of serum thymosin α_1 and serum lysozyme. These findings are important because they may lead to a better understanding of the etiology and pathogenesis of the syndrome and also because they will allow us to identify patients who may be candidates of immunorestorative immunotherapy prior to the development of the full fledged syndrome.

Several of the findings are worthy of special comment. First, four of the parameters were abnormal in essentially all of the patients. This indicates that by carrying out only these four, relatively simple assays, we can identify virtually all subjects with the prodrome. These parameters include the level of helper cells, the helper: suppressor ratio, the serum thymosin α_1 level, and the serum lysozyme. In contrast, if we would have to depend for identifying patients with the prodrome on the basis of skin test reactivity, total T cells or lymphocyte blastogenic responses, which are also abnormal but only in a fraction of the patients, we would miss certain individuals with the prodrome of this syndrome.

While the skin test reactivity of the patients was definitely subnormal, and indeed eight of the individuals were anergic to our battery of five skin test antigens, it is of interest to note that 52% of the patients were reactive to candida. This may reflect the heavy incidence of candida infection in these patients. Many of them have manifested mild to severe thrush, esophageal candidiasis, or fungal infection of the nails or skin.

As noted above, the OKT 4 positive cells are low in essentially all of the patients. Indeed, in some of the patients there are less than 5% detectable OKT 4 positive cells. The etiology of this phenomenon is obscure at the moment. However, it is characteristic, not only of patients with this syndrome, but also patients with various viral infections, in patients with graft versus host reactivity after bone marrow transplantation, and most recently has been reported to be present in at least a subpopulation of otherwise normal pregnant women. Whether this represents impaired cell maturation, redistribution of a cell subpopulation, accelerated utilization of this population or sequestration at a particular site, such as the gastrointestinal tract or lymph nodes, is not known at present. Immunohistological studies of various tissues may shed light on this.

Another surprising finding was the elevated level of thymosin $\alpha 1$. We actually anticipated finding the level of this hormone to be depressed. We attribute the elevated level to possible end organ failure and failure of feedback control of its level.

The constellation of monocyte associated parameters, namely diminished monocyte adherence, normal monocyte mediated ADCC (to HRBC), and the markedly elevated serum lysozyme, also warrents comment. We speculate that there are fewer numbers of circulating monocytes, that the residual circulating monocytes may be activated to be more effective in ADCC and that the elevated serum lysozyme further reflects this activation. Thus, cells are being recruited from the peripheral blood to the tissues, reducing the number in the periphery and elevating the level of serum lysozyme.

The findings of normal NK cell and ADCC activity is also of interest. Apparently in patients with more advanced degrees of acquired immunodeficiency, these parameters are depressed. It may be that ultimate depression of these parameters is a poor prognostic sign and is either causally related to the acquired opportunistic infection or may be the result of it.

Finally, it is clear that the opportunistic infection which occurs in some of the patients with the acquired immunodeficiency syndrome, is the result of the immune deficiency and, while not proven, it may be that the Kaposi's sarcoma and other malignancies are also the result of an impaired immunosurveillance mechanism. Therefore, the logical next step in the development of research in this area is the pre-clinical and ultimate clinical study of immunorestorative immunotherapy. A number of immunorestorative agents, such as thymic hormones, are available to specifically restore deficient T cell functions. Others, such as isoprinosine, affect both T cell and monocyte functions and have antiviral activities as well, while others, such as indomethacin and cimetidine are directed at monocyte and lymphocyte mediated suppressor cell activity. We speculate that an in vitro study of the immunorestorative effects of these and other agents on the leukocyte functions of patients with the prodrome of the syndrome will lead to a rational development of immunorestorative immunotherapy which may prevent full expression of the disease syndrome.

SUMMARY

Homosexual patients who mainly had the prodrome of the syndrome of opportunistic infection and Kaposi's sarcoma were studied immunologically. Patients showed diminished delayed hypersensitivity to recall antigens, diminished lymphocyte blastogenic responses, a suppressor cell for lymphocyte proliferative responses, low helper cells and an inverted helper:suppressor ratio. The patients had low levels of adherent monocytes. NK cell activity and antibody dependent cellular cytotoxicity were normal. Virtually all patients showed elevated serum thymosin α_1 levels and elevated serum lysozyme levels. The most consistent findings were the low helper cells, inverted helper:suppressor ratio and elevated serum thymosin α_1 and lysozyme. The patients with the prodrome should be subjected to therapeutic research with immunorestorative drugs.

REFERENCES

1. Gottlieb, M.S., R. Schroff, H. M. Schanker, J. D. Weisman, P. T. Fan, R. A. Wold, and A. Saxon. 1981. Pneumocystis carinii pneumonia and mucosal candidiasis in previously healthy homosexual men. Evidence of a new acquired cellular immunodeficiency. N. Engl. J. Med. 305: 1425-1430.

2. Masur, H., M. A. Michelis, J. B. Greene, I. Onorate, R. A. Vande Stouwe, R. S. Holzman, G. Wormser, L. Brettman, M. Lange, H. W. Murray and S. Cunningham-Rundles. 1981. An outbreak of community-acquired Pneumocystis carinii pneumonia. Initial manifestation of cellular immune dysfunction. N. Engl. J. Med. 305: 1431-1438.

3. Siegal, F. P., C. Lopez, G. S. Hammer, A. E. Brown, S. J. Kornfeld, J. Gold, J. Hassett, S. Z. Hirschman, C. Cunningham-Rundles, B. R. Adelsberg, D. M. Parham, M. Siegal, S. Cunningham-Rundles, and D. Armstrong. 1981. Severe acquired immunodeficiency in male homosexuals, manifested by chronic perianal ulcerative herpes simplex lesions. N. Engl. J. Med. 305: 1439-1444.

4. Vilaseca, J., J. M. Arnau, R. Bacardi, C. Mieras, A. Serrano, and C. Navarro. 1982. Kaposi's sarcoma and Toxoplasma gondii brain abscess in a spanish homosexual. Lancet I: 572.

5. CDC. 1982. Pneumocystis carinii pneumonia among persons with hemophilia A. Morbid. and Mortal. Weekly 31: 365-367.

6. Conant, M.A., P. Bolberding, V. Fletcher, F. I. Lozada and S. Silverman. 1982. Squamous cell carcinoma in sexual partner of Kaposi sarcoma patient. Lancet I: 286.

7. CDC. 1982. Diffuse undifferentiated non-Hodgkin's lymphoma among homosexual males - United States. Morbid. and Mortal. Weekly 31: 277-279.

8. Morris, D. L., E. M. Hersh, J. U. Gutterman, M. Marshall and G. M. Mavligit. 1979. Recall antigen delayed type hypersensitivity skin testing: standardization of self reading by patients. Cancer Immuno. Immunother. 6: 5-8.

9. Lewinski, U. H., G. M. Mavligit, J. U. Gutterman and E. M. Hersh. 1977. Interaction between skin testing with recall antigens and temporal fluctuations of in vitro lymphocyte blastogenesis in cancer patients. Clin. Immuno. Immunopath. 7: 77-87.

10. Muchmore, A. V., J. M. Decker and R. M. Blease. 1977. Spontaneous cytotoxicity of human peripheral mononuclear cells toward red blood cells targets in vitro. Characterization of the killer cell. J. Immunol. 119: 1680.

11. Poplack, D. G., G. D. Bonnard, B. J. Holiman and R. M. Blease. 1976. Monocyte-mediated antibody dependent cellular cytotoxicity: a clinical test of monocyte function. Blood 48: 809-816.

12. Currie, E. A. and G. W. Hedley. 1977. Monocytes and macrophages in malignant melanoma. Peripheral blood macrophage precursors. Brit. J. Cancer 36: 1-6.

13. Hoffman, R. A., P. C. Gung, W. P. Hansen and G. Goldstein. 1980. Simple and rapid determination of human T lymphocytes and their subclasses in peripheral blood. Proc. Natl. Acad. Sci. 77: 4914-4917.

14. Gmelig, M. F., A.G.C.H. Uyt de Haag and R. Ballieux. 1977. Human B cell activation in vitro. T. cell dependent pokeweed mitogen - induced differentiation of blood B lymphocytes. Cell. Immunol. 33: 156.

15. McClure, J. E., N. Lemeris, D. W. Wara and A. L. Goldstein. 1981. Immunochemical studies on thymosin: radioimmunoassay of thymosin α_1. J. Immunol. 128: 368-375.

16. Hersh, E. M., Y. Z. Patt, S. G. Murphy, K. Dicke, A. Zander, M. Washington and R. Goldman. 1980. A radiosensitive thymic hormone sensitive suppressor cell in the peripheral blood of cancer patients. Cancer Res. 40: 3134-3140.

A LONGITUDINAL STUDY OF A PATIENT WITH ACQUIRED IMMUNODEFICIENCY SYNDROME USING T CELL SUBSET ANALYSIS

R. Lawrence Siegel[1] and Roger W. Fox[2]

Department of Pediatrics[1] and Department of Internal Medicine[2], University of South Florida College of Medicine, Tampa, Florida (USA)

INTRODUCTION

The Centers for Disease Control in 1981 reported an epidemic of *Pneumocystis carinii* pneumonia and Kaposi's sarcoma in young previously healthy homosexual men (1,2). Additional reports have been published identifying viral, bacterial, fungal, and protozoan infections in this and other patient groups (3-5). Clinical observations and immunologic evaluations have defined an Acquired Immunologic Deficiency Syndrome (AIDS) in these patients (3-7).

In many of the initial cases described, five major features were found. They were opportunistic infections (1), such as *Pneumocystis carinii* pneumonia, Kaposi's sarcoma (2), cytomegalovirus infections (3), recreational drug use (4), and homosexual or bisexual activities (5). Several of these reports have presented evidence for an acquired T cell defect in these patients. These patients are usually anergic, lymphopenic, and have decreased lymphocyte proliferation to mitogens and antigens *in vitro*. Analysis of peripheral blood T cell populations has revealed decreased numbers of the T helper/inducer population (Leu 3+ or OKT4+) subset and an increased percentage of T suppressor/cytotoxic cells (Leu 2+ or OKT8+)(3,6,7). These studies have not reported any changes in T cell subsets during the course of the disease. Thus, we undertook a four month longitudinal study of a patient with this syndrome using T cell subset analysis.

METHODS

Patient case report

VB was a 30 year old, black, male who was well until January 1981, when he began to have intermittent fevers up to 103°F, with chills, sweats and 8 to 10 watery, brown, non-greasy, non-foul-smelling stools daily. Fever and diarrhea persisted, but the patient did not seek medical attention until April, 1981. At this time, he was seen for a sore throat and was told he had a viral infection.

He was diagnosed as having Candida esophagitis in July, 1981 and was treated with nystatin with a good response. However, he continued to have fevers and diarrhea. He underwent a fissurectomy and excision of anal nodules in September, 1981. Pathology reports were unremarkable, but he had a lymphogranuloma venereum titer of 1:1240 (normal <1:256). He was hospitalized for diarrhea, dyspnea, and dysphagia in November, 1981.

Physical examination was normal except for a white exudate with serpiginous margins on his hard palate, decreased breath sounds in both bases, and healing rectal surgical scars. Chest X-ray was normal, but radiographic studies revealed extensive esophageal candidiasis with a speckled white pattern in the proximal second part of the duodenum. Endoscopic examination disclosed esophageal candidiasis, gastritis, and duodenitis. A small bowel biopsy revealed shortening and widening of the villi and inflammatory infiltrates of plasma cells and occasional macrophages. Cultures of duodenal aspirates were negative for ova and parasites but positive for yeast.

Mumps, PPD, Candida, and SKSD (Streptokinase-Streptodornase) skin tests were negative ANA was positive with a 1:40 speckled pattern. LE prep was negative and FTA was positive. Immunoelectrophoresis showed a polyclonal gammopathy. HAA was negative, but antibodies to the surface and core components of the hepatitis B virus and to the hepatitis A virus were present. Liver function tests and liver biopsy were normal. Zinc and magnesium levels were normal. His pulmonary status began to decline on 12/12/81 when evaluation disclosed a blood gas of PO2=50 torr on room air, bilateral infiltrates on chest X-ray, and a normal lung perfusion scan. Bronchoscopy was performed; biopsy brushings were positive for Pneumocystis carinii and he was started on trimethoprimsulfamethoxazole. T cell number (E rosettes) was 10% (normal 60-70%) on 12/18/81. Ophthalmology consult found flat retinal lesions compatible with an inactive Candida infection.

He became hypotensive and hypoxic on 12/26/81. Worsening of his pneumonia was noted on X-ray and he was started on pentamadine and and broad spectrum antibiotics. He required assisted ventilation for the next 5 days. Antibiotics were discontinued and he was extubated on 1/1/82. Pentamadine was discontinued due to several hypoglycemic episodes. He was then transferred on 1/8/82 to James A. Haley Veterans Hospital, Tampa, Florida.

Past medical history is significant in that the patient was a known bisexual who had documented infections with gonorrhea in 1970, 1972 and 1981 and syphilis in 1975. He had frequent homosexual contacts up to July, 1981. Surgical history included a tonsillectomy and adenoidectomy at age 7, a hemorroidectomy in 1970, and the recent fissurectomy. He claims to have been in good health until his illness started and missed only a few days of work each year. He denied IV drug use, but had used amyl and butyl nitrite and marijuana.

At transfer, his problems included *Pneumocystis carinii* pneumonia, *Candida* esophagitis, diarrhea, malabsorption, and low T cell numbers. Physical examination revealed an alert, active, cachetic, male in no acute distress. Small flat white lesions were present in the peripheral retinal fields. Several small scattered white exudates were noted on the posterior pharynx. Neck was supple without adenopathy. Chest exam was normal except for decreased breath sounds in both bases. Cardiac exam revealed a normal S1 and S2 without murmurs. Abdominal exam was unremarkable. The neurologic exam was intact.

Admission laboratory tests were as follows: WBC was 5,800 with 46 polys., 20 bands, 8 lymphs., 15 mono., 2 eos., 2 myleos. and 2 metamyelos.. Hemoglobin was 11.1 and hematocrit was 33.2. Monospot test was negative. Blood chemistries were normal except for T.P=5.3, Alb=2.2, ALK Phos=678, SGOT=245, LDH=551, gamma GT=272, and Globulin=3.1. A CXR was still abnormal. EKG showed a normal sinus rhythm. Upper GI showed a normal esophagus, stomach and duodenum. A repeat small bowel biopsy was normal except for slightly shortened villi. Right upper quadrant sonogram revealed cholelithiasis. C3 was 137 mg% (70-176), C4 was greater than 62 mg% (17-45 mg%), IgM was 66 mg% (40-120 mg%), IgD was 2.75 mg% (0.5-3.0 mg%), IgA was greater than 450 mg% (50-250 mg%) and IgG was 1820 mg% (800-1600 mg%).

The patient continued to develop worsening hypoxia in association with pulmonary infiltrates despite treatment with trimethoprim-sulfamethoxazole and other antibiotics. His chronic diarrhea was unresponsive to different forms of therapy and his esophageal candidiasis persisted despite therapy with ketoconazole and nystatin. He remained lymphopenic and anergic. However, for approximately one week the patient had marked clinical improvement while off most medications; a period which coincided with improved *in vitro* immunologic laboratory results. He later developed disseminated herpes simplex which responded to an initial course of acyclovir

(250 mg/M^2 q8 hours), but a relapse two weeks later did not respond to a second course of acyclovir.

He continued to deteriorate clinically and developed mental status changes, ataxia, and lethargy, in association with worsening hypoxia. A computerized axial tomography scan revealed bilateral frontal lobe densities. The patient died on 4/26/82 of a sudden intracerebral hemorrage despite extensive medical supportive care.

Autopsy revealed a malignant lymphoma present in the left and right basal ganglia and focal nodules (1.0 to 1.5 cm) in the liver; an intracerebral hemorrhage (4.0 cm in greatest dimension) involving the deep left frontal lobe and the anterior portion of the left and right basal ganglia; an acute and focally organizing pan-lobular bronchopneumonia (post mortem cultures were positive for Klebsiella pneumoniae); bibasilar pulmonary infarction; a cytomegalic virus pneumonitis; mucosal ulcerations and muscular necrosis with cytomegalic virus inclusions involving the esophagus, stomach, jejunum, ileum, and colon; lipid depletion, fibrosis, hemorrhage, and cytomegalic virus inclusions of both adrenals; fungal organisms consistent with Candida albicans in the esophagus; herpetic lesions of the hands, feet, ankles, face, and lips; chronic cholecystitis and cholelithiasis with stones present in the hepatic duct; pulmonary congestion and edema; fatty change of the liver; hemosiderin deposition in the liver and spleen; pleural adhesions of the left upper lobe; and a focal granuloma (1.5 cm) in the liver.

Immunological tests

Peripheral blood mononuclear cells were isolated from heparinized blood by ficoll hypaque density gradient centrifugation as previously described (9). Monoclonal antibodies anti-T3 (T3), anti-T4 (T4), and anti-T8 (T8) were obtained from ORTHO Pharmaceutical Corporation (Raritan, NJ). Anti-T3 reacts with 100 percent of peripheral T cells or 55-60% of peripheral lymphocytes. In contrast, the T4 antigen is expressed on approximately 40-45% of peripheral lymphocytes and the T8 antigen is present on 15 to 20% of peripheral lymphocytes. Functionally, the T4 antigen defines the helper cell population and the T8 antigen defines the suppressor/cytotoxic population. Analysis of T lymphocyte subset population was performed by means of indirect immunofluorescence using the mouse monoclonal antibodies to the T cell antigens T3, T4, and T8 and fluorescein-conjugated goat anti-mouse IgG (G/M FITC) obtained from Tago Laboratories (Burlingame, CA) as previously described (9).

Stimulation of peripheral blood lymphocytes by mitogens was assayed by mixing the mitogens with 1 x 10^5 ficoll-hypaque purified peripheral blood lymphocytes in 0.2 ml of RPMI 1640 supplemented with L-glutamine, streptomycin, penicillin, and 10% heat activated fetal calf serum in round bottom microtiter plates. Final concentrations were pokeweed mitogen (PWM) 1:100 w/v, phytohemagglutinin (PHA) 1:50 w/v, and concanavalin A (Con A) 10 micrograms/ml. Mitogens were previously titrated to obtain maximal stimulation.

Mixed lymphocyte cultures were set up in round bottom microtiter plates. One x 10^5 cells from each individual were suspended in RPMI 1640 supplemented with L-glutamine, streptomycin, penicillin and 10% heat inactivated fetal calf serum and placed in wells. Cells were treated with mitomycin C (25 micrograms per ml) for 30 minutes at 37°C. Mitomycin C treated cells serve as targets and do not participate in proliferative response. Mitomycin C treated cells had counts equal to or below that of unstimulated cells in one and two way MLC. The same individual was used throughout the study.

RESULTS

Table 1 shows the results of the patient's T cell subsets over a 4 month period. In general, decreased peripheral T cell numbers (T3+ cells), decreased numbers of T helper cells (T4+ cells) and increased numbers of T suppressor cells (T8+ cells) were found.

The patient's initial T cell evaluation was done on 1/14/82. At this time T cell mitogen stimulation studies were done and are shown in Table 2. Depressed responses to pokeweed and concanavalin A are noted with minimal response to phytohemmagglutinin.

Table 1. T cell subset analysis

Date	%T3+	%T4+	%T8+	MLC
1/14/82	6	3	7	ND
1/21/82	38	4	34	-
1/28/82	32	1	31	ND
2/22/82	28	0	28	ND
3/11/82	49	37	33	+
3/26/82	66	7	59	-
4/06/82	55	2	52	ND
4/26/82	46	12	48	ND
Normal Range	55-70%	35-45%	15-25%	

Table 2. T cell mitogenic index.

Date		PWM	PHA	Con A
1/14/82	Patient	2	11	2
	Control	14	79	33
1/28/82	Patient	2	90	26
	Control	37	265	179
2/22/82	Patient	4	100	23
	Control	22	144	101
3/26/82	Patient	2	36	9
	Control	6	19	14

Subsequent T cell analysis done on 1/21/82 revealed an improvement in T cell subsets associated with minimal clinical improvement in the patient. At this time, a mixed lymphocyte culture (MLC) was done. As can be noted, the patient showed an inability to respond in a mixed lymphocyte culture to an unrelated individual.

T cell subsets were repeated on 1/28/82. A depressed T cell number was still present; T helper cells were virtually absent; and an increased number of T suppressor cells were noted. Mitogen studies showed some improvement. Similar results were obtained on 2/22/82.

However, during a period of clinical improvement from 3/8/82 - 3/15/82 the previously abnormal T cell subsets approached near normal levels. At this same time, his previously negative mixed lymphocyte culture became positive. However, the patient subsequently deteriorated clinically and this was reflected in his abnormal T cell subsets and his negative lymphocyte culture done on 3/26/82. Additional T cell studies remained abnormal prior to the patient's death.

DISCUSSION

This study showed that the patient had consistently abnormal T cell subsets with the exception of the studies done in mid-March. At this time, the previously negative mixed lymphocyte culture was positive. During this spontaneous recovery to near normal T cell subset numbers and ratio, the patient improved clinically. However, he later deteriorated clinically and immunologically on the same treatment modalities.

Thus, T cell subset analysis may be clinically useful in following patients with this disorder; particularly, in a prospective study to determine individuals at risk for AIDS, their clinical course, and their response to future therapeutic agents. Understanding the pathogenesis and latency periods of this disease is an immediate goal, since its incidence and affected patient population are increasing. The appearance of this new disease is associated with a number of unproven factors. The fact that the initial cases were found predominantly in male homosexuals and bisexuals suggests that this is a sexually transmitted disorder. Perhaps, this new disease has resulted from recent changes in the lifestyle of homosexuals and bisexuals, such as more anonymous sexual encounters and the use of recreational drugs such as amyl and butyl nitrite. Multiple infections with cytomegalovirus, herpes simplex, hepatitis, syphilis, gonorrhea, and other sexually transmitted diseases in individuals with the proper genetic predisposition may be necessary for the production of this syndrome. Frequent and intense exposure to these agents may be one of the factors responsible for this disease. Transmission of an infectious agent by blood products, intravenous drug use, or sexual contact may explain cases in previously healthy heterosexual individuals.

Further immunologic data would provide valuable information regarding the pathogenesis, clinical course and response to treatment of this disease. Therefore, additional T cell subset monitoring studies need to be done in this population of AIDS patients.

SUMMARY

Acquired Immunodeficiency Syndrome (AIDS) has recently been documented in patients in association with opportunistic infections, Kaposi's sarcoma, cytomegalovirus infections, and recreational drug use. AIDS is characterized by cutaneous anergy, diminished peripheral lymphocyte responses to mitogens and antigens, and abnormal T cell subpopulations. These patients have been described as having decreased total T (T3+) cell numbers, virtual elimination of the T helper (T4+) cell population, and an increased percentage of the T suppressor-cytotoxic (T8+) cell population. T cell subset monitoring has not been performed during the course of this disorder. A four month longitudinal study of the T cell subsets of a 30 year old bisexual male with AIDS revealed changes in his T cell subpopulations and in his ability to respond in a one way mixed lymphocyte culture (MLC). The results indicated that the patient's previously abnormal T cell subpopulations returned to near normal values during a period of spontaneous clinical improvement. The patient's MLC response also returned to normal in association with the return of the T helper cell population. The patient's T cell subpopulation and MLC response subsequently became abnormal and remained abnormal until the patient died. Thus, it appears that T cell subpopulations may spontaneously improve during the course of this disorder. T cell subset analysis may offer a means of monitoring the clinical course of this disorder as well as the response to therapeutic agents.

ACKNOWLEDGEMENTS

This work was supported by BRSG Grant 2 SO7 RRO5749 awarded by the Biomedical Research Support Program, Division of Research Resources, National Institute of Health. The authors would like to acknowledge the excellent technical assistance of Mrs. Debbie Conarroe and the excellent secretarial assistance of Mrs. Ruth Hand.

REFERENCES

1. Centers for Disease Control. 1981. Pneumocystis pneumonia-Los Angeles. Morbid. Mortal. Weekly. 30: 250.

2. Centers for Disease Control. 1981. Kaposi's sarcoma and Pneumocystis pneumonia among homosexual men-New York City and California. Morbid. Mortal. Weekly. 30: 305.

3. Gottlieb, M. S., R. Schroff, H. M. Schanker, J. D. Weismann, P. T. Fan, R. A. Wolf, and A. Saxon. 1981. *Pneumocystis carinii* pneumonia and mucosal candidiasis in previously healthy homosexual men: evidence of a new acquired cellular immunodeficiency. N. Engl. J. Med. 305: 1425.

4. Masur, H., M. A. Michelis, J. B. Greene, I. Onorato, R. A. V. Stouwe, R. S. Holzman, G. Wormser, L. Brettman, M. Lange, H. W. Murray and S. Cunningham-Rundles. 1981. An outbreak of community-acquired *Pneumocystis carinii* pneumonia: initial manifestation of cellular immune dysfunction. N. Engl. J. Med. 305: 1431.

5. Siegal, F. P., C. Lopez, G. S. Hammer, A. E. Brown, S. J. Kornfeld, J. Gold, J. Hassett, S. Z. Hirschman, C. Cunningham-Rundles, B. R. Adelsberg, D. M. Parham, M. Siegal, S. Cunningham-Rundles and D. Armstrong. 1981. Severe acquired immunodeficiency in male homosexuals, manifested by chronic perianal ulcerative herpes simplex lesions. N. Engl. J. Med. 305: 1439.

6. Dent, P. B. 1972. Immunodepression by oncogenic viruses. Prog. Med. Virol. 14: 1.

7. Woodruff, J. F. and J. J. Woodruff. 1975. The effect of viral infections on the function of the immune system. In A. L. Notkins (ed.) Viral immunology and immunopathology. Academic Press, New York.

8. Centers for Disease Control Task Force on Kaposi's Sarcoma and Opportunistic Infections. 1982. Epidemiologic aspects of the current outbreak of Kaposi's sarcoma and opportunistic infections. N. Engl. J. Med. 306: 248.

9. Siegel, R. L., T. Issekutz, J. Schwaber, F. S. Rosen and R. S. Geha. 1981. The cellular defect in transient hypogamma-globulinemia of infancy. N. Engl. J. Med. 305: 1307.

WORKSHOP SUMMARY: CLINICAL EVALUATION OF IMMUNOMODULATING AGENTS IN CANCER WITH EMPHASIS ON NEW APPROACHES

B. Serrou[1] and J. L. Touraine[2]

Laboratoire de'Immunopharmacologie des Tumeurs[1]
INSERM U 236 and ERA-CNRS N° 844, Centre Paul Lamarque-
B.P. 5054, 34 033 - MONTPELLIER - Cedex - France

Clinique de Nephrologie - Pavillon P.[2]
Hopital Edouard Henriot - Place d' Arsonval
69 374 -LYON - Cedex 2 - France

Clinical evaluation of immunomodulating agents is a new approach which should be considered separate from that associated with chemotherapeutic agents. A few very important points must be made concerning these new agents modulating the immune response in order to avoid mismanagement and fatal errors associated with their use. To begin with, the agents should be chemically well defined compounds. Mixtures of complex molecules (for example BCG and *Corynebacterium parvum*) should be avoided. Chemically characterized drugs are a prerequisite for an accurate pharmacological profile concerning its metabolism in the body, the blood and urine. In our opinion, this approach is essential to be able to establish a correlation between drug blood levels and its effects on the immune response. The immunological target will also have to be identified in both animal models and *in vitro* in order to apply the best adapted and the most significant *in vivo* tests to the human situation. It is essential to identify not only the immunological target cells, but also the target function(s). Criticism concerning the results presented for many immunomodulating agents has centered around the fact that no placebo was used. It is an accepted fact that the placebo effect can profoundly modify immune response in 30 to 40% of patients. We believe that this sort of control is essential to the evaluation of new immunomodulating agents. The last point which we wish to underline concerns the evaluation of side-effects vis a vis not only the immunological system but also different organ systems and their functions.

With these remarks in mind, the results concerning a few such compounds were presented. TP-1 or thymostimulin is a thymic extract which is not yet available as a purified compound. Ambrogi and Davis presented data suggesting that this kind of extract was able to normalize purine catabolism and thus could be useful in CLL, and to improve E-rosette percentage and PHA response of immunodepressed Hodgkin's patients independent of clinical and histological stage. In our opinion, Har and Layer studies are needed using a chemically characterized TP-1 in double blind studies with placebo. The same remarks can be made concerning the evaluation of mycobacterial cell wall substances such as those presented by Vosika et al. even though no toxicity was observed at the doses employed and few responses were observed in trials with tumor patients.

Among the chemically defined agents, three immunomodulating agents require more complete evaluation. The first is C 1821 a purified glycoprotein extract from _Klebsiella pneumoniae_ serotype 2. Compared to placebo this agent significantly enhances skin reactions to several antigens and restores lymphocyte levels of cAMP and cGMP in untreated cancer patients (Lary et al.). Along the same lines, Blomgren has shown that Bestatin, a low molecular weight metabolite from _Streptomyces olivoreticuli_, increases the capacity of lymphocytes to bind sheep red blood cells and augments their NK cell activity as well as the release of interleukin 2. Clinical evaluations for these drugs are now underway using placebo. Preliminary results confirm animal and _in vitro_ data.

Morin et al. clearly demonstrated in a placebo controlled study that Isoprinosine was able to retard the evolution of breast, uterus and head and neck cancers and can be used with curative intent for viral infections in immunodepressed patients with food tolerance. These results are sufficiently convincing as to justify the use of this drug in the treatment of certain viral infections within a clearly defined context.

Chihara and Tajeuhi presented a complete study on Lentinan, a purified glucan from the edible mushroom _Lentinus edodes_. T cells are the main target for this compound which demonstrates antitumor activity. Randomized controlled studies support the clinical activity of this agent as an adjuvant to chemotherapy for advanced gastric and colo-rectal cancers. However, it is still too early to come to any definite conclusions and the adjuvant approach has yet to be evaluated fully.

Among the newer approaches being evaluated in cancer treatment is the use of monoclonal antibodies. The animal data presented by Feinerman and Paul suggest that Chlorambucil bound to monoclonal antibody can efficiently eliminate murine leukemia. These results attest to the possible use of monoclonal antibodies as a drug carrier to decrease nonspecific cell cytotoxicity. However, many problems remain unresolved concerning modulation of circulating antigens and ineffective immune response.

All of the presented data were both of interest and promising. However, these results will have to be considered by the scientific community in the field of immunopharmacology to precisely define the criteria to be used for the evaluation of the new compounds in clinical trials in order to avoid uninterpretable or erroneous studies which would be to the detriment of the patient as well as the immunopharmacologist. With this in mind, we wish to re-emphasize the necessity of chemically characterized and potentially dosable drugs having a precise, known immunological target. Under these conditions, double blind studies with placebo are preferable for phase 1 and 2 studies, not only for cancer patients but also other diseases. A particularly attractive candidate within the latter category would be viral disease.

WORKSHOP SUMMARY: ANIMAL TUMOR MODELS FOR EVALUATING CHEMICALLY DEFINED IMMUNOMODULATORS

John W. Hadden[1] and Federico Spreafico[2]

Immunopharmacology Program[1], University of South Florida College of Medicine, Tampa, Florida (USA)
Instituto Mario Negri[2], Via Eritrea, Milan, Italy

Efforts to establish an immunopharmacology for cancer immunotherapy have been frustrated by the lack of animal tumor models which directly relate to human cancer. Initially, emphasis was placed on transplantable tumors which were often inadvertently immunogenic by nature of infection with murine viruses or were of nonsyngeneic origins. The easily demonstrated effectiveness of BCG, _C_. _parvum_, and high molecular weight polysaccharide preparations led to the erroneous conclusion that such therapy in man would be equally effective. Considerable clinical trials since have not generally supported this conclusion. The relative failure of these agents in the human can be attributed to a number of factors including the inadequacy of the models. Complexity and ambivalence of their actions in humans have played a major role. The evolution of immunotherapy in human cancer has increasingly moved away from the complex agents towards the use of biologicals and chemically defined agents. It is clear that seldom are the agents effective in cancer therapy when used as a monotherapy. The apparent rule, both in murine tumor systems and in human cancer trials, has emerged that these agents act to increase the number of individuals remaining in remission following effective cytoreductive therapy with chemotherapy, surgery or irradiation. They have not been particularly active in treating progressive disease. Levamisole offers a case in point. In 34 animal tumor models in which it was used as a monotherapy no effect was observed; however, following cytoreductive therapy it was active in 13 of 21 systems. The experience in human cancer generally parallels these results. If one accepts the contention that levamisole is the only agent whose animal experience correlates with the human then logically the models in which it has been effective are the most appropriate for considering related agents. One of the difficulties in this consideration is that very little is known about the detailed antitumor mechanisms of the action of levamisole in either the animal models or in human cancer.

Animal tumors like human tumors involve immunosuppressed hosts and since cytoreductive therapy may contribute further to the immunosuppression, it is essential to know something about the immune status of the host prior to intervening with an immunotherapy. The first goal of immunotherapy should be to determine if immunologic reconstitution is effective. Secondary goals should include not only whether decreased growth of the primary tumor or of metastases and increased survival result but also whether increased resistance to secondary infection occurs. Finally, if survival is increased, it is important to determine whether resistence to rechallenge with the tumor indicates that specific antitumor mechanisms are involved. In designing combined therapy in these animal models it is important that the degree of antigenicity of the tumor be determined and to ensure that the tumor is syngeneic to the host and uninfected with antigenic pathogens so that only tumor antigenicity will determine specific host resistance.

In organizing this workshop our intent was to invite participants whose experience with animal, particularly murine, tumor models would shed light on the search for meaningful models and methods for studying the actions of chemically defined immunotherapeutic agents. The lack of time and participation allowed only a few to be presented. Notably absent were investigators to describe the models employed by the Biological Response Modifier Program of the NCI, particularly, the B16 melanoma and the ultraviolet irradiation cutaneous tumor models.

Dr. Vincent J. Merluzzi (Sloan-Kettering Institute) reported on the recovery of immune reactivity after chemotherapy-induced immunosuppression. Specific immunological and hematopoietic functions were studied during treatment with anti-neoplastic agents in mice bearing leukemias of defined immune origin. Both B- and T-lymphocyte functions (antibody-forming cells and cell-mediated lympholysis toward alloantigens) were suppressed in spleen cells of mice bearing these lymphoid tumors. Hematopoietic functions (granulocyte, macrophage, and megakaryocyte progenitors) were variably influenced by growth of the selected lymphoid tumors. Actinomycin D was effective in reducing tumor and restored immune functions suppressed by tumor growth to control levels, in the absence of evident toxicity to hematopoietic function or clonable B cells. 1-β-D-Arabinofuranosylcytosine and Polyinosinic-polycytidylic acid suppressed immune effector function in the absence of evident toxicity to hematopoietic function or clonable B cells. Mitomycin C on the other hand, was very toxic to hematopoietic functions and clonable B cells, while not significantly suppressing immunological functions.

High doses of cyclophosphamide (CY) inhibited cytotoxic T-cell (CTL) generation due to the elimination of accessory T cells and their corresponding helper factors. The results indicate that helper cells, required for development of CTL responses to alloantigens are eliminated by CY in the absence of evident toxicity to CTL precursors.

5-fluorouracil (5-FU) administered in daily injections to mice was differentially toxic to helper T cells. Precursors for both antibody forming cells and CTL were spared. 5-FU suppressed the *in vitro* T-cell-dependent antibody response to sheep red blood cells (SRBC). This low response was restored to normal levels by the addition of T-cell-replacing factor (TRF) or mixed lymphocyte culture (MLC) supernatants to the culture system. T-cell-independent antibody responses to TNP-LPS were not eliminated by 5-FU but, in contrast, were elevated two to four-fold. These results indicate that precursors for antibody-forming cells for T-cell-dependent and T-independent antibody responses were not eliminated by 5-FU. 5-FU administration in the same regimen did not reduce the number of CTL precursors as shown by limiting dilution analysis, but did cause a reduction in the capacity of lymphocytes from pre-treated mice to generate a CTL response *in vitro*. This low CTL response was restored to control levels by adding Lyt $1^{+}2^{-}$ T cells or sources of interleukin 2 (IL2) to the culture system, indicating that 5-FU similarly eliminated helper cells for CTL precursor differentiation as well as helper cells of antibody synthesis. This study showed that tumors of immune origin can differentially inhibit immune response and that in certain instances tumor-induced immune suppression could be reversed by chemotherapy. While reversal of tumor-induced immunosuppression did not always coincide with increased survival, in no case did chemotherapy increase survival unless immunorestoration occurred. Understanding such relationships are important in developing effective combination protocols for use in humans.

Dr. Gerard Renoux (University of Tours College of Medicine) recounted his experience with the Lewis lung model. He initially reported that levamisole was effective in reducing lung metastases in this model; however, was unable to repeat these observations at Sloan-Kettering with Dr. George Tarnowski. Others have also reported negative results with levamisole in this model and the basis for the differences between laboratories was never resolved, although it is known that sublines of the Lewis lung tumor exist differing in relavent aspects such as growth rate and capacity to metastasize. Dr. R. L. Fenichel (Wyeth Laboratories) presented that levamisole was significantly active in his Lewis lung system which employed not B6 but the BDF_1 hybrid. In his system, six to eight week old male BDF_1 mice were injected in the axillary region with Lewis lung tumor cells prepared from tumors grown in C57BL/6 mice. Regardless of the dosage schedule followed, intraperitoneal injections of 3-(p-chlorophenyl)thiazolo[3,2-a]benzimidazole-2-acetate acid (Wy-18,251, NSC 310533) or levamisole were always given in a solution composed of one part carboxymethyl cellulose and two parts of 0.9% NaCl 24 hours after the initiation of tumor growth. Control mice in all experiments received vehicle alone. Fifteen days after tumor implantation, the mice were sacrificed by cervical separation and the lungs excised. The best reduction of metastases occurred with one dose per week at one and five mg/kg of Wy-18,251. Levamisole evinced statistically significant reduction of lung metastases at three mg/kg, given once per week, but not at 25 mg/kg. It may be that use of the F hybrid or the carboxymethyl cellulose contributes to the activity. Dr. Lionel Simon (Newport Pharmaceuticals International) reported that NPT 15392 (0.1 mg/kg) was significantly active to reduce metastases in the Lewis lung model using B6 mice. Dr. Michael Osband (Boston University School of Medicine) presented that cimetidine (approximately 2 gm/kg) was active to reduce metastases in this model. These observations with NPT 15392 and cimetidine were confirmed by Dr. Irene Florentin ICIG Villejuif, France) in B6 mice. In no case did the chemically-defined immunotherapeutic agents reduce the primary tumor.

Drs. Osband and Florentin presented information on immune mechanisms in this system. Within three days following inoculation of the tumor in the foot pad, cytotoxic lymphocytes (CTL) and increased natural killer (NK) cell activity are apparent in the spleen. Beginning at 7 days concurrent with micrometastasis formation there is a progressive decline in CTL and NK cell activity in association with a progressive increase in the number of suppressor T lymphocytes in the spleen. To date, none of the immunotherapeutic agents have been analyzed in this system to see if they modify the progression of these immune events. Such would appear to be desirable.

Dr. Sharad D. Deodhar, (Cleveland Clinic Foundation) reported on studies on inhibition of lung metastases in mice bearing a malignant fibrosarcoma. This syngeneic tumor, originally induced by dibenzanthracene, (Sarcoma T241 in C57BL/6 mice) has been kept alive by serial transfers in live C57BL/6 mice. This animal tumor model is clinically relevant since (1) the tumor is poorly immunogenic as are most human tumors, and (2) it spontaneously metastasizes to the lungs, a common site of metastases for most human tumors. In studies with this model, the tumor cells are implanted in the subcutaneous tissue of one hind foot on day 1 of a given experiment, and the tumor is allowed to grow for 14 to 17 days. At this point, macro and/or micrometastases occur in the lungs in virtually all of the tumor bearing animals. To study the effect of a given therapeutic agent on lung metastases, the tumor bearing foot is amputated between day 14 to day 17 and appropriate treatment instituted after amputation. Agents such as BCG, *C. parvum*, levamisole, NPT 15392 or complete Freund's adjuvant are partially effective in inhibiting metastases provided these agents are administered very early in the course of tumor development. The most significant effects have been observed with liposome-encapsulated crude lymphokine or liposome-encapsulated human C-reactive protein.

Dr. Hideo Ishitsuka (Nippon Roche Research Center) presented on the protective activity of thymosin α_1 against opportunistic infections and tumor progression in immunosuppressed mice. Animal models for opportunistic infections were established in mice immunosuppressed by daily treatment with 5-FU for 8-10 days (25 mg/kg/day, ip). Thymosin α_1(4 - 400 μg/kg/day, ip), given concomitantly with 5-FU, protected mice against lethal infections by various opportunistic pathogens. The protective activity against *Candida* was abrogated by antithymocyte serum or carrageenan, while that against *Pseudomonas* was not affected by these agents. Thus, thymosin α_1 seems to exert its effect not only on T-cells and macrophages but also on other cells, e.g. neutrophils. In mice inoculated with L1210 leukemia or with B16 melanoma, immunosuppression by cytostatics or x-ray caused more rapid death or increased the incidence of pulmonary metastasis, respectively. Thymosin α_1 given concomitantly with the cytostatics or x-ray prevented the rapid death and the increase of metastases. The protective activity of thymosin α_1 against the rapid death could be transferred by inoculation of spleen cells from the donor mice treated with 5-FU and thymosin α_1, but not from the donor mice treated with 5-FU alone. The effector cells were suggested to be NK cells by treating with antisera against NK surface antigens. In fact, treatment with 5-FU reduced NK activity in spleen, but the combined treatment with thymosin α_1 prevented such reduction. In 5-FU treated mice, distribution of ^{125}I-L1210 cells inoculated was higher in blood and lung, but lower in liver and spleen as compared to that in normal mice. On the other hand, when thymosin α_1 was given with 5-FU the pattern of the tissue distribution was almost the same as that in normal mice. Similar phenomena were also observed when ^{125}I-B16, ^{51}Cr-lymph node or bone marrow cells were inoculated. Thus thymosin α_1 protected mice treated with immunosuppressive therapies from deleterious side effects of the treatments on surveillance systems against tumor. Furthermore, in therapy of P388 leukemia in mice, thymosin α_1 allowed the use of higher doses of 5-FU than in single therapy through prevention of side effects of 5-FU.

Dr. Allan Goldstein (George Washington School of Medicine) re-reported on the work of Dr. Marion Zatz who has studied the MOPC-315 tumor system in C57BL/6 mice. In this model, cyclophosphamide 20 mg/kg) was effective at reducing tumor load yet did not yield cures. The addition of thymosin α_1 (.01-1 μg/mouse 3 times per week) increased mean survival time and led to long term survivors. Thymosin fraction V was also reported to be active in the model. Rechallenge of long time survivors with tumor indicated immune resistance. All these results indicate that thymosin α_1 may be useful as an adjuvant in cancer therapy.

Transplantable murine tumors have been used as experimental models in cancer chemotherapy research for many years. However, in the common, repeatedly transplanted tumor systems, genetic drift in either the host or the tumor is likely to have occurred during the years, and it is reasonable to assume that resulting antigenic disparity between tumor and host may result in transplantation immunity that participates unduly in the killing of tumor cells leading to overly optimistic evaluation of therapeutic manipulations in such models. Therefore, a more appropriate animal model system is necessary for preclinical therapy studies, and this is particularly true for those studies involving immunotherapy.

Dr. Robert L. Stolfi (The Catholic Medical Center of Brooklyn and Queens) presented on the spontaneous $CD8F_1$ breast tumor model for experimental immunotherapy. This model developed for use in experimental cancer therapy, recently has been made available for general use through the Division of Cancer Therapy of the National Cancer Institute. These tumors share many characteristics with the human disease counterpart. Histologically characterized as adenocarcinomas, they are slowly evolving, with a relatively slow growth rate. Tumors become detectable in mid-to-late middle age and they are highly metastatic. They show a pattern of heterogeneity of many characteristics including growth rate and chemotherapeutic sensitivity which is analogous to human breast tumors, and distinctly different from the relatively more homogeneous long-transplanted murine tumors. Further, $CD8F_1$ breast tumors have been shown to be sensitive to all of the chemotherapeutic drugs that are considered to be effective clinically against breast cancer.

These spontaneous breast tumors are considered to be weakly antigenic in that attempts to immunize syngeneic mice against transplantation of spontaneous tumors are usually unsuccessful. Nevertheless tumor-specific cell-mediated cytotoxicity, complement-dependent and lympocyte-dependent antibody mediated cytotoxicity, as well as lymphocyte blocking and antibody blocking activities are measured in mice with the smallest of detectable tumors. As the tumor increases in size, the balance between the potentially beneficial and the potentially unfavorable immune components changes so that the titer of blocking activity increases, while cytotoxic antibody activity becomes undetectable and eventually cell-mediated cytotoxicity becomes undetectable. This ineffective immune response appears to be a likely candidate for therapeutic manipulation.

Several lines of evidence suggest that immunity is a relevant therapeutic consideration in this tumor system. Therapeutic synergism has been demonstrated between innate host antitumor immunity and a regimen consisting of enucleative tumor surgery and combination chemotherapy. Further, splenectomy, performed in conjunction with tumor enucleation and combination chemotherapy, resulted in a significant decrease in the number of tumor recurrences during a 6 month observation period than that observed in control mice treated with tumor surgery and chemotherapy. Analysis of tumor-specific immune reactivity revealed a more rapid decline in circulating blocking complexes and a more rapid return of cytotoxic antibody reactivity following enucleative tumor removal in mice that had been splenectomized at the time of tumor surgery compared to sham splenectomized controls. In addition, significant inhibition of the growth rate of spontaneous $CD8F_1$ breast tumors was observed following weekly administration of immunpotentiating agents such as *C. parvum* vaccine, or the maleic anhydride-vinyl copolymer, MVE-2 (15,000 m.w.).

Because of the slow and variable growth rate of this spontaneous murine tumor model, it is costly and more time consuming than available transplantable tumor models. Nevertheless, the most critical feature of an animal model for cancer therapy is the likelihood of its relevance to the human disease. Even aside from demonstrated analogies, the spontaneous, autochthonous nature of the murine breast tumor must be considered a priority evidence of its suitability.

The general discussion in this workshop session made it apparent that there is considerable interest in the selection and improvement of animal tumor models. It was generally thought that insufficient time has been allocated to this discussion and that there is need in the future for a several day workshop in this area.

INDEX